LIMEYS

For
Andrew Davidson Harvie
and
Helen Jane Skinnider Harvie

LIMEYS

The Conquest of SCURVY

DAVID I. HARVIE

SUTTON PUBLISHING

This book was first published in 2002 by
Sutton Publishing Limited · Phoenix Mill
Thrupp · Stroud · Gloucestershire · GL5 2BU

This paperback edition first published in 2005

Copyright © David I. Harvie, 2002

All rights reserved. No part of this publication may be reproduced, stored in a retrieval system, or transmitted, in any form, or by any means, electronic, mechanical, photocopying, recording, or otherwise, without the prior permission of the publisher and copyright holder.

David I. Harvie has asserted the moral right to be identified as the author of this work.

British Library Cataloguing in Publication Data
A catalogue record for this book is available from the British Library.

ISBN 0 7509 3993 1

Typeset in 10/13pt Iowan.
Typesetting and origination by
Sutton Publishing Limited.
Printed and bound in Great Britain by
J.H. Haynes & Co. Ltd, Sparkford.

Contents

Acknowledgements		vii
Introduction		1
1	'Death's Dire Ravage'	11
2	'Soe Many of the Best Chirurgeons'	20
3	'The Vain and Chimerical Belief'	42
4	'A Learned Man'	59
5	'I Shall Confirm All by Experience and Facts'	83
6	'The Province Has Been Mine'	95
7	'But the Power is in Others'	115
8	'My Attendance was Never Again Asked'	145
9	'Policy as Well as Humanity Concur'	164
10	'Every Ship Shall Have on Board a Sufficient Quantity'	198
11	'Lime Juice and Wine Merchants'	218
12	'The British Army Were Allowed to Rot of Scurvy'	228
13	'The True Antiscorbutic is Purity of Food'	238

14 'A Sufficient Explanation of the Anomaly'   253

Epilogue   276

Notes and References   280
Bibliography   306
Index   313

Acknowledgements

LIKE anyone writing an account such as this, I have relied heavily on much that has been written by others. In particular, I have drawn upon, and recommend highly, two very readable academic works. The four-volume *Medicine and the Navy, 1200–1900* by Keevil, Lloyd and Coulter is a magnificent and highly accessible work; and *A History of Scurvy and Vitamin C* by Kenneth Carpenter is excellent for anyone wishing to pursue the medical detail.

The Navy Records Society, whose Herculean work in researching, editing and publishing a vast range of naval documents is a remarkable benefit to historical enquiry, as well as being a fine testimony to those who wrote the original papers, and I gratefully acknowledge the society's permission to quote from a number of volumes. I also appreciate the permission of the late Sir John Clerk to quote from the private Clerk of Penicuik Papers deposited in the National Archives of Scotland.

I am grateful to the staffs of a number of libraries and archives: The Public Record Office at Kew; The Caird Library of the National Maritime Museum at Greenwich; The Wellcome Trust Library; The National Archives of Scotland; The National Library of Scotland; Glasgow University Library (particularly the Special Collections Department); and the Mitchell Library, Glasgow. I am also grateful for the generous help of the library of The Royal College of Physicians of London. These and similar institutions contain a humbling range of early original manuscripts, books and documents. The care and accessibility of such a vast range of material amounts to nothing less than one of the country's greatest cultural testimonials.

I owe particular gratitude to Professor Mike Lean, Head of the

Department of Human Nutrition at Glasgow University, who very generously and enthusiastically read the manuscript with a view to alerting me to inadvertent errors and misinterpretation of medical matters. This chore came to him out of the blue at a time when he had more than enough on his plate, and his efforts on my behalf are much appreciated. Needless to say, any remaining infelicity is mine and assuredly not his.

I would also like to acknowledge the help of a number of correspondents, and those who have enabled me to trace illustrations. In particular, Camilla Seymour of Bonham & Brooks in London enabled me to use the previously unseen miniature portrait of James Lind; Matthew Wheeler of the Dacorum Heritage Trust found me the portrait of Lauchlan Rose, and Elaine Munding at Cadbury Schweppes arranged permission to use it.

My wife Rose has shown typical resilience and forbearance in observing me ignore 'real work' in order to pursue this particular project. My thanks to all of those, and others unmentioned. I hope they will feel that this has been a tale worth the telling.

David I. Harvie
March 2005

Introduction

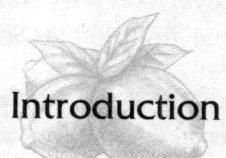

SCURVY was a hideous disease that killed thousands of men, mainly sailors, every year for at least four centuries before a remedy was found. For every man killed, three or four were severely incapacitated. In every seafaring nation, potential treatments were continually tried, discarded and replaced. Some of these therapies seem idiotic to us; some were worthy in theory but useless in practice; others were dangerous, and a few fatal. The longest-serving treatment in medical history, the bleeding of the patient, was forlornly and often dangerously used against scurvy. When the efficacy of acidic 'medicine' came into favour, spices were added to poisons such as mercury and sulphuric acid for internal consumption. A more aggressively physical treatment took the form of burial up to the neck in sand.

Mystique, absurd rationalisation and plain ignorance often characterised the subject. Sometimes, attempts at treatment were accidentally close to being successful, but there were too many unrecorded and casual remedies to allow proper judgement. Often, the physicians who wrote about scurvy observed that there appeared to be no-one of sufficient stature to adjudicate from the standpoint of scientific observation. The scientific method of hypothesis generation and testing was centuries away.

Lemon juice as a remedy was finally proved in the 1740s in the first controlled clinical trial, carried out on a ship-of-the-line at sea, by James Lind, a young Scottish naval surgeon. Initially misinterpreted and mistrusted, his work was of truly pioneering, international significance, and his findings were momentous in their potential for bringing to an end one of the greatest obstacles to national prosperity. In 1753, four years after resigning from the Royal Navy as a surgeon, James Lind introduced his definitive *A Treatise of the Scurvy* by saying:

> The subject of the following sheets is of great importance to this nation; the most powerful in her fleets and the most flourishing in her commerce of any in the world. Armies have been supposed to lose more of their men by sickness than by the sword. But this observation has been much more verified in our fleets and squadrons where scurvy alone, during the last war, proved a more destructive enemy, and cut off more valuable lives, than the united efforts of the French and Spanish arms.[1]

Today we regard medicine as a sophisticated science that offers us assurance that when we are ill we can reliably expect relief or even a cure. In the wider field of public health, we anticipate a similar outcome, even if there are instances that should make us question whether our collective health is perhaps more fragile than we suppose. Such justified confidence in medicine could hardly have been common in the eighteenth century, yet even 250 years ago, James Lind was scathing of what he called the 'vain and chimerical belief' – the ease with which people spoke of the certainty of cure. These were times when medicine and natural magic were synonymous.

In medieval times, the great public executioner was the Black Death, known as 'The Great Mortality'. This began in 1348, and in the first two years it is reckoned to have killed 30 million people in Europe – a third of the population. Another of the world's greatest killers is much less well known, despite the fact that its effect on the nation's economic and military capabilities was critical and long lasting. Scurvy has plagued mankind since prehistory. Until the sixteenth century it remained nameless. Hippocrates recognised it, found it difficult to cure and knew that most victims were condemned to an awful death. Pliny also recognised and described what was clearly scurvy.

Unlike the plague, scurvy did not produce panic in the streets, for its behaviour was not to attack as a sudden epidemic, but to

INTRODUCTION

be a constant and deadly companion, particularly to those at sea. While this disgusting, painful and deadly disease imposed its pitiless effects in all kinds of settlements and populations, its worst effects were seen among sailors. In practice, scurvy was extremely difficult to distinguish from the other sea diseases. As often as not, contracting scurvy exposed the sufferer to the full catalogue of medical disorder. It inflicted havoc on the body's immune system, and while it was common for death at sea to be blamed on 'the bloody flux' or 'ague' or 'the pox', the victim had often been brought down by an initial attack of scurvy. It was sometimes known as *Purpura Nautica* and (like many other diffuse conditions) was commonly thought of as a venereal disease – an implication attributed to the supposedly vile habits of sailors. Queen Anne's Physician, Martin Lister, was convinced that scurvy had not appeared until after the voyage of Columbus to the New World. He was equally persuaded of the connection with venereal disease, writing in 1694:

> I have placed scurvy adjacent to the chapter on venereal disease, because of the newness of the disease, and because both are so closely related and have so many symptoms in common that they are not readily distinguished from each other, except by an experienced physician.[2]

Many of the physical symptoms of scurvy and venereal disease were indeed similar, and a great many physicians claimed to specialise in both. Indeed, James Lind wrote his formal Latin thesis for Edinburgh University on aspects of venereal disease.

All the early maritime trading nations suffered from the effects of scurvy. Britain suffered particularly badly in the seventeenth and eighteenth centuries, after the Royal Navy began to embark on very long voyages. Not only did the country's economic and trading abilities suffer, but the increasing need to wage war at sea was dramatically compromised. Scurvy was bad enough during Britain's wars with the Dutch, French and Spanish, when squadrons in the Channel or the Mediterranean had to return to port after six weeks at sea due to the ravages of scurvy. When the Royal Navy followed the private merchant companies such as the East India Company in extended voyages around the world, the effects were often disastrous. There was no running for home during a three-year voyage. Often, during the several months of assembling a fleet, disease would take hold in the home port and on departure half the ships would have to be left behind due to the incapacity of crews and accompanying marines. Scurvy killed more men and destroyed more naval and military operations than did the totality of enemy action.

The conquest of scurvy by ill-resourced and professionally despised naval surgeons is one of the great triumphs of eighteenth-century medicine. The men who went to sea as naval surgeons were not paragons; these often ill-trained men practised their craft in the most difficult of physical circumstances. Although their commonest duties were to staunch blood and straighten broken limbs, theirs was not just the bloody business of the after-effects of battle. As voyages became extended they had to deal with a vast range of hitherto unknown and deadly diseases acquired in alien climates. The physician of shore life was generally a well-to-do gentleman of university training and some standing in society. In the eighteenth-century Royal Navy, physicians as such were extremely rare and retained the status of their shore-bound brothers. Most 'doctors' at sea were known as naval surgeons, and they did not enjoy high standing. The usual route into naval medicine was for a relatively untrained man (often an assistant to a physician on shore) to enlist as a surgeon's mate, and to gain promotion by observation, imitation and – if he was lucky – a touch of patronage.

During his sea experience James Lind witnessed not only the awful conditions in which sailors existed, but the lack of care by the Admiralty in providing decent food and clothing. He was dismayed by their lordships' lack of interest in adequately addressing how to combat the enormous range of diseases contracted by seamen both on board ship and in foreign climates.

INTRODUCTION

He could not know, of course, about vitamin C, or realise that scurvy was due to its deficiency, although he did recognise that dietary factors were crucial. He was not always correct; and he was probably not vigorous enough in promoting his central ideas. But he swept aside centuries-old prejudice, misinformation and plain ignorance and relied on his own rigorous experiment, observation and interpretation to provide him with facts – 'the surest and most unerring guides'. Lind's unique investigative approach, and his insistence on the need for prevention rather than simply cure, proved the definitive treatment against a disease that was generally treated by the use of simple but useless palliatives or dangerous quack medicines.

The success that would rid the seafaring nations of such a scourge, and pave the way for greater economic prosperity should have seen Lind's work celebrated. However, it was to be another half-century before the Admiralty agreed the compulsory daily issue of lemon-juice as an antiscorbutic in the Royal Navy; even longer for the Merchant Navy. Although Lind held a senior position, he had no influence with the Lords of the Admiralty – a hierarchy of patronage and arrogance which was more inclined to favour society physicians and their often fraudulent remedies. Other naval surgeons, some promoting useless nostrums, were better connected socially, with the result that the Admiralty not only allowed but actively encouraged treatments that were pointless and even fatal. The great Captain Cook, who was a brilliant and humane commander, could do no wrong in the eyes of some of his supporters in London society. However, he made a negative contribution to the treatment of scurvy by following the fruitless remedy of the protégé of one of the powerful Admiralty cliques. In doing so, he happily accepted the entirely inappropriate public soubriquet of 'the man who conquered scurvy'. Lind, a scholarly man who despised self-promotion, and whose sole patron within the Admiralty had died, did not retaliate.

Lind wrote further important volumes on naval hygiene and tropical medicine, and made endless recommendations for the improvement of the health of sailors based on practical observation and research. Meanwhile, the Admiralty dithered and continued to allow scurvy to be casually treated with the same old variety of doubtful remedies. If it had initially been the corrosive result of misguided patronage that undermined Lind, attitudes became more suffused with the smell of conspiracy when he later developed a system for producing fresh water from sea water on board ship. The Admiralty first ignored him, then forced him reluctantly to endorse the activities of another surgeon who had stolen his distillation process and who was eventually handsomely rewarded with finance by Parliament.

Decades later, two of Lind's brother surgeons, Gilbert Blane and Thomas Trotter, recognised the value of Lind's work, and worked tirelessly to have his recommendations for the use of lemons officially adopted. They formed a perfect double act. Blane moved in society circles, was well connected socially and had appointments to several royal households; Trotter was more outspoken and much less likely to bend the knee to authority. Together, their influence with a rather more enlightened group of Admiralty lords enabled them to achieve what Lind could not. In 1795, the Royal Navy was issued with orders to carry lemon juice on every ship, to be issued daily for the prevention of scurvy. James Lind had died the year before. This delay in implementing his recommendations – which cost thousands of naval lives – has been described as one of the most tragic in the history of medicine, and a criminal episode caused by deviousness.[3]

Sir Gilbert Blane wrote in 1830 of the improvements in the health of seamen in the late eighteenth century, and related these improvements to Britain's maritime prowess:

> It now remains to be mentioned, through what means these mighty results have been brought about. Are we to thank for it a guardian angel, presiding and watching over the dearest and most valuable interests of our country? Or is it more rationally imputable to some of those profound and exquisite discoveries in science, mathematical, chemical, mechanical or

pharmaceutical, with which the present age abounds above all others? No such thing. The scurvy has been prevented, subdued and totally rooted out, by the general use of lemon juice, supplied for the first time at the public expense in the year 1795, and which operated so speedily that in less than two years afterwards it became extinct, and has remained so.[4]

The delivery of similar victualling orders to the Merchant Navy was to take a further fifty years, by which time ships sailing from Britain began to be irreverently referred to as 'lime-juicers'. This allusion was later modified in the USA to the rather more provocative 'limeys' as an insult directed at British seamen.

The application of the new victualling regime in Britain did not proceed successfully. Confusion and corruption entered the system of supplying fruit. The Admiralty's parsimony, and a political impetus to promote British commerce led to disaster. Lemons had been purchased from foreign suppliers in the Mediterranean, but in about 1840 it was decided to support English lime-growers, who were establishing estates in the West Indies. By this time the words 'lemon' and 'lime' were being used indiscriminately, with disastrous consequences. By 1860, limes took the place of lemons as the antiscorbutic of choice. And scurvy returned. It was another sixty years before it became known that, compared to lemons, limes contained about a quarter of the still-mysterious antiscorbutic agent. By that time, confidence in Lind's remedy had waned, although nobody recognised that he had never mentioned limes, and had confined his recommendations to the more efficacious oranges and lemons.

Naval expeditions in the Arctic in the second half of the nineteenth century had varying success using citrus juice, and two expeditions in particular, in 1850 and 1875, experienced dramatically different outcomes. Parliament ordered an urgent inquiry, the results of which led eventually to comprehensive chemical investigations in laboratories across the world. Eventually, the existence of 'accessory food compounds' and 'vital amines' was recognised, and the dedicated branch of organic chemistry that concerns itself with diet and nutritional deficiencies was born.

More momentous than the later introduction of copper sheathing, steel hulls and steam power, the conquering in the eighteenth century of scurvy and the solving of the longitude problem were the two great achievements of maritime history. These two triumphs enabled safer seafaring and vastly increased economic and military benefits to be obtained by the world's maritime nations. There was even a spin-off industry. Where the appropriate fruit could be procured for the victualling of ships, there was still a major problem of its preservation on long voyages. That problem led directly to the foundation of the world's soft drinks industry.

Edinburgh's seaport of Leith became the birthplace of that industry when Lauchlan Rose devised an improved method of preserving lime juice without using any of the existing methods, which produced serious adulteration. After successfully perfecting a system of bottling for the Navy, Rose decided that he would try to interest the public in buying a sweetened version of his lime juice. One of the world's most lucrative industries was born.

The story of the defeat of scurvy at sea is an intriguing mix of pioneering achievement, bureaucratic inertia, wilful neglect and the corrosive poison that patronage induced in society. Much of the medicine in Hanoverian Britain was undertaken by practitioners obsessed by 'the state of the blood' and similar seemingly mystical notions. Many of these men became extremely wealthy by doing little more than 'cupping' or inducing the leakage of blood from deliberately induced blisters. The majority of the population – if it had access to medicine at all – made do with a doubtful and sometimes dangerous array of pills, potions, philtres and charms. Dubious medical opinion and influence was writ large in the confused background of medicine at sea.

The 'social history' of scurvy and its interlinked political

INTRODUCTION

context has more than one resonance that can be recognised in today's often complex public affairs. The story of James Lind and scurvy illustrates perfectly the fact that what Herbert Spencer called the 'perversity of officialism' can lead to the apparent paralysis of government, despite all the means of progressive action founded on facts and intelligent analysis.

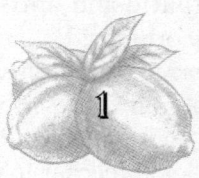

'Death's Dire Ravage'

SCURVY. The disease itself lived up to all the innuendo of the word, which appeared to sum up the sense of disgust that the scourge evoked in those who witnessed its progress. It is difficult to be sure when scurvy was first recognised as a condition in its own right, distinct from the many other forms of fever, ague, flux and pox which afflicted sailors and other victims. Confusion with the symptoms of other diseases ensured vague and unlikely treatment. Apart from the many fraudulent pills and potions, there was a range of 'internal remedies' from the ingestion of spiced sulphuric acid, vinegar and molasses, to spruce beer and sauerkraut. In the sixteenth and seventeenth centuries desperate external attempts at treatment included bathing in animal blood, and that perennial standby of the early physicians – phlebotomy, or bloodletting. Violent 'purging' of the belly was also considered appropriate. It is almost beyond the bizarre to include the preferred treatment in some quarters, that of burial up to the neck in sand. The word scurvy itself was left to carry all the threat and horror that confirmed it as one of the most potent symbols of dread in any community.

According to the *Oxford English Dictionary*, the first account of the disease itself which actually used the word *scurvy* came in 1565: 'Our legs now . . . swolne every joint withal With this disease, which, by your leave, the Scuruie men doe call.'[1] Other variant spellings in use at that time were scurvie, skirvye, scurvey, scurby, skyrby, scorbie and scorby. Another common archaic name for the disease was *Scorbutus*, which has given us the medical terms scorbutic and antiscorbutic: vitamin C is properly referred to as ascorbic acid.

No sooner was the horror of the disease recognised than the adjective *scurvy* was employed to describe some thing or person as disreputable, vile or contemptible. The *OED* gives the first such usage by the writer and preacher John Northbrooke in 1579, 'Looke that thou flee and eschewe this scabbed and scuruie company of Dauncers'. This was a common usage that appeared in the literature of such writers as Swift, Shakespeare, Smollett, and Scott, who in *Peveril of the Peak* writes:

> Take your hand from my cloak, my Lord Duke. . . . I have a scurvy touch of old puritanical humour about me. I abide not the imposition of hands.[2]

Scurvy – known since the early twentieth century to be a vitamin C deficiency – results in an inability of the body to produce collagen, a connective tissue that binds the body's muscle and other structures together. It maintains the immune system and is part of the means of building and protecting blood vessels. Vitamin C acts as an antioxidant, it assists in the healing of wounds, and works to detoxify the body's organs and processes. It is not manufactured in the human body and has to be acquired either by dietary means or by supplement. (Most species can synthesise vitamin C; humans and guinea-pigs are unusual exceptions.) Scurvy – often described as 'a fatal wasting disease' – induced internal and external haemorrhaging, mental fatigue and physical weakness. In classic sea scurvy, the first signs were usually bleeding of the gums and teeth, accompanied by a revolting smell. Cuts, bruises and injuries failed to heal, and old wounds reopened (one case is recorded of wounds sustained at the Battle of the Boyne reopening fifty years later).[3] The immune system broke down, leaving the body at risk of other infections; hallucinations and blindness often accompanied the more extreme stages. While the disease was neither infectious nor contagious, in circumstances where the community was 'closed' and everyone's diet similarly restricted – as in a ship – the death rate could be extremely high. Early medical purists were likely to differentiate between 'land' and 'sea' scurvy, but it was the latter that inflicted the most awful physical damage to sailors and economic damage to a country that prided itself on its maritime prowess and foreign trade.

James Lind spoke of the origins of the word scurvy as being either from the Danish *schorbect* or the Dutch *scorbeck*, both words referring to ulcers of the mouth. Alternatively there was the Saxon word *schorbok*, meaning a griping or tearing of the belly. Lind favoured the Slav word *scorb* as the derivation, being aware that the disease was especially endemic in Russia and the northern countries.[4] In the countries bordering the Baltic and the North Sea, poor living conditions and dietary deprivation were severe problems, especially in the long, dark, wet winters. In some countries, there was a sense of indigenous possessiveness as in *The Disease of London*[5] or *The Dutch Distemper*[6]. Scotland was more down-to-earth, referring to scurvy simply as *Blacklegs*.[7] Lind, when researching all the previous writers on scurvy, was clear that Hippocrates, 'The Father of Medicine', who probably died in 357 BC, may have made the first sufficiently clear description of the unnamed disease. He had noted that those who were afflicted 'have a foetid breath, lax gums, and an haemorrhage from the nose'.[8] Hippocrates also recorded that the disease required a tedious cure that often 'accompanied a patient to his death'. Lind was surprised that, by and large, the ancient Greek, Roman and Arab authors were silent on the disease, beyond relying on the description by Hippocrates. Indeed Lind was strongly critical of suggestions that some of the ancients had actually described scurvy, insisting that 'such opinions deserve no serious confutation.' He was forthright in the preface to his *Treatise* in refuting earlier dogma and erroneous opinion:

> ... it is no easy matter to root out old prejudices, or to overturn opinions which have acquired an establishment by time, custom, and great authorities.[9]

Lind was interested in early descriptions of the disease before it acquired its own identity and name. Convincing reports came from the Crusades in the mid-thirteenth century, when 'the barber surgeons were forced to cut away the dead flesh from the gums to enable the people to masticate their food.' The disease had broken out at Lent, when soldiers ate no meat except a species of eel which their superstitious beliefs led them to think 'ate dead people' and was therefore seen as the cause of the disease.[10]

In 1497 Vasco da Gama sailed from Lisbon with three small 200-ton ships and a 400-ton store ship to discover a passage to the East Indies via the Cape of Good Hope. It is thought that scurvy was the cause of death of 100 out of a total of 160 men. This was the first occasion on which scurvy was described during a sea voyage. The Portuguese soldier/poet Luis de Camoëns described conditions en route for Goa, and commemorated the deaths of so many sailors in his epic 'The Lusiad':

> A dread disease its rankling horrors shed,
> And death's dire ravage through mine army spread.
> Never mine eyes such dreary sight beheld,
> Ghastly the mouth and gums enormous swell'd;
> And instant, putrid like a dead man's wound,
> Poisoned with foetid streams the air around.
> No sage physician's ever-watchful zeal,
> No skilful surgeon's gentle hand to heal,
> Were found: each dreary mournful hour we gave
> Some brave companion to a foreign grave.[11]

Presumably in some desperation, Vasco da Gama gave instructions for the use of urine as a mouthwash against 'death's dire ravage'.

One of the best of the early descriptions of the anonymous scourge comes from the sixteenth century, when the French were colonising the east coast of Canada – the Maritime Provinces as we know them. In the summer of 1535, Jacques Cartier set sail from St Malo in Brittany with three ships. This was his second such expedition, and was better equipped than his voyage the previous year. However, despite the useful experiences of the earlier expedition, he made a calamitous mistake by setting off later in the season. They had time to do little more than explore part of the St Lawrence River before the unforgiving Canadian winter set in:

> the unknowen sicknes began to spread itselfe amongst us after the strangest sott that ever was eyther heard of or seene, insomuch as some did lose all their strength, and could not stand on their feete, then did their legges swel, their sinnews shrinke as black as any cole. Others had all their skins spotted with spots of blood of a purple coulour: then did it ascend up to their ankles, knees, thighes, shoulders, armes, and necke: their mouth became stincking, their gummes so rotten, that all the flesh did fall off, even to the roots of the teeth, which also almost fell out. With such infection did this sicknes spread itself in our three ships, that about the middle of February, of a hundred and ten persons that we were, there were not ten whole.[12]

Cartier had sufficient concern and foresight to have his surgeon conduct a post-mortem on one of the dead, hoping forlornly to discover the cause. By the time the winter ended, twenty-five sailors were dead and only three men were fit enough to go below to draw their probably unpalatable drinking water. Cartier's expedition was only saved from total disaster by taking the advice of friendly Indians, who made them take a concoction made from 'the juice and sappe of the leaves of a certain Tree.'[13] The account of Cartier's voyage shows how desperate was their need for relief:

> The tree is in their language called *Ameda* or *Hanneda*. After the medicine was found and proved to be true, there was such strife about it, who should be first to take of it, that they were ready to kill one another.[14]

As was commonly the case, no attention was paid to either the lack of fresh fruit or vegetables, or to what had been the 'certain tree' that the Indians had used. Pointless speculation was the habitual response. James Lind later concluded:

> I am inclined to believe, from the description given by Cartier of the *ameda* tree, with a decoction of the bark and leaves of which his crew was so speedily recovered, that it was the large swampy American spruce tree. For although the pines and firs, of which there is a great variety, differ from each other in their size and outward form . . . yet they seem all to have analogous medicinal virtues, and great efficacy in this disease.[15]

The Dutch were great and early explorers of the world's oceans, and were the first to acquire a great merchant fleet with which they dominated trade to the East Indies. As a result of their extended voyages, they were also among the earliest to record many of the sea diseases, and to attempt the use of remedies. James Lind acknowledged the efforts of the Dutch physician Ronsseus of Gonda, who as early as 1564 had used citrus fruit as a remedy for scurvy, and who wrote the first book written specifically about the disease.

A few years later, in 1604, another French expedition headed for *Nova Francia*, or what we would call the state of Virginia. Their story was the same – without the saving grace of the *ameda*:

> Briefly, the unknown sickness like to those described by James Cartier, assailed us. As to remedies, there were none to be found. In the meanwhile, the poor creatures did languish, pining away by little for want of meats to sustain their stomach; which could not receive hard food, by reason of a rotten flesh which grew and over-abounded within their mouths; and when one thought to root it out, it grew again in one night's space, more abundantly than before. As to the tree called *ameda*, mentioned by the said Cartier, the savages of these lands know it not.[16]

The savage Virginians instead used 'frequent sweatings' as a treatment, and claimed that a singular preventative was mirth and a cheerful humour – a recommendation that was to feature widely in later years. Sweating, bloodletting and purging were to remain favourite 'remedies' for the next three centuries. The great naval surgeon John Woodall wrote in 1639 in his famous volume, *The Surgeon's Mate*:

> . . . some are troubled with an extreme costiveness [constipation] that for fourteen daies together they do not go to stoole once, wherefore the Chirurgeon is constrained with an instrument to take out the excrements to avoide death.[17]

Woodall was one of the first to recommend the use of citrus fruit against scurvy. The writer John Coltbatch had also heard of the idea in 1699:

> I have frequently been told by some seamen and surgeons, that have had long voyages at sea, especially towards China and the Indies, that of a hundred men in a ship, not two of them but have been almost eaten up with the scurvy, their skin squalid and full of blotches, their gums eaten away, and their teeth ready to drop out, pains and aches all over their bodies, and yet on their landing at Cadiz, or thereabouts, where is plenty of oranges and lemons, eating large quantities of them, in one fortnight's time at farthest scarce one has failed of being perfectly cured. This is not a relation of one or two persons only, but what is generally agreed upon, and allowed by all to be truth.[18]

Since medieval times the disease affected settled communities, where it was seen as virtually another plague; it appeared in closed communities such as prisons and asylums for the insane it ravaged armies on the move and towns under siege. It is recorded that from 1556 to 1877 there were 143 epidemics on land alone. The interesting thing about this statistic is that the incidence of epidemics increased throughout the period, from 2 outbreaks in the sixteenth century to 104 in the nineteenth.[19] This increase is probably explained by an increase in travel during the period before remedial treatment was available. However, the worst effects of scurvy were seen at sea, and it is as a sea disease that it is characterised.

By the eighteenth century scurvy was a major problem. The Royal Navy, which had hitherto sailed mostly in home waters, was beginning to undertake long transoceanic voyages in pursuit of colonial aspirations, and in support of the great merchant companies. The Admiralty casually encouraged, and in some cases ordered, the use of unproven and often useless remedies from 'quack' pills to sulphuric acid, the smoking of tobacco and the burning of tar as fumigants. As a consequence of such uncertainty there was little expectation of successful treatment or cure. Outside the Royal Navy, medicine was similarly sidelined, even in some of the extremely wealthy merchant trading companies. The East India Company, whose first surgeon-general was John Woodall, did nevertheless try to use lemons against scurvy. With its much earlier and greater experience of long voyages than the Navy, it was at least in theory in a better position to build practical knowledge. However, difficulties of supply and preservation of fruit were apparently enough to prevent any proper analysis of the relative efficacy of citrus fruit and other potential remedies. In practice, East India Company men probably suffered less from scurvy than Royal Navy sailors because their diet was better, and their living conditions were less overcrowded.

Other than passive indifference, there was one overriding explanation for the Admiralty's lack of motivation in seeking a cure for this most pernicious disease, which was having a disastrous economic effect on the country. It had been easier and cheaper to press-gang new recruits than to take care of the crews of the ships which crossed the oceans and charted the world for the glory of the Crown. 'When we recall that the naval manning problem arose principally through losses from disease, that much of this was scorbutic or intestinal,' wrote J.J. Keevil in *Medicine and the Navy, 1200–1900*, 'the failure to obtain fresh provisions at every opportunity can be accounted for only on grounds of economy. It was in fact cheaper to replace seamen than to replace stale victuals.'[20]

James Lind was driven to tackle scurvy in the aftermath of one of the greatest and most adventurous naval expeditions. In 1740, Commodore George Anson had left Portsmouth with 7 ships and 2,000 men intending to circumnavigate the world; he returned from the Chinese coast with one ship and 188 scared sailors accompanying a fabulous, glittering Spanish treasure. Although affected by scurvy, not one of the officers succumbed; of the 1,400 men who died, only 4 were killed by enemy action. Scurvy claimed the lives of almost all the others. Anson returned to a hero's welcome and subsequently, as First Lord, became one of the great Admiralty reformers. He may have been responsible for Lind's promotion within naval medicine, after his *A Treatise of the Scurvy* was published in 1753. However, before achieving that initial success, Lind had to try to dismantle the obstacles of bureaucratic inertia and prejudice. In addition, there was a long history of ignorance and confusion surrounding the disease itself. The young Edinburgh doctor would discover that antiquated traditions and mystique were to prove easier antagonists than contemporary power and patronage.

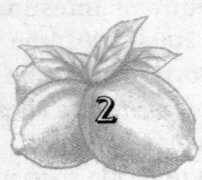

'Soe Many of the Best Chirurgeons'

JAMES Lind was born in Edinburgh on 4 October 1716, the second child of James Lind and Margaret Smellum. During the reign of Mary Queen of Scots in the early part of the sixteenth century the family had moved from their 240-acre estate at Dalry in Ayrshire to Edinburgh, where they bought land at Gorgie. This move into business in Edinburgh appears to have been highly rewarding. In the seventeenth century, James's father, also James, was one of five brothers in business in Edinburgh and London. He and his brother John had settled as merchants in Poland. After John died there, James returned to Edinburgh in 1705 to marry Margaret Smellum. The Lind and Smellum families appear to have been well-to-do. Margaret Smellum's father was a 'Burgess and Merchant' and a brother was a Fellow of the College of Physicians of Edinburgh. One of the Linds was an Edinburgh town councillor and bailie; a later eighteenth-century Lind was an advocate and the first sheriff-depute of Edinburgh, while another was Lord Provost of the city and Member of Parliament in the 1760s. Other cousins of James Lind were in medicine, the Army and diplomacy (as privy councillor to the King of Poland).

There has been confusion between 'our' James Lind and a younger well-known physician of the same name, a cousin born in Edinburgh in 1736, who sailed to China as a surgeon with the East India Company. He sailed with the botanist and explorer (Sir) Joseph Banks, and became Physician to the Royal Household of George III at Windsor. There is no record of the

'SOE MANY OF THE BEST CHIRURGEONS'

two Linds having any professional contact, although some personal relationship no doubt existed. The younger James Lind died in London in 1812. (At this period, there was also yet another unrelated James Lind in the register of surgeons in the East India Company).

When James Lind was born in 1716, Edinburgh was a place of some political agitation, with no sign yet of the famous Georgian New Town which is such a visually strong aspect of the city today. The 30–40,000 inhabitants lived in crowded tenements down the length of the Royal Mile from the Castle to the Palace of Holyrood. The Act of Union of 1707 was widely derided, and its origins attributed to deeply undemocratic plotting – aided by the activities of Daniel Defoe. He broke off from his various other roles as diarist, novelist and pamphleteer and acted as a spy for the Tory minister, Robert Harley, the Earl of Oxford, to ensure that the Scots commissioners for Union toed the required Westminster line.

Living conditions in the city when Lind was growing up were variable. For the poor, existence could be harsh indeed, but the 'merchant classes' enjoyed considerable comfort, and no doubt welcomed the fact that the port of Leith was the major British port for the import of the best French claret. Travel was difficult; it took a week's boneshaking to reach London by coach. Most roads in Scotland were little more than dirt tracks, although largely as a result of the forfeiture of estates after the 'Forty-Five' (the Jacobite Rising of 1745–6), roads were steadily improved, often on the basis of existing military roads. Edinburgh, then as now, was a city whose most prosperous activities centred around the law, banking and the university – each of these kingpins of society retaining independence after the Union.

The beginning of the eighteenth century saw the first stirrings of what has become known as the Scottish Enlightenment, and Edinburgh in particular became the 'hotbed of genius'. This was a time of intellectual and philosophical inquiry and achievement which was the envy of Europe. The movement was ironically born in what was thought of as a rather backward country, only half a dozen years after a student at the university was hanged for blasphemy. But Scotland overcame a period of introverted, romantic self-destruction and started out on a new road of open democratic perspective, quite at odds with the greedy squalor of much of the society that Walpole created in London. A wide variety of radical philosophical societies nurtured new empirical ways of thinking, and bred a new democratic insistence on sceptical enquiry and practical experiment. The theory and practice of science, economics, medicine and painting were all transformed by the new approach.

In 1503, Edinburgh town council elevated the city's barber-surgeons into a craft incorporation. Edinburgh University was founded in 1583 as the first civic university in Britain, and the Medical School opened in 1720, based on those at Padua and Leyden. The latter, in particular, had close connections with Edinburgh, and students of the humanities moved between those two universities in great numbers. The greatest seventeenth-century Scottish physician, Archibald Pitcairne, was appointed Professor of Medicine at Leyden in 1692 and had the equally great Hermann Boerhaave as a pupil. Boerhaave was an early writer on scurvy, exponent of the use of crab apples and other fruit in its treatment, and was notable for teaching medicine as a practical skill.

The Edinburgh Medical School grew rapidly and soon the annual enrolment in anatomy was over 400: all males, of course – women were not admitted until 1886, following bitter battles with the medical fraternity and the law. Apart from the high quality of the teaching and the liberal organisation, the Edinburgh Medical School became popular with students from abroad because courses were relatively cheap and there were no religious tests directed at candidates. Indeed, the atmosphere was so open that ordinary members of the public were able casually to attend lectures. The Medical School was also progressive in that although important written work still had to be completed in Latin, lectures were given in English.

Few details are known of James Lind's childhood, but it is clear that he enjoyed a good schooling, because in later life he was adept at Latin and Greek, and probably to a lesser extent, French and German. The extensive reading of early medical texts which is revealed in his *A Treatise of the Scurvy* is proof of considerable language ability. Even in the lowliest of Scottish schools, Latin at least would have been all but compulsory, given its universal importance in academic professions. Lind did not go directly to Edinburgh University, which is a little odd for four reasons. Firstly, he seems to have had a good school education; secondly, his family was not poor; thirdly, an uncle by marriage was a Fellow of the College of Surgeons; and lastly, Edinburgh University had such a worldwide reputation for its medical training. For whatever reason, James Lind was apprenticed in December 1731, at the age of fifteen, to George Langlands, a member of the Incorporation of Surgeons. Langlands, who had studied at Leyden under Boerhaave, was a well-known figure in Edinburgh medical circles.

Lind's apprenticeship to Langlands would not have been unusual for a boy of fifteen. The apprentice would do all the running and fetching and cleaning and general chores, but would have progressed to mixing chemical compounds, bleeding patients and dressing wounds. The novelist Tobias Smollett paints a picture of his hero Roderick Random's approach to Dr Launcelot Crab, in the hope of becoming his apprentice, at about the same time that Lind started with Langlands:

> That I may be as little burthensome as possible, I would willingly serve in your shop, by which means I may save you the expense of a journey-man, or porter at least, for I understand a little pharmacy, having employed some of my leisure hours in the practice of that art, while I lived with Mr Potion: neither am I altogether ignorant of surgery, which I have studied with great pleasure and application.
>
> 'Oh ho! You did?' (says Crab). 'Gentlemen, here is a compleat artist! Studied surgery! What? In books I suppose. I shall have you disputing with me one of these days, on points of my profession. You can already account for muscular

motion (I warrant) and explain the mystery of the brain and nerves – ha! You are too learned for me, d—n me. But let's hear no more of this stuff, can you bleed? And give a clyster, spread a plaister and prepare a potion?'[1]

A keen apprentice with a good physician would have made a skilful twosome, and an able pupil could expect to learn a great deal by observation and experience. Opportunity for informal and formal study would also be available, and it is entirely likely that Lind would have attended occasional medical lectures and demonstrations. The apprenticeship would probably have been contracted in the common manner; it would last for three years, and the youth would agree

> . . . to bind himself to his master by day and by night, holy-day and weekday; to reveal no secret of master or patient; to commit no filthy crimes or sins; to go to no professor of medicine, chyma, anatomy, surgerie, or materia medica during the first two years; to pay £50 sterling as apprentice fee, in return for which the chirurgeon obliges himself to instruct him in the said airtes of surgery and pharmacy, and shall conceal nothing of the same, and entertains him sufficiently in bed and board.[2]

It is not clear how long James Lind remained with Langlands, but eight years after he became apprenticed, he decided to go to London. This would have been no easy decision – the rigours of the journey alone would ensure that the issue would have been well thought out in advance. It seems likely that he had decided in advance to enter the Navy. He had a younger brother who was already a naval officer, so that fact may have been an influence. On the other hand, his family connections, together with the standing of George Langlands in the profession, could have secured him a good future in Edinburgh. There was a strong tradition of men trained at Edinburgh University joining the naval medical service, and it is possible that the start of yet another war in October that year, this time with Spain, provided the final incentive. Whatever combination of reasons prompted Lind's decision, his move was made at a time when Britain was moving into a period of great colonial and trading expansion. The private merchant companies, such as the Hudson's Bay, the South Sea and East India Companies, were thriving, and exerting consequent pressure on the Navy to provide worldwide protection both for their extended voyages and colonial settlements. The relationship between the Royal Navy and the country's economic development had become critical.

When James Lind entered the Royal Navy in 1739, another Scot, Tobias Smollett, born in Renton in Dunbartonshire, entered as a second surgeon's mate. *Roderick Random* was Smollett's first novel, published anonymously in 1748 to great acclaim. This satire hilariously records the wildly fluctuating experiences of his hero who, among other adventures, joins the Royal Navy as a surgeon's mate. Roderick's adventures are regarded as an accurate account of Smollett's own experiences, which clearly included dealings with much hypocrisy and incompetence. Such was the willingness of people to recognise the accuracy of the account that Smollett was advised to publish disclaimers stating, perhaps tongue-in-cheek, that 'no Person living is aimed at'.[3]

Roderick is given advice on how to proceed with the Navy Office at Crutched Friars, near the Tower of London:

> I must first go to the Navy Office, and write to the Board, desiring them to order a letter for me to the Surgeons' Hall, that I may be examined touching my skill in surgery; that the surgeons, after having examined me, would give me my qualification sealed up in form of a letter, directed to the Commissioners; which qualification I must deliver to the Secretary to the Board, who would open it in my presence, and read the contents. After which, I must employ my interest to be provided for as soon as possible. That the expense of this qualification for a second mate of a third rate, amounted to thirteen shillings, exclusive of the warrant, which cost half

a guinea and half a crown, besides the present to the Secretary, which consisted of a three pound twelve piece.[4]

When Roderick is finally summoned to Barber-Surgeons' Hall for examination and reveals that he is from Scotland, he gets the tart reply, 'We have scarce any other countrymen to examine here – you Scotchmen have overspread us of late as locusts did Egypt.' His interrogator proceeds to insult him and tells him that 'it was a shame and a scandal to send such raw boys into the world, as surgeons; that it was great presumption in me, and an affront upon the English, to pretend to sufficient skill in my business.'[5] Heaped upon these insults was the suggestion that it would have been better if he became a weaver or shoemaker. After further nonsense, including a question about how to treat a man whose head has been blown off, the fifteen-minute examination was over, and Roderick had his qualification.

When a Surgeon is warranted to serve in any of H.M. ships, he is to provide himself with instruments and a chest of medicine and present the same to be viewed by the Physician in the Commission of Sick and Wounded or (if there be none) by the Physician of Greenwich Hospital, in conjunction with the Surgeons' Company. When the survey is over, the chest is to be locked and the seals of the Physician and of the Surgeons' Company to be affixed thereto in such a manner as to prevent it being afterwards opened before it comes on board; nor is the Captain to admit any chest into the ship without these marks upon it.[6]

So read the first of the *Instructions for Surgeons* that were in force when Lind and Smollett joined the Navy. On finally stepping aboard ship, the conditions to be found in the sick bay, as described by Smollett, were nauseous:

I was much less surprised that people should die on board, than that any sick person should recover. Here I saw about fifty miserable distempered wretches, suspended in rows, so huddled one upon the other that not more than fourteen inches space was allotted for each with his bed and bedding; and deprived of the light of the day as well as of fresh air; breathing nothing but a noisome atmosphere of the morbid steams exhaling from their own excrements and diseased bodies, devoured with vermin hatched in the filth that surrounded them, and destitute of every convenience necessary for people in that helpless condition.[7]

That first sentence carries a resonance that was to haunt naval surgeons for the best part of another two centuries. The surgeon's main responsibilities were to visit the sick at least twice a day, and keep the commander informed. He was also required to recommend changes to hasten recovery, prevent the spread of disease, and improve the health of the ship's crew. There was also a responsibility to maintain journals of medical and surgical procedures.

The Royal Navy of the seventeenth and eighteenth centuries was a very, very large business indeed, with a huge turnover of ordinary seamen. By the mid-eighteenth century, the Navy comprised roughly 230 ships of various sizes, 85,000 seamen, 880 lieutenants and 500 captains. As for medical officers, Smollett had it that, 'the Captain is too much of a gentleman to know a surgeon's mate by sight.' Their professional equals ashore always regarded the status of the naval surgeon as decidedly inferior. They certainly were not at sea for the money. Prior to 1795, surgeons received derisory basic pay augmented by a fixed bonus per case of venereal disease treated;[8] this was a discriminatory process that was eventually stopped by the demands of the surgeons themselves. New regulations entitled them to 11s a day, rising to 18s for those with twenty years service.[9]

Rates of pay were also a significant disincentive for able seamen. In the mid-eighteenth century, the Navy paid 24s a month, as against 70s a month offered by private shipowners or merchant companies such as the East India Company.[10] The use of impressment was strictly intended to apply only to those men whose employment was, or had been in the past, connected to the water. The abduction of 'landsmen' (or even seamen who were officially in possession of a temporary 'protection certificate') was illegal, although it happened frequently.[11] Eventually, the press gangs were subject to control, and Regulating Captains were brought in, largely to put an end to disputes with local authorities. Later still, the Impress Service was formalised under an admiral. The inducement of prize money was often used in an effort to recruit, but more often than not led to disputes. The prize money resulting from the capture of foreign vessels and bounty was usually divided into eight shares. Three shares went to the captain; one share was divided equally between all captains of marines, lieutenants, master and physician; one share was divided equally between all lieutenants of marines, admiral's secretary, principal warrant officers, master's mates and chaplain; one share was divided equally between all midshipmen, inferior warrant officers, principal warrant officer's mates and marine sergeants; and two shares were divided equally between all other crew. The room for dissatisfaction was substantial, and there are many examples of flag officers, squadron commanders and captains amassing fabulous wealth from the proceeds of prizes. One account records the case of the naval and military commanders after the capture of Havana in 1762 gaining over £120,000 each; this is a large amount in today's terms, but in 1762 it would have been breathtaking.[12]

From the seventeenth century, the prevailing conditions resulted in increasing desperation to obtain qualified medical staff. As early as April 1665, the Privy Council ordered the Barber-Surgeons' Company 'forthwith to Imprest & take up for His Majesties Service soe many of the best, ablest and Most Experienced Chirurgeons, Mates and Barbers as shal be requisite.'[13] Later that year one captain wrote to Samuel Pepys,[14] then Secretary to the Admiralty, pleading that attention be given to his urgent demands for a surgeon and a surgeon's mate, as he had much sickness aboard.[15] The demand was hardly outrageous, given that the surgeon's mate would be essentially untrained, and the surgeon himself largely self-taught. Wholly untrained ordinary seamen carried out much of the physical care of sick and wounded sailors, and young boys known as 'loblolly boys' were often available as general labour. There is conflicting evidence about the numbers of surgeons serving. In the war years from 1739–44 the annual intake varied between 139 and 440; there was felt to be such a shortage that impressment from the civilian population was considered.[16] Britain was a maritime nation, and recruitment of both seamen and naval surgeons was critical to the country's well-being. However, in a letter of 1726 John Cockburne, Lord of the Admiralty, says in response to an enquiry about a vacancy as a surgeon's mate:

> There are such numbers soliciting for such employment that as ships is no sooner ordered to be fitted but twenty candidates appear where there is only room for one.
> ... I had for answer ... that all were now full and they had a list of above a hundred who had apply'd lately for whom there was no room.[17]

The wealthy merchant companies were also subjected to pressure from the patrons of young men seeking appointment. One letter of March 1729 from the East India Company to Clerk of Penicuik suggests that applicants who have not been to university in Paris or Holland should work for a year in an apothecary's shop to gain experience of making up medicines:

> ... and something of their smartness and language which I find your nephew much in want of and consequently not so ready for his examination at Surgeons' Hall which must afford him a certificate of qualification before he can either be admitted into a man of war or in an India ship.[18]

As late as the 1790s, there were only three properly educated doctors of medicine (all trained at Edinburgh) in the entire naval service.[19] One indication of the status of naval surgeons is illustrated by the fact that when surgeons were ashore they were on greatly reduced pay; this had been normal for many grades, but surgeons were only included in this largesse after 1805. Between appointments there typically ensued a stream of letters to individual Lords of the Admiralty, lobbying for favours in obtaining new or improved appointments for individual surgeons.

The level of naval activity was substantial; in Britain there were huge naval dockyards, mostly in southern England, at places such as Deptford, Woolwich, Chatham, Portsmouth, Plymouth and Sheerness. In addition, there were important bases established abroad; Port Royal at Kingston, Jamaica; English Harbour, Antigua; in the Mediterranean there were dockyards at Gibraltar, at Port Mahon on Minorca, and at Malta. There were wars to be fought, mostly against France, Spain, Holland and America and their colonies. In prosecuting these wars, the Navy had to be prepared to help establish and support military and civilian colonies; and expeditions were regularly mounted to explore and chart new territories and foreign waters. Ship construction and repair, together with the supply of chandlery and provisions were large, thriving industries – many of them privatised.

A first-rate ship of 100 or more guns might have a crew of about 1,000 men; a third-rater of 74 guns perhaps 700 men. The living conditions for ordinary seamen, especially in hot climates, were a significant deterrent. As Dr Johnson pointed out:

> No man will be a sailor who has contrivance enough to get himself into a jail; for being in a ship is being in a jail, with the chance of being drowned. . . . A man in a jail has more room, better food, and commonly better company.[20]

This was a sentiment recognised 150 years earlier by Sir Walter Raleigh, who understood that seamen served in the Jacobean Navy as readily as if they were galley slaves. However, he was always keen to get his men:

If yow had geven the order to the cunstables of the country to lay [search] the villages yow might have taken thos marines agayne that ranne away, for wee shalbe undun if wee miss them.[21]

Aboard ship, lighting was by candles, and there was little or no ventilation, except on the gun deck, and then only if gun ports were permitted to be opened. On decks below the waterline, ventilation was non-existent. Water penetration was constant, soaking every surface; the lack of fresh air meant that nothing dried, and the air became even more rancid. Hammocks were slung at the regulation distance of fourteen inches apart. Even without the presence of sickness, the pungent smell derived from such close and rough living was often gut-wrenching. In these humid, stinking conditions, the possibilities for the incubation and spread of disease were endless. There were rats, weevils, maggots and other pests living in populations as dense as those of the humans; there was poor and often bad food; and water, which, if the crew was lucky, was only stagnant. Uniforms were lacking, and there was no discipline in the washing of clothes, sailors habitually wearing the same, filthy and often wet clothing for long periods. It is hardly surprising that sailors in such conditions might, perhaps after enduring harsh punishment, make desperate escape attempts. One account from 1793 tells of a small group of men on a Navy ship off Cape Town who – seeing the approach of an East India Company fleet – climbed down the lines towing wooden gratings which were being washed. Hoping to be picked up by an East Indiaman, they cut the ropes and took to the high seas off the Cape of Good Hope on their unseaworthy and unsteerable lumps of wood. However, the captain of the following merchantman ignored their pleas and left them to an unknown fate.[22]

In port, the only consolation was often the discretion that enabled the captain to permit women aboard. The rules were that only sailors' wives, signed aboard as such, were given dispensation to come aboard. Unfortunately, the incidence of prostitution was high, and the rules were widely flouted. One account tells that of 450 women coming aboard a ship docked at Portsmouth only 50 were wives. The result of that kind of situation was often extended misery in the form of venereal diseases. It was the kind of behaviour that did not go down well in most ports; the citizens of Aberdeen were not being particularly radical in their demands when they petitioned the Admiralty to stop allowing prostitutes on board Navy ships.[23] Even in home ports, seamen who had been pressed were sometimes confined to their quarters to prevent escape. John Nicol, a ship's cooper from Edinburgh, had been impressed to serve on HMS *Edgar* of 1794 under Captain Sir Charles Henry Knowles:

> We went upon a cruise to the coast of Norway, then touched at Shetland for fresh provisions. Afterwards we sailed for Leith Roads. I now felt all the inconveniences of my confinement. I was at home in sight of the place where I wished all my wanderings to cease. Captain Barefoot of the *Nottingham* had wrote to Sir C.H. Knowles in my behalf, and he was very kind to me. I asked leave to go on shore to see my friends which he consented to, but Lieutenant Collis would not allow me, saying 'it was not safe to allow a pressed man to go on shore at his native place.'[24]

Punishment was another factor affecting morale and life in general. Over the years there may have been an overemphasis on some of the more lurid accounts of cruel and inhuman treatment. While punishment in the closed community of a ship on a long voyage was a necessary feature, there were cases of inhuman treatment in an age when personal violence was more commonly accepted than it is today. There was indeed a clause in regulations which indicated that particularly harsh sea traditions might apply: 'all other faults committed at sea should be punished according to the customs of the sea.' The death penalty was available for a large proportion of offences; in addition, there were other savageries such as flogging, the stopping of rations, keelhauling, ducking and tongue-scraping. There was little consistency of punishment from ship to ship and from fleet to fleet. Through the various accounts, contradictions and capricious behaviour by individual officers abound. There were generous, humane captains such as Cook, Nelson and Cuthbert Collingwood. The compassionate and very outspoken Admiral Vernon (who was also a Member of Parliament) said that, 'our Fleets, which are defrauded by injustice, are first manned by violence and maintained by cruelty.'[25] Following the mutiny at the Nore anchorage off the coast of Kent in 1797 (when its leader Richard Parker, was hanged from the yardarm) Collingwood was offered a larger ship and an increased salary. He refused them on the grounds that 'I know and am known here, which in these ticklish times, I hold to be of much consequence.'[26] There were also monsters such as Hugh Pigot, whose desperate crew in 1797 murdered him in order to escape his cruelty.[27] The leaders of the Nore mutiny wrote an *Address To The Nation* in which they complained of 'the unbounded oppression and cruelty that has from time immemorial been shown to us.' The ship's cooper, John Nicol, witnessed one not untypical but harrowing event while sailing in HMS *Surprise* in the American War in the early 1780s. Under Captain Reeve, he reports:

> One of our men was whipped through the fleet for stealing some dollars from a merchant ship he was assisting to bring into port. It was a dreadful sight: the unfortunate sufferer tied down on the boat and rowed from ship to ship, getting an equal number of lashes at the side of each vessel from a fresh man. The poor wretch, to deaden his sufferings, had drunk a whole bottle of rum a little before the time of punishment. When he had only two portions to get of his punishment, the captain of the ship perceived he was tipsy and immediately ordered the rest of the punishment to be delayed until he was sober. He was rowed back to the *Surprise*, his back swelled like a pillow, black and blue. Some sheets of thick blue paper were steeped in vinegar and laid to his back. Before he seemed insensible. Now his shrieks rent the air.[28]

No doubt hard-pressed surgeons were required to deal with the consequences of such punishments, as they had to deal with the results of accidents and the most traumatic battle wounds.

One of the unique features of Lind's approach to scurvy, and to naval medicine in general, was his insistence that what mattered above all was the *prevention* of disease. This required an innovative way of thinking, and may have partly caused wariness and inertia by the Admiralty. To Lind, curative measures were important but distinctly of secondary concern. He stressed this approach in the preface to his important *An Essay on the most effectual means of preserving the Health of Seamen in the Royal Navy*, published in 1757:

> The *Prophylactic* or preventive branch of medical science does, in many instances, admit of as much, or even more certainty, than the curative part. . . . A medicine, which effectually prevents, deserves to be more esteemed than that which removes a Fever.[29]

This remains the prevailing philosophy of human nutrition within medical practice.

Scurvy was one of the most critical features of life aboard ship. The problem was exacerbated by the uncertainty of the length of voyages due to the inability to measure longitude accurately – a problem not solved until the end of the eighteenth century. The length of voyage particularly affected the supply of fresh food and drink. Without the ability to preserve by refrigeration or chemicals (other than salt and occasionally alcohol), crews were exposed to widespread deficiencies, disease and outright poisoning, especially when sailing in tropical climates. The humid hold of a wooden sailing ship at sea was no place to store food. James Lind, deeply interested in all aspects of naval hygiene and conditions, was clearly convinced that scurvy had its incidence rooted in atmospheric conditions and diet. One of his earliest ideas was that salt was unlikely to be a cause. Salt was a significant feature of naval diet, since it was the main means of preserving meat, and most theorists blamed the incidence of more than one disease on its eternal presence. Others, in contradiction, recommended the use of salt water against scurvy.

The Navy, through the Commissioners of the Victualling Board set up in 1692, controlled a vast system supplying provisions to ships and foreign dockyards. The board operated bakeries, slaughterhouses, breweries and specialist facilities such as the Soup Houses for the production of Portable Soup. This took the form of huge, solid cakes of offal, vegetables and salt which were taken aboard ship in large quantities and were boiled with water and peasemeal; they were essentially industrial-sized stock cubes. Meat was supplied salted and stored in brine barrels; most other foodstuffs were dried. Beer, wine and water were carried in barrels. In addition, some ships carried a limited number of live pigs and poultry, and many surgeons encouraged the growing of fresh mustard and cress. A ship on a lengthy voyage could not carry enough food for the whole passage; even if it could have been preserved, there was insufficient storage space. Some foodstuff could be preserved using alcohol, and attempts were often made to distil fresh water from seawater. Whichever part of the globe was being traversed, arrangements had to be made to obtain fresh supplies – often at the cost of introducing further disease; water and other supplies obtained abroad were not always reliable or safe.

In theory, officers ate the same food as men. In practice, they were able to buy additional and better quality supplies. In most ships, the officers contributed jointly to funds for the enhancement of their own mess supplies. In every sense, including the availability of servants, the officers were much better provided for than ordinary seamen. The normal crewman's daily diet consisted of heavily salted meat, biscuit, cheese, peasemeal, unleavened bread and small beer or water. The cheese was apparently as excellent for making trouser buttons as was the dried, salted beef for fashioning tobacco boxes. Not only was the diet monotonous, day after day, but it was wholly lacking in vitamin C and was hard to digest. Later, there was made available 6 ounces of sugar per man per week, and fresh vegetables 'when they can be procured and not at any time exceeding the value of the pease saved.' In foreign parts, there was wine rather than beer, which did not keep; and raisins, rice and olive oil if available locally. Two days each week were meat-free; they were known as 'banyan days' after a Hindu vegetarian sect, and on these days fish was eaten if available. The Victualling Board was unconcerned with the healthiness of the diet; they were conservatively interested in maintaining a workforce at little cost. One protestor wrote in 1703:

> A hot country, stinking meat, maggoty bread, noisome and poisonous scent of the bilge-water, have made many a brave sailor food for crabs and sharks . . . Where we had one man dyed by shot in the navy, we had ten dyed by means of bad provisions.[30]

In the summer of 1703, Sir Cloudesley Shovell led his Mediterranean Fleet from Spithead. To begin with, he had to leave eight ships behind because of sickness. The fleet became becalmed off the North African coast and soon ran short of water in an area where there was no prospect of supply. By the time the fleet returned to England in November, there had been no contact with the enemy, and yet more than 1,500 men had died (probably from scurvy, exacerbated by lack of water) and three-quarters of the remainder were too ill to work. Shovell was appointed Admiral, and the blame was laid at the door of the Victualling Commissioners by one of his fleet captains, 'because the sickness was amongst our men at Portsmouth, before they left England.'[31] Attitudes did not improve markedly. In 1740, when Anson was preparing his circumnavigation, the two victualling agents appalled the board when they revealed that they had budgeted 18*d* per day per man for food. The Victualling Board replied tartly that this sum 'farr exceeded the price given on any Contract subsisting with this Board.'[32] Their retort was probably relevant, since the value of 18*d* in 1740 would have been substantial.

'SOE MANY OF THE BEST CHIRURGEONS'

The table below shows the typical weekly provisions allowed for each man aboard a Royal Navy ship in the earlier part of the eighteenth century.

BASIC WEEKLY PROVISIONS FOR EACH MAN[33]

	Biscuit	Beer	Beef	Pork	Pease	Oatmeal	Butter	Cheese
Sunday	1 lb	1 gall.	–	1 lb	½ pint	–	2 oz	–
Monday	1 lb	1 gall.	–	–	–	1 pint	2 oz	4 oz
Tuesday	1 lb	1 gall.	2 lb	–	–	–	–	–
Wednesday	1 lb	1 gall.	–	–	½ pint	1 pint	2 oz	4 oz
Thursday	1 lb	1 gall.	–	1 lb	½ pint	–	–	–
Friday	1 lb	1 gall.	–	–	½ pint	1 pint	2 oz	4 oz
Saturday	1 lb	1 gall.	2 lb	–	–	–	–	–

At this time the Victualling Board did little more to improve the dietary aspects of their responsibilities. They concentrated on securing a worldwide supply network, although the Admiralty Board often refused them funds for some of their more radical improvements even in that area. Improvements in the provision of fresh meat and beer were made, although these changes may have been brought in to improve morale rather than diet. By the middle of the century, the Victualling Board was undoubtedly spending vast sums of money on provisions, and it was dealing with a logistical problem of awesome complexity. Central to the way things worked was the role of the purser, who was essentially a freelance agent aboard ship responsible for ordering supplies. However, he was also accountable for payment, credit and for any losses, theft or wastage due to decay or battle action. As part of the complex accounting system, the purser was entitled to a personal eighth share of all provisions issued. The scope for fraud among all those suppliers and contractors with whom the purser had to deal was extremely wide, although pursers themselves probably had most interest in ensuring that crews were reasonably well provisioned. Figures giving the total volumes of foodstuffs issued between 1750 and 1757 make clear the formidable size of the victualling process. (A tun equalled 216 gallons, and a bushel was a dry measure equal to 8 gallons):

Bread	54,642,437 lbs	[24,837,471 kg]
Beer	110,049 tuns	[23,770,584 gallons or 108,061,075 litres]
Brandy	351,692 gallons	[1,598,791 litres]
Beef	4,498,486 lbs	[2,044,766 kg]
Pork	6,734,261 lbs	[3,061,027 kg]
Pease	203,385 bushels	[1,627,080 gallons]
Flour	6,264,879 lbs	[2,847,672 kg]
Suet	809,419 lbs	[367,917 kg]
Raisins	705,784 lbs	[320,811 kg]
Oatmeal	138,504 lbs	[62,956 kg]
Vinegar	390,863 gallons	[1,776,863 litres]
Stockfish	166,943 lbs	[75,883 kg]
Oil	71,668 gallons	[325,802 litres][34]

Despite all the stories about bad food, it is likely that the majority of sailors in the eighteenth century ate a better diet most of the time than they would have done ashore. Given that they were regularly entitled to meat perhaps four times a week, with a reasonable supply of vegetables, fruit and beer, spirits and occasionally exotic foodstuffs, their lot was often not as bad as has often been painted.

It was a court-martial offence to 'stir up any disturbance' over food. The Articles of War made it a requirement that any complaint about victuals had to be made to a senior officer, and that such complaints had to be remedied. By and large, however, the Admiralty was unresponsive to demands for improvements even from surgeons. Ironically, when fresh vegetables or fruit could be obtained, some sailors would resist eating them since these items were not normally available to them ashore either. Their natural conservatism is easy to understand. Sauerkraut for example, which was commonly used to some effect against scurvy, was universally loathed. Some captains – even better ones such as James Cook – ignored their crew's preferences and imposed fresh food on peril of severe punishment. He once had two seamen flogged for a refusal to eat fresh meat.[35] Cook, who was known for his ability to obtain better supplies than other captains, was frustrated that his well-intentioned efforts on behalf of his sailors were difficult to bring into effect:

'SOE MANY OF THE BEST CHIRURGEONS'

Every innovation whatever tho ever so much to their advantage is sure to meet with the highest disapprobation from Seamen, Portable Soup, and Sour Krout were at first both condemned by them as stuff not fit for human being[s] to eat. Few men have introduced into their Ships more novelties in the way of victuals and drink than I have done; indeed few men have had the same opportunity or been given the same necessity. It has however in a great measure been owing to such little innovations that I have always kept my people generally speaking free from that dreadful distemper the Scurvy.[36]

In the mid-eighteenth century an employee of one of the great victualling yards became a powerful proponent of better supplies. William Thompson had ironically been sacked for sharp practice, but for years he maintained a constant attack on the authorities for what he saw as a grossly fraudulent trade that consigned seamen to cruel despair and illness:

... the bread so full of large black-headed maggots that the men have so nauseated the thoughts of it as to be obliged to shut their eyes to confine that sense from being offended before they could bring their minds into the resolution of consuming it. That the beer has stunk as abominably as the foul stagnant water which is pumped out of many cellars in London at midnight hour.[37]

The supply of fresh water for both drinking and hygiene purposes was a particular problem. It was stored in barrels deep down in the ships, but even at the start of long voyages, it was not wise to rely on the quality of what was supplied. It often remained there serving only as ballast when its wholesomeness had clearly gone, and the men would drink small beer or watered wine instead. Leonard Gillespie, joining Nelson's fleet at Yarmouth in 1788, was not the only naval surgeon to complain of the six-months-old Thames water, 'putrefaction has made it fetid and stinking.'[38] During the course of a voyage, supplies of fresh water were vital, from wherever a ship could put in to port. Taking on water was, however, a slow business, and what was available could produce more problems than were solved. Off the Mexican coast Anson's fleet took a month to restock with water, which had to be ferried to the ships in small canoes. The water was found to be brackish and 'full of nauseous live worms.' Water was always collected on board ship from rainfall, but this could hardly be relied upon, and in terms of quantity was practically meaningless. There were attempts to preserve water by adding chemicals, but the results were unpalatable. Crude distillation of sea water was also tried. The addition of chemicals such as silver nitrate, calcined bones and even chalk, made water undrinkable.

For hundreds of years, sailors complained of dozens of diseases which fitted themselves into four everyday words – 'scurvy', 'ague', 'flux' and the inevitable 'pox'. One of the great melancholy ballads of the eighteenth century commemorates 'Admiral Hosier's Ghost' and the incidents of the war with Spain in 1726. It is also a powerful reference to the fact that the nation was powerless in the face of disease on a catastrophic scale. Hosier's squadron mounted a blockade in the Caribbean to prevent the movements of Spanish treasure ships. A staggering 4,000 men from a complement of 4,750 (including Hosier himself) died of disease. It is probable that most succumbed to yellow fever, but of the few details that remain, there is one comment from Hosier himself that refers to 'scorbutic and other distempers'.[39] The ballad was written by Richard Glover in 1740 to celebrate the victory of Admiral Vernon at the same location, and conjured the image of the ghosts of Hosier's seamen warning Vernon's fleet. Thereafter, the possibility of being sent to the West Indies was always regarded by sailors as deeply undesirable. Second only to scurvy, 'Yellow Jack' – the shipboard name for Yellow Fever – was probably the most feared ship disease. It was prevalent off the coast of South America and the West Indies, and was so infectious that even a single case occurring on board ship might easily wipe out the whole crew. The infectious agents of these diseases were unknown, although in retrospect it is likely that impaired immune function as a result of scurvy contributed to the high infectivity and high mortality among sailors.

What persuaded the Admiralty of the need for dramatic action to protect national interests was a typhus outbreak in 1740. After 15,000 new recruits had been rapidly signed up for war, only 1,000 were fit for duty six months later: throughout the Navy 25,000 men fell ill; 2,500 died, and another 2,000 deserted. In the Seven Years War (1756–63), ten times as many men died from disease as were killed in action. In the twenty years of wartime from 1793, 6.3 per cent were killed in action and 81.5 per cent died from disease and accident.[40] The eighteenth century saw the Royal Navy involved in almost constant wartime activity, and the ravages of disease on such scales was a national disaster. Without any doubt, as shown by diaries and journals, and most of all by the fervent wishes, pleas and demands of surgeons that someone would find the answer, scurvy was the most loathsome and feared disease of all.

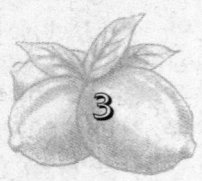

'The Vain and Chimerical Belief'

THE diseases that afflicted sailors in the eighteenth century were often not clearly diagnosed, and this impeded their treatment considerably. Lind was certain that this fundamental uncertainty had been historically damaging:

> The common names of fevers, as I have elsewhere shewn, are too unsatisfactory to be regarded in practice; being founded chiefly on vague and theoretical opinions of their causes and effects. Physicians, who have had the most frequent opportunities of seeing numerous patients in fevers, have always found great difficulty in arranging their cases under the common appellations. An attempt of this sort has frequently led them into absurdities, as it is certain, that almost all these fevers may proceed from one and the same cause.[1]

The treatments used and promoted for scurvy, both sworn by and tried in desperation, ranged from the accidentally sensible to the outlandish and fraudulent. To an extent the Admiralty connived at the confusion by promoting the use of one or other of the latest theories by fashionable physicians; and many of the Navy's own surgeons were publishing extensive but conflicting reports and treatises on the subject. From the times of the earliest recorded outbreaks, there matured a long inventory of favoured recommendations. Lind was contemptuous of the simplistic notion of any kind of assumed 'right' to a cure for disease. He spoke of 'the vain and chimerical belief' in the concept of 'an infallible remedy' that had for so long 'rendered the art of healing as variable and unconstant as our dresses'. He was inclined to characterise diet and confinement as two main targets of the fight against scurvy:

> Many diseases have been well known and accurately described for above a thousand years, yet for which of them have we an infallible remedy? What medicine can counteract the continued influences of improper diet, air and confinement, the last of which in particular I may judge to be a principal cause of the great obstinacy and frequent mortality of the scurvy in long voyages at sea?[2]

From the time of Henry III there had been rational sailors who gave wholly sensible advice on diet as a means of combating disease. In 1227 Gilbertus de Aquila travelled to Palestine in the course of writing a huge work on medicine. Probably largely by intelligent guesswork rather than anything else, he recommended exercise, cleanliness, fresh clothing and bedding and a moderate diet including apples, pears, pomegranates, cucumbers, citrons, lemons, muscatels and vegetables pickled in brine.[3] That extraordinary advice constituted perhaps the best remedy for the prevention of scurvy for several centuries, and James Lind would unhesitatingly have endorsed each one of those recommendations.

Most remedies were in the form of 'medicine', but there were also preventative procedures used aboard ship against disease in general. These included swabbing the decks with vinegar and the widespread burning of both tar and tobacco as fumigants. Bleeding the patient was popular in the mid-eighteenth century as a panacea for almost any disease, when many physicians, ashore and at sea, promoted a view of medicine based on theoretical states of the blood. The public also took the view that, healthy or otherwise, a gentleman could not preserve his constitution at certain seasons of the year unless he was 'let blood'. It was said that more blood was shed in peace than in time of war, and that 'there is no more frequent charge in medical bills than for phlebotomising.'[4]

During the circumnavigation by Ferdinand Magellan's expedition in 1521, eating ship's rats was apparently the answer (more likely the answer to old-fashioned hunger rather than the claimed scurvy). Another eccentric remedy employed against scurvy, especially by pirates apparently, was burial up to the neck in sand. Surgeon Robert Crosfield referred to this absurd notion in 1797:

> It is said to occasion great pain on being first used, but in a few repetitions the pains wear off, and the whole habit quickly amends. How far this is the case I am unable to determine; but as the earth-bath can only be practised on shore, the change of diet which may be supposed to obtain at that time may perhaps effect the cure. The application of the fresh earth may perhaps palliate the symptoms, but it must strike everyone as a manifest absurdity to imagine that the morbid effects can permanently cease when their cause (bad and insufficient food) remains.[5]

James Lind recounted an even more bizarre instance of this practice, told to him by a friend:

> One day hunting in Newfoundland, he discovered what appeared to him at a distance to be a number of graves, with a man's head fixed to each. Struck with the novelty of the sight, he went to the place; where he was further surprised to find the men alive; they informed him they belonged to a ship which lay in the road, and that having been reduced to unspeakable misery by the scurvy, they were thus interred in order to obtain a cure.[6]

When Cartier's expedition was saved by the Canadian Indians in 1535, they were drinking one of the commonest standard remedies – spruce beer. This old favourite had pride of place for

'THE VAIN AND CHIMERICAL BELIEF'

centuries in various parts of the world, and it *was* an antiscorbutic. Essentially, spruce beer was a strong tea made by stewing spruce leaves in water; later, spruce sprigs would be added to the standard naval-issue small beer. Much later, as we shall see, there was an insistence on a fermentation process to prevent putrefaction. Over the years, there were teas, beers and infusions of all sorts of fruit, herbs, roots and vegetables, according to which was currently favourite. One formula published in 1656 used a multitude of herbs, many of them lost to us, including the famous scurvy grass or spoonwort (*cochlearia officinalis*), a botanical relation of cabbage and swede turnip (and all of them usefully antiscorbutic):

> Dr Deodates Scurbuttical Drink:
> Take Roman Wormwood, Carduus Benedictus, Scurvy-grasse, Brooklime, Water-cresses, Water Trifoil, of each one handful, Dodder, Cetrach, Scolopendria, Burrage, Buglos, Sorrel, Vervain or Speedwell, of each one handful, Elicampane root one ounce, Raisons of the Sun three ounces, slices of Oranges and Lemmons of each fifteen, boil, or rather infuse these in a double glasse, with so much white Wine, as will make a pint and a halfe of the liquor when it is done.[7]

Scurvy grass held pride of place in the list of remedies for centuries, and consequently has attracted a wealth of folk imagery. It is a small, low-growing plant with egg-shaped leaves that thrives in gritty soil by rivers in northern areas, in the Arctic Circle and often at high elevations. It contains vitamin C and is antiscorbutic and diuretic. In his 1734 analysis of the causes of scurvy, J.F. Bachstrom illustrated the accidental discovery of the efficacy of scurvy grass by 'a sailor in the Greenland ships . . . so over-run and disabled with the scurvy'. The unfortunate man had been taken ashore by his comrades and abandoned to his fate. Unable to make any use of his limbs, he had been crawling around helplessly on the ground:

... this he found covered with a plant, which he, continually grazing like a beast of the field, plucked up with his teeth. In a short time he was by this means fully recovered; and, upon his returning home, it was found to have been the herb scurvy-grass.[8]

A chemist from Leipzig, Dr Andreas Valentinus Moellenbrok, made a special study of scurvy grass in the mid-seventeenth century. He produced and analysed many different medical preparations which had been developed from dozens of domestic concoctions and potions used in the kitchen. It is probable that, in the course of making his *pièce de résistance*, which he called the 'Volatile Salt of Scurvy-grass', he may entirely unconsciously have produced crystals of ascorbic acid:

> Let the thick leaves of *Scurvygrass*, and full of juice, be boiled a little while in water, and afterwards press out the juice, or which is better, if only the juice pressed out of the fresh gathered leaves be purified, and a little evaporated till it be somewhat thickened, and so set by, till of its own accord the Salt shoot in the juice. The chief efficacy of *Scurvygrass* is from the volatile Salt.[9]

Moellenbrok offered as an encouragement a Latin verse from a much earlier writer, Johannes Joachim Bechorus:

> Spoonwort doth warm, and also doth dry,
> In the Scurvy, 'tis a great Remedy,
> It sends out all corrupt humours by sweat
> With this your mouth gargel often, and wet,
> This plant which deserves so much of your praise
> The Apothecaries use six several wayes,
> It's Spirit, Syrup, Water procures health,
> So doth its Salt conserve, and the Herb itself.[10]

Scurvy grass ranks along with spruce beer as one of the oldest antiscorbutics. It made a popular tonic drink and diuretic, and its

'THE VAIN AND CHIMERICAL BELIEF'

'essential oil' was also recommended in cases of paralysis and rheumatism. While oranges and lemons were incorporated into treatments for scurvy long before James Lind's time, as further accounts will show, no-one could really be sure what worked and what did not in the desperation to use just about every possible substance available.

Another standard early remedy was cinchona, or 'Peruvian Bark' or 'Jesuits Bark'. The supposed curative powers of this rare material were discovered by a Jesuit priest in 1633, and within a few years its popularity was assured. The bark contained the alkaloids cinchonidine, quinidine and quinine, giving it particular value against malaria; perhaps because of this it assumed almost supernatural status against scurvy and all forms of fever. Cinchona was extremely expensive, growing only in Peru and Bolivia. By the mid-nineteenth century, the East India Company alone was spending the enormous sum of £100,000 annually on cinchona, and the British Army in India required 750 tons.[11] Its widely claimed successes – Admiral Nelson was a keen supporter – were apparently matched by an equally long list of potentially serious side effects. As ever, there was no-one properly able to quantify its value.

At the beginning of the seventeenth century, the first connections between citrus fruit and scurvy were independently made by four notable men – two great sailors and two physicians. Sir Richard Hawkins, a veteran of the battles with the Spanish Armada, sailed for South America in 1593. At sea near the Equator, his crew began to suffer scurvy:

> The signes to know this disease in the beginning are divers, by the swelling of the gummes, by denting of the flesh of the leggs with a mans finger, the pit remayning without filling up in a good space.[12]

After weeks becalmed they were able to go ashore in southern Brazil, where they traded under truce with the Portuguese for oranges and lemons to add to the mysterious nostrum that Hawkins also carried with him:

> That which I have seene most fruitfull for this sicknesse, is sower Oranges and Lemmons, and a water which amongst others (for my particular provision) I carryed to the Sea, called *Doctor Stevens his Water*, of which, for that his vertue was not well knowne unto me, I carryed but little, and it tooke end quickly, but gave health to those that used it.[13]

The distilled water peddled by Dr Stevens contained twenty-one ingredients, and had been concocted in Paris. This nostrum tasted strongly acidic, and therefore fell into the first and most popular category of remedies for scurvy. It was described in 1588 as, 'good juice somewhat hoate, thinne, piercing and cleansing.'[14] Hawkins goes on to say that until encountering the 'wonderful secret' he had used one of the other early remedies – 'oyle of vitry' or sulphuric acid. However, he was completely certain of the superior efficacy of oranges and lemons, and was one of the first both to declare that reliance and to recognise something unknown about the source of the benefit:

> Coming aboord of our Shippes, there was great joy amongst my Company, and many with the sight of the Oranges and Lemmons, seemed to recover heart; this is a wonderful secret of the power and wisedome of God, that hath hidden so great and unknowne vertue in this fruit, to be a certaine remedie for this infirmitie.[15]

Despite appearing to recognise the value of citrus fruit, Hawkins seems to have had a blind spot. He could not make the connection between the efficacy of the fruit obtained at a foreign port and used as a curative, and the wisdom of carrying that same fruit on board ship as a deliberate preventative measure. What Hawkins did realise was that it would need someone rather special to examine the issue on a proper scientific basis:

> I wish that some learned man would write of it, for it is the plague of the Sea, and the spoyle of Mariners' doubtlesse, it

would be a meritorious Worke with God and man, and most beneficiall for our Countrie, for in twentie years, since that I have used the sea, I dare take upon me to give accompt of ten thousand men consumed with this disease.[16]

Another important Elizabethan surgeon was William Clowes. He was very knowledgeable about scurvy, and wrote in 1596 that it was related to diet, and advised one containing fruit and vegetables, including watercress; he also recommended that freshly picked scurvy grass should be steeped in ship's ale. The connection that Hawkins missed was made a few years later with the first expedition to Sumatra by the newly formed East India Company in 1601 (the English company that is; the Dutch East India Company had been founded six years earlier). Sir James Lancaster commanded the three ships that made passage towards the Cape of Good Hope:

> . . . by this time many of our men were fallen sick of the scurvy in all our ships, and unless it were in the general's ship only . . . our weaknesses of men was so great that in some of the ships the merchants took their turns at the helm, and went into the top to take in the topsails, as the common mariners did.[17]

But it was noticed that those on board Lancaster's own ship were much less affected by the scurvy:

> And the reason why the general's men stood better in health was this; he brought to sea with him certain bottles of the juice of lemons, which he gave to each one, as long as it would last, three spoonfuls every morning, fasting; not suffering them to eat anything after it till noon. This juice worketh much the better if the party keep a short diet and wholly refrain from salt meat; which salt meat, and long being at the sea, is the only cause of the breeding of this disease.[18]

Lancaster clearly understood the preventative role of citrus juice. Some people wondered how he 'stumbled upon the cure for scurvy'. The truth is that he probably didn't think he had. There is one account that refers to a chronicler of an earlier voyage having noted the magical recovery of a crewman after consuming oranges and lemons obtained on the island of St Helena.[19] However, it was the most common belief at the time that the consumption of salt meat was implicated in the incidence of scurvy. Lancaster simply couldn't have quantified the possible effects of one administration of lemon juice against the possible effects of any of the other supposed remedies that could be in use at the same time. Hawkins' 'learned man' was still missing.

Accounts suggest that Lancaster had carried lemon juice preserved by a mysterious secret process.[20] Sir Hugh Platt, son of a London brewer, was an inveterate inventor and something of a self-publicist. He experimented in mechanics, agriculture and horticulture, and wrote extensively on such diverse subjects as dyeing the hair, distilling and, significantly, preserving fruit. He also wrote classical poetry and cookery books for ladies. While advising Sir Francis Drake some years earlier, he had recommended a novel food for use when fresh was unavailable – 'a cheape, fresh and lasting victual, called by the name of "Macaroni" amongst the Italians.'[21] His methods of preservation were published in a pamphlet entitled *Certaine Philosophical Preparations of Foode and Beurage for Sea-men, in their long voyages* in 1607. In this he described his method of preservation of fruit juice by the use of 'philosophical fire' or heat. This would not have been successful; even if the juice had been successfully 'preserved' by heat, the antiscorbutic factor, in the form of vitamin C, would have been destroyed. It must be remembered that nothing was known of vitamin C. Platt also promoted his methods of preserving fresh water, which he guaranteed 'to last sweete, good, and without any intention to putrefaction, for two, three or four yeeres together'.[22] Later critics have suggested that Platt used 'secret powders' and suchlike alchemical substances. Platt apparently denied that he had made any claim to have prepared the juice for Lancaster, only that 'the juice of lemons was found (by him) to be an assured remedy for the scurby'. Platt's only assertion was that such juice, 'by fortifying it with [my] own fire, it will be lasting and durable' while if it were not so treated it would 'lose much of its first manifest nature, which it had while it was contained within its own pulp and fruit'.[23] In any case, after the first flurry of publicity, nothing more was heard of it all. Lemons and oranges continued to be used sporadically at sea when they were obtainable, but no more than was any other popular nostrum.

The fourth significant character in the early scurvy trail was a medical man. John Woodall had been a military surgeon; he was appointed the first surgeon-general to the East India Company in 1612, and was a surgeon at St Bartholomew's Hospital in London from 1616 until 1643. He was the first of the truly great naval surgeons, and in 1617 he published the first edition of *The Surgeon's Mate* in which he laid out his recommendations on surgery, medicines, instruments and therapeutics and the whole sweep of matters medical for aspiring naval surgeons. His extraordinary volume reads as if it was written precisely for the individual reading it. In addressing scurvy, he says that

> ... there are few diseases at sea happeneth to seamen but the scurvy hath a part in them; the fluxes which happen chiefly proceed from the scurvy, and I suppose if seamen could be preserved from that disease, few other diseases would endanger them.[24]

He confesses that the causes of scurvy are infinite, and that, 'they far pass my capacity to search them all.'[25] He echoes the lament of Sir Richard Hawkins for the missing 'learned man':

> It is strange in so many ages past, that no one Chirurgeon of our countrymen hath out of his experience taken in hand sincerely to set down to posterities the true causes, signs and cures thereof; neither left any instructions, caveats or experiences, for the prevention or cure of the same.[26]

Woodall was quite clear as to the main reasons why the disease attacked seamen so readily:

> . . . the chief cause whereof is the continuance of salt diet, either fish or flesh, as pork and the like, which is not to be avoided at sea; another cause is want of sufficient nourishing food, and of sweet water, and also for want of *aquavitae*, wine, beer, or other good water to comfort and warm their stomachs.[27]

He also blamed inadequate clothing and unhygienic accommodation. He gave instructions for treatment at different stages of the disease, and wrote with a clarity and certainty that was not equalled until James Lind proved the case:

> The use of the juice of lemmons is a precious medicine, and well tried, being found and good; let it have the chief place, for it will deserve it, the use whereof is; it is to be taken each morning, two or three spoonfuls, and fast after it two hours, and if you add one spoonful of aquavitae thereto to a cold stomach, it is the better. Also if you take a little thereof at night it is good to mix therewith some sugar.[28]

Woodall is interesting for his very positive views, and for his willingness to distinguish between the cure and the day-to-day use of citrus fruit as a preventative. Neither is he above suggesting that some subterfuge might be necessary:

> Some Chirurgeons also give of this juice daily to the men in health as a preservative, which course is good if they have store, otherwise it were best to keep it for need. I dare not write how good a sauce it is at meat, lest the chief in the ships waste it in the great Cabins to save vinegar.[29]

Woodall suggested that in the absence of lemons, limes, oranges or tamarind pulp, the ship's surgeon should resort to the old standby, '... oyle of vitriol, as many drops as will make a cup of beer or water sower a little.'[30]

Ralph Stockman, Professor of Materia Medica and Therapeutics at Glasgow University wrote, perhaps over critically, of Woodall in 1926 that 'a great deal of his advice is trivial, and he proposes too many alternative cures and treatments.'[31] The ability to quantify the alternative cures and treatments lay at the heart of the scurvy problem for centuries, and Woodall was certainly not above suggesting other remedies. Some seem to us absurd, such as the recommendation that:

> ... where you can have it, a good bath of the blood of beasts, either cows, horses, asses, goats or sheeps blood is exceeding good, namely, to put the legges of the patient, yea and his bodie too, if it may be, into a tub made fitting, and the blood kept warm.[32]

However, Woodall was giving practical advice to less experienced men ('babes in Chirurgery' as he describes them) not attempting a definitive theory, and reiterated his (and Hawkins') hopes that someone would tackle the scientific analysis:

> I must constrain myself to go briefly to the business in hand, namely to inform the Chirurgeons Mate how he should demean himself to comfort his Patients at Sea in that most dangerous disease, neither will I here strive to give the curious reader other content than this, that if he like it not, let him amend it himself, which I should heartily rejoice to see any good man do, knowing mine own weakness. A learned Treatise befits not my pen, and to declare those good medicines, which cannot be had at sea, is but time lost.[33]

That learned treatise would still be some time away. Meanwhile, Shakespeare's son-in-law, John Hall, a Warwickshire doctor, was one of the first to promote the use of antiscorbutics – the first hint of specific cures for scurvy. In a book published in

1657 he claims as a remedy for scurvy a beer brewed from 'Scorbutick hearbs, viz.: scurvy-grass, water-cresses and brook lime.' There were others who advocated the use of mustard, radish and balsam; calomel, opium, mercury, rice, rhubarb and 'train oil' – a thick, oily substance obtained by boiling seal carcasses. In 1572, King James VI of Scotland (and later James I of England) addressed a diatribe to 'all Taverns, Inns, Victualling-Houses, Ale-Houses, Coffee-Houses, Strong-Water-Shops and Tobacco Shops in England, Scotland or Ireland'[34] attacking the use of tobacco. He appended a 'Learned Discourse' by Dr Everard Maynwaringe, 'proving that Tobacco is a procuring Cause of The Scurvy'. He threatened all manner of ill effects from 'the taking of some kind of Poyson' and claimed that the 'dulcid good juyce of the body' would be exhausted. Maynwaringe wrote:

> I observed in Virginia, being for some time in that Colony, that the Planters who had lived long there, being great Smokers, were of a withered, decayed Countenance, and very Scorbutick, being exhausted by this immoderate fume; nor are they long-lived, but do shorten their days by the intemperate use of Tobacco and Brandy.[35]

Lind accused Maynwaringe of being a bit of a *poseur* who condemned all the recommendations of other writers while claiming that he had all the answers, 'which, however, he does not make public.'[36]

There was a multitude of claims for the causes and remedies, some of them obviously associated with attempts to market pills and potions, as Maynwaringe was doing. There was a theory of copper poisoning as the cause of scurvy, which will be looked at later. From time to time, in the midst of the confusion, individual physicians 'came out'. In 1672, John Fryer was a surgeon in the East India Company, sailing for Madras. By the Cape of Good Hope, half the fleet of ten ships was sick. Putting into an island off Mozambique, Fryer noted:

'THE VAIN AND CHIMERICAL BELIEF'

... the first care was to send the Sick Men ashore when it is incredible to relate how strangely they revived in so short a time, by feeding on Oranges and Fresh Limes, and the very Smell of the Earth; for many that were carried from the ship in Cradles, and looked upon as desperate, in a days time could take up their Beds and walk.[37]

Another, a progressive, practical surgeon named John Moyle, with a reputation as a clever, perceptive observer, wrote twenty year later:

... when the Succulent Herbs and Roots, and Fruits, as Lemmons and Oranges are freely taken, and good wine drank, there's no fear of the Scurvy.[38]

But confusion and uncertainty reigned. In only the first five years of East India Company expeditions, 800 out of a total of 1,200 sailors died of either scurvy, typhoid or 'the bloody flux', and a third of their ships had been sunk. The company was very progressive, in that its surgeons were required to provide detailed medical records to a central administration, and was therefore in a position to make recommendations founded on practical experience. However, in the confusion over treatments for scurvy, the company abandoned its early provision of citrus juice.[39] The Dutch East India Company had never even tried it.

As still often happens today with controversial issues, a 'contra' faction arose, and a dissenting party of 'anti-fruiters' developed. The impetus came after a disastrous expedition to colonise Hispaniola and Jamaica in the 1650s. The expedition was ill-planned and ill-supplied, and everything that could possibly have gone wrong did. General Venables, who was in charge of the huge force of fighting soldiers carried by the fleet, began the attack on fruit:

Our men the last fortnight at sea had had bread, and little of it or other victuals, notwithstanding General Penn's order [Penn was the sea commander], so that they were very weak at landing, and some instead of three days provision at landing had but one, with which they marched five days, and therefore fell to eat limes, oranges, limons etc, which put them into fluxes and fevers.[40]

In the minds of ordinary sailors and soldiers, the wisdom of Hawkins, Lancaster and Woodall (had they been aware of it) would have been dashed in an instant. But there was an issue of politics here, and a range of explanations was being devised which would help to maintain public face after the national disaster of the expedition. A target for blame was required.

Some years later a surgeon named James White was court-martialled on board ship in the harbour at Lisbon for 'mutiny and disaffection' because of his political views. He was dumped ashore with no resources, but soon prospered as a local physician. In 1712 he published an account of an epidemic of flux in the fleet in which he laid the blame on lemons. This was a view that gained some support, and it is thought to have been responsible for a subsequent increase in scurvy. About the same time a Bristol physician, Thomas Dover, sailed to South America with the Bristol Society of Merchant Venturers. Scurvy broke out rounding the Horn, and the sick were landed on the island of Juan Fernandez in early 1709, where they discovered Alexander Selkirk, the marooned sailor from Fife in Scotland who was the model for Defoe's *Robinson Crusoe*. With Selkirk's help it was soon reported that by means of fresh goat meat and 'Greens and Goodness of the Air they recover'd very fast of the Scurvy.' Dover declared that green fruit was a vermifuge [a drug expelling worms], but "Tis Ripe Fruits that breed Worms.'[41]

The 'anti-fruiters' did not gain very much credence; they added to the general confusion by failing to offer any evidence either way. Another confusion, which due to the attitude of the Admiralty had more serious repercussions, was the credibility given to doubtful peddlers of 'secret potions'. One mixture of antimony and phosphate of lime was sold as

'Dr James's Powder'. Despite the fact that this secret compound allegedly killed Oliver Goldsmith the Irish playwright,[42] and the fact that several physicians, including James Lind, advised against its use, the Admiralty ordered its trial in the Channel Fleet. It was reported that it killed many men. The Admiralty nevertheless persisted. Later, the self-assured Dr James recommended 'a German dish known by the name of Sour Kraut, which is nothing but cabbage cut up small, pressed down and preserved in a manner so as to keep it a long time.'[43] James Lind had recommended the Navy's use of sauerkraut some years before, but the Admiralty, for perverse reasons unknown, preferred to wait upon the pronouncement of a charlatan.

About the same time the Admiralty also bestowed its favours on another medical con man, Dr Joshua Ward (known as 'Spot Ward' due to a large claret birthmark on his cheek). It seems that Ward, who had no medical training, was given the secret formula for his infamous pills in Paris. He promoted himself avidly, while at the same time trying to avoid the enquiries of the College of Physicians. Despite being held up to ridicule by the medical profession, he successfully advertised both himself and his dangerous pills. Ward was depicted in 1736 by the brilliant satirist William Hogarth, who had a fascination for medical affairs, in a drawing entitled 'The Company of Undertakers, or Consultation of Quacks'. Ward was attacked professionally in 1736 by a Mr Clutton, a Holborn apothecary who condemned Ward in a pamphlet whose title is so bizarre that it deserves mention: *A True and Candid Relation of the Good and Bad Effects of Joshua Ward's Pill and Drop; Exhibited in Sixty-eight Cases; quotations from the Writings of Learned Physicians concerning Arsenick; some Cases of Persons who have taken it; and Experiments to shew what are the component Principles of these Pills; introduced with Occurrances shewing the Rise and Progress of this Controversy; The Whole being an Essay to discover how far this Random Practice of Physic is really useful.* Clutton claimed that 16,380 of the pills could be made for the small sum of 1s 3 1/2d. Ward responded to this campaign by hiring 'puffers to go about the town into coffee houses and elsewhere to cry up to the skies this great and most wonderful cure.'[44] This successful use of spin doctors was apparently enough to have Ward adopted by the Admiralty in the 1750s as a physician of great esteem. The Pill and Drop acted as a violent diuretic, killed many who took it and made very many more extremely ill. In 1753 the Admiralty ordered its use in the Channel Fleet, twenty-five powders per ship, and on the West Indies station. Ward became very wealthy. After his death, his executor, John Page MP, revealed that the secret 'Pill and Drop' was a useless but dangerous compound of antimony, balsam and wine.

Popular confidence in quack medicines, both at home and at sea, was entirely misplaced, and often led to dangerous complications and even death. Sir Samuel Garth, the seventeenth-century physician to George I and physician-general to the Army, was also a poet and satirist. In his 1699 burlesque poem 'The Dispensary' he satirised fraudulent medicine, and showed that while soldiers and sailors might expect to die in battle, they could nevertheless succumb to the actions of the likes of Dr Joshua Ward:

> Some fell by laudanum, and some by steel,
> And death in ambush lay in every pill.

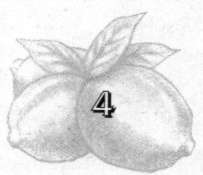

'A Learned Man'

LIND spent eight years at sea, from 1739 to 1748, sailing in a number of ships and progressing from surgeon's mate to surgeon. He was sent on voyages to the Mediterranean, West Africa and the West Indies, and spent long periods on patrol in the English Channel during the complex War of the Austrian Succession (1740–8), which, despite its prosaic name, involved a large part of the world. Apart from the normal surgeon's duties, Lind's main interest while at sea was in recording everything that related to disease and hygiene in great detail. This was the period during which he built the experience and gathered the knowledge that was to enable him to produce with such clarity the prodigious written works of later years. This detailed medical observation was not achieved in the rather relaxed manner of the wealthy gentleman-scientist (such as his younger half-cousin) invited to join a well-endowed expedition. Lind was still the surgeon's mate in a service which neither rated him highly nor gave him adequate resources to do his job, far less the facilities for scientific research. However he may not, like Roderick Random, have encountered a difficult or incompetent surgeon:

> Captain Oakhum, having received sailing orders, came on board, and brought along with him a surgeon of his own country, who soon made us sensible of the loss we suffered in the departure of doctor Atkins; for he was grossly ignorant, and intolerably assuming, false, vindictive, and

unforgiving; a merciless tyrant to his inferiors, an abject sycophant to those above him.

Or an impossible, choleric captain:

> In the morning after the captain came on board, our first mate, according to custom, went to wait on him with a sick list, which when this grim commander had perused, he cried with a stern countenance, 'Blood and oons! Sixty-one sick people on board of my ship! Harkee you, sir, I'll have no sick in my ship, by G–d.' The Welchman replied, he should be very glad to find no sick people on board; but while it was otherwise, he did no more than his duty in presenting him with a list. 'You and your list may be d—ned', said the captain, throwing it at him 'I say there shall be no sick in this ship while I have command of her.'

The year after joining the Navy, Lind sailed with Admiral Sir Nicholas Haddock, commander-in-chief of the Mediterranean Fleet. They attacked the Spanish coast, blockaded Barcelona and Cadiz and took two Spanish treasure ships. This expedition was to provide Lind with his first experience of a major sea epidemic. Typhus raged throughout England during 1740–1, and it probably spread from Portsmouth to the Mediterranean Fleet due to an influx of pressed sailors. One captain had put sick seamen ashore in a large barn at Ryde on the Isle of Wight, since the hospital at Portsmouth was full. He claimed nevertheless that the infamous Dr Ward's pills had worked wonders on 'rheumatic, scorbutic, itchy and venereal diseases.'[1] All achieved by one magical pill . . . no wonder the Admiralty was happy to promote the amazing Dr Ward.

When they arrived at Gibraltar, Haddock discovered that the hospital there consisted of 2 sheds accommodating 30 men. He hired houses to cope with a further 160, and demanded that the Admiralty build a hospital capable of dealing with up to 1,000 men. Lind witnessed the worst ravages of the disease at the main Mediterranean naval base at Port Mahon on the island of Minorca. The naval hospital there was little better than the one at Gibraltar, and had been largely ignored by the Board of the Sick and Wounded. Even the board's official agent complained about the conditions and pointed out that seamen there went to hospital with the same reluctance as a prisoner going to Newgate Jail.[2]

Lind wrote of Port Mahon:

> When a malignant fever, in the late war, was brought from England into the hospital at Mahon, the house being found insufficient for the reception of so great a number of patients, tents were erected in the fields for many of the men. These poor men were thought to be badly accommodated, but it was observed, that most of those, who lay in the tents, recovered; when the mortality in the house was so great, that in some wards, not one in three escaped.[3]

This seemed, confusingly, at odds with other experiences of men accommodated in tents and suffering fever. Lind had recommended that nights spent ashore in tents should be avoided. He maintained that tent flaps should face seawards, and that fires should be kept burning; in that circumstance, what his instructions might have partly prevented was not contact with the infected body lice that caused typhus, but contact with malarial mosquitoes.

In the same year that Lind first experienced typhus in the Mediterranean, a huge expedition was mounted by Commodore George Anson. This was the important but ill-fated circumnavigation that was to give James Lind the impetus to make a detailed study of scurvy. Anson's voyage – despite its disastrous features – is regarded as one of the great feats of naval adventure and heroism. It had been decided to mount the expedition against Spanish colonies when the war with Spain began in 1739, but the plan soon appeared to gain the character of a voyage of discovery and colonial probing as much as a military campaign.

It is probable that the voyage was decided upon after the success of Admiral Vernon in capturing Porto Bello in 1739. The case for further harassing Spanish interests in the West Indies was impossible to ignore politically. History has suggested that there was probably a hidden intention of attacking Spanish influence in Chile and Peru and substituting British colonial authority. Anson was ordered to attack Callao (the port of Lima in Peru), destroy Panama and return home by either Cape Horn or the Cape of Good Hope. However, the voyage was a disaster of unrealistic objectives, widespread fatal disease in the form of scurvy, mutiny, hardship and almost superhuman endurance. The return of Anson's flagship to London (the only one of the eight ships that had left four years earlier) was presented as a triumph of courage, tenacity and brilliant leadership. Anson himself later became First Lord of the Admiralty, and was a humane and renowned naval administrator.

The expedition was the result of debate at various political levels, with the inevitable intervention of parties whose interests were directed at the commercial exploitation of South America. The plan was eventually promoted by Sir Charles Wager, then First Lord of the Admiralty, and Admiral Sir John Norris. While the main intention was to attack Spanish interests in the Caribbean, there was the added appeal of intercepting a Spanish treasure ship thought to carry silver worth £2 million on its annual trip from Acapulco to Manila in the Philippines. Anson was given command of the squadron of 6 heavily armed ships, 2 store-ships and just under 2,000 men. The logistics involved in planning for such an adventure were complex, and Anson spent almost a year in preparation, during which time his masters at the Admiralty changed his orders, dithered, and generally added confusion and indecision to an already difficult situation.

This was to be the first great circumnavigation by the Royal Navy – many years after the private merchant fleets had first undertaken such adventurous voyages. However, there was little evidence that the experiences of men such as Hawkins and Lancaster in combating scurvy on long voyages would be heeded.

'A LEARNED MAN'

The likelihood of outbreaks of scurvy was nevertheless addressed, and the Admiralty took the advice of Dr William Cockburn, who had recently retired as Physician at Greenwich. Cockburn – trained at Edinburgh and Leyden – was a very influential, conservative snob who had been physician to the fleet and who had made a great deal of money in private practice, largely by promoting his 'Electuary' – a doubtful cure for dysentery. This potion, which he kept secret, had been obtained in Italy. He claimed that it had been used to cure Pope Clement XI in 1731, and despite complaints from Admiralty Commissioners, his patron, Admiral Sir Cloudesley Shovell, promoted its widespread use in the Navy. Despite his influence, his dull, inflexible approach resulted in a lack of conspicuous medical progress during his career. He was described as 'an old, very rich quack' and is ironically the only naval physician to be buried in Westminster Abbey.[4] Cockburn's big contribution to the professional discussion of scurvy was that it was caused by congenital laziness among the sailors. He did admit that fresh vegetables might help those already sick, and had even witnessed the efficacy of lemons, but on serious preventative measures he had nothing new to say.

Hanoverian Britain, and London in particular, was beset by quack medicine, much of it practised by rank amateurs. There were pills, potions, lotions and devices being peddled for all sorts of conditions, some real and some imagined. Some of these products were harmless, but others were dangerous or fatal. There were society favourites who specialised in nothing more than the popular procedure of 'blood-letting', an ancient means of maintaining the body's four humours 'in balance'. Many of the 'practitioners' became extremely wealthy, and sustained celebrity status in society. When asked for advice on avoiding scurvy for the Anson voyage, Cockburn self-confidently recommended the use of vinegar; this was an old-fashioned nostrum which at least had the merit of encouraging some degree of cleanliness. He consulted with the surgeons of the Royal Caroline, Woolwich and Deptford yards and suggested that the ships' interiors should be swabbed down with it, and that in addition each sailor should be given 2 oz per day, to be diluted and drunk 'on flesh days'. The Navy Board noted:

> We are humbly of opinion that the washing of the ships with vinegar should be continued, as their Lordships have been pleased to direct and that the constant issuing of vinegar to the ships' companys, both at home and abroad, in petty warrant as well as in Sea Victualling, to mix with their food by at least one quart a week to four men may greatly contribute to their health, and be very instrumental in preventing scurvy, fluxes and fever. The charge whereof we have estimated at two pence a man a month.[5]

Instead of trusting the judgement of its own experienced sea surgeons, the Admiralty decided to seek confirmation from the Royal College of Physicians and its leading light. Dr Richard Mead [1673–1754] was one of the greatest physicians of his time. Trained at Leyden and Oxford, he was in practice at Stepney and was appointed to the staff of St Thomas's Hospital. He became Physician to George II in 1727, and was famous for his personal library, which contained an extraordinary collection of works on anatomy.

The College, led by Mead, decided that instead of vinegar, 'elixir of vitriol' or sulphuric acid (to be mixed with alcohol, sugar and spices) should be given internally – 'it would be a very great Means to preserve them from that disorder.'[6] Mead himself was also in favour of vinegar, but he was specific about what kind of vinegar:

> . . . a quantity of wine-vinegar should be allowed to the company of every ship. This qualifies the salt of the food, and makes some amends for the want of sub-acid fruits. But I must remark, that the vinegar of strong beer has neither the flavour nor the virtue of that from wine; and ought indeed to be forbidden our tables.[7]

'A LEARNED MAN'

The Navy Board, with typical arrogance, went beyond the College of Physicians and Richard Mead and insisted on the supply of Ward's Pill and Drop, almost certainly because of favouritism towards Ward, since there was no supporting medical evidence whatsoever. As far as the treatment of scurvy was concerned, everyone involved seemed willing to proclaim the definitive approach; one Admiralty instruction at this time actually took on the more eccentric 'anti-fruit' mantle:

> . . . one must, when ships reach countries abounding in oranges, lemons, pineapples, etc., ensure that the crew eat very little of them since they are the commonest cause of fevers and obstruction of the vital organs.[8]

Anson himself wrote from Spithead asking for tamarinds, which had been successfully used against scurvy by the East India Company:

> As His Majesty's ship *Centurion* under my command is ordered a foreign voyage, I desire you to order me a supply of surgeons' necessaries for twelve months, as the fruit will keep but a little time in a hot country. I desire the following alteration to be made, in lieu of currants and raisins, to have 50 of sago, double of quantity of tamarinds, if remainders to be in sugar, to have but one half of quantity of nutmeggs & mace that is allowed, and to have cinnamon added in lieu of them.[9]

There had never been a means of preserving tamarinds for any length of time (or lemons, or other fresh fruit for that matter), and Anson was in no better position to do so than anyone before him, so his sensible suggestion would have had limited value in practice. Despite that, he restated his demand more than once (as he was in the habit of having to do for most of his other requirements). That the East India Company had much longer and earlier experience of extended voyages than the Admiralty was apparently irrelevant. There is no evidence that the Navy

Board was active in seeking the benefit of the merchant company's acquired knowledge.

Anson demonstrated the general uncertainty over medical measures by making a further demand for supplies:

> I desire you'd please to order the surgeon of His Majesty's ship *Centurion* to be supplied with the usual quantity of Doctor Cockburn's Electuary for fluxes, for a foreign voyage.[10]

In another letter seeking assurance that enough bricks were to be available 'in case by any accident our coppers should give way', Anson added the more unusual request: 'please to order *Centurion* to be supply'd with a Jack in the Box.'[11]

Having ensured protection from scurvy, the Admiralty worked its way towards equally convenient solutions of other vital issues. There was controversy over the employment of two victualling agents who were to sail with the expedition. Both men had considerable experience of South America with the South Sea Company. The intention was to carry provisions for at least twelve months – a huge undertaking, given the number of ships involved. As was common practice, the agents were acting in a freelance capacity, and disquiet arose over their 'perk' of also being responsible for the procurement of extremely valuable trade goods for bartering purposes. The Admiralty authorised their advance payment of £10,000 for the purchase of such items – this was two-thirds of the value of the goods, and a massive amount of money for the period. It was widely suspected that the agents' main interest was in maximising private profit on their own account. Normally, a captain in a friendly port would use commonly accepted bills of exchange to acquire provisions; in unfriendly areas, he would simply mount an attack and seize what goods were required. The victualling agents were allowed to bring several members of their own staff on board, while Anson himself was refused the normal assistance of a secretary to deal with his considerable volume of official paperwork.

Throughout the whole period of preparation for sailing, the

Admiralty was naturally enough preoccupied with the fact that yet another war was under way, and new ships were being hurriedly constructed and fitted out. It does seem perverse, nevertheless, that such a huge undertaking as Anson's was given short shrift during the whole fitting-out period. Even the central purpose of the expedition seems to have been subject to change and counterchange. Initially two separate, smaller, squadrons were to be employed, one to attack Manila and the other to strike South America. Later, a single squadron was favoured and Anson was told to ignore Manila and concentrate on attacking the South American targets. It was six months after this major change in plan before Anson actually received his orders in writing. Indecision on such a scale had a disastrous effect on the logistics and practical preparation for the voyage. There were major repairs required to the ships; refitting to accommodate several companies of soldiers; more detailed refitting to satisfy the demands of the many Army officers; and endless other small but nevertheless important matters, which even Anson had trouble manoeuvring through the bureaucracy.

One of the biggest problems – and one with disastrous consequences – was manning. The Admiralty was slow to comply with the manning arrangements, and Anson complained that he was short of 300 seamen and the full complement of soldiers. Instead of the expected regiment of red-blooded marines, 500 pensioners from Chelsea Hospital were drafted. Many of these invalids were nevertheless fit enough and had sufficient natural guile to desert into the backwaters of Portsmouth, and only half that number was received by the fleet. As Anson's chaplain aboard the flagship, Revd Richard Walter, recorded for the account published under Anson's name:

> . . . all those who had limbs and strength to walk out of Portsmouth deserted, leaving behind them only such as were literally invalids, most of them being sixty years of age, and some upwards of seventy.[12]

Most of this decrepit band were ill and some were so sick that they had to be carried aboard ship; none of them was to survive the voyage. Anson was outraged and managed to discharge the most unfit cases, but worse was to come. In replacement for those who had deserted or were discharged, he was supplied with over 200 untrained recruits. In addition there was an uncertain number of pressed men, whose state of training and health are unknown. The last group to join the fleet was a contingent of young ships' boys. These children – for children they undoubtedly were, from about the age of seven or eight upwards – were sufficient in youth and number to warrant the appointment of a teacher. A large percentage of the total complement remained sick on board ship at Portsmouth for months before the fleet even sailed. In truth, this situation may not have been entirely unusual, but it was exacerbated by the fact of war. Fitting out at Portsmouth at the same time as Anson's was a fleet destined for the West Indies – a fleet of thirty ships-of-the-line accompanied by store-ships. The logistics of preparing such huge fleets must have been extremely daunting. However, it is hard to avoid concluding that the manning of Anson's ships was conducted incompetently. The age and state of health of the various sailors, 'marines' and soldiers must have been critical factors in the horrific toll of disease that was looming.

The fleet left St Helen's on the Isle of Wight, on 18 September 1740, almost a year after the decision was taken to mount the expedition. There were two immediate consequences of the delay; many of the crew and troops were already weak or sick, and the Spanish had gained warning of the impending assault on their South American colonies. The expedition's aims were supposedly secret, but French spies in London had passed accurate intelligence to Madrid. Within weeks of departure, two invalid captains had died, and the son of Admiral Norris, Captain Richard Norris of the *Gloucester* returned sick to England from Madeira, apparently convinced of the expedition's impending failure. The flagship's senior surgeon and purser both contracted typhus and died. By the time the fleet had crossed the Atlantic, men were dead of fever and dysentery, and eighty were put ashore at the island of St Catherine's off the Brazilian coast. There the fleet regrouped, the ships were fumigated and the decks washed with vinegar; but mosquitoes plagued the healthy, the sick and the convalescents alike. En route for Port St Julian on the Patagonian coast, elements of the fleet became separated; there were violent storms; more men died, including one of the captains, and one ship had a close escape from a Spanish squadron.

On the extremely dangerous passage round Cape Horn, the fleet was dispersed. Scurvy was already taking hold, and the Revd Walter's account paints a vivid picture as well as showing how diffuse and obstinate were the signs of the disease:

> As we did not get to land until the middle of June, the mortality went on increasing; so that, after the loss of above 200 men, we could not at last muster more than six foremast men in a watch, capable of duty. However, though it frequently puts on the form of many other diseases, and is therefore not to be described by any exclusive and infallible criterions; yet there are some symptoms which are more general than the rest, and occurring the oftenest deserve a more particular enumeration. These common appearances are, large discoloured spots dispersed over the whole surface of the body; swelled legs; putrid gums; and above all, an extraordinary lassitude of the whole body, especially after any exercise, however inconsiderable: and this lassitude at last degenerates into a proneness to swoon, on the least exertion of strength, or even on the least motion. This disease is likewise usually attended with a strange dejection of spirits; and with shiverings, tremblings, and a disposition to be seized with the most dreadful terrors on the slightest accident.[13]

Rounding the Horn was a feat of extraordinary endurance and seamanship. The seas were mountainous and the fleet was battered by freezing wind, sleet and snow. Sails were ripped, rigging destroyed, yards smashed, decking torn up and every vessel damaged in an awful assortment of ways. Men were flung from the yards into the tumultuous seas, and many others were badly injured. Below decks everything was soaking, and nothing could be done in the way of preparing food or maintaining hygiene. Pascoe Thomas, the instructor to the ships' boys, wrote a detailed account of his experiences and of the landscapes and cultures which they encountered. He did not stint in his descriptions of the storms or the horrors of scurvy:

> 10th March 1741:
> The ship rolled almost gunnel-to continually, the sails were almost always splitting and blowing from the yards; the yards themselves frequently breaking; the shrouds and other rigging cracking and flying to pieces continually. It was indeed a signal mercy that none of our masts gave way, but all stood firm; had we lost them, or even any of them, of which there was great danger, I fear we should have inevitably perished. And now as it were to add the finishing stroke to our misfortunes, the people began to be universally afflicted with that most terrible, obstinate, and at sea incurable disease, the Scurvy, which quickly made a most dreadful Havock among us, beginning at first to carry off two or three a day, but soon increasing, and at last carrying off eight or ten a day very often.
>
> I have seen four or five dead bodies at a time, some sown up in their hammocks and others not, washing about the decks for want of help to bury them in the sea; and this melancholy situation we had but little hopes of getting out of, being at last reduced to that lamentable pass that I believe there were not above twelve or fourteen men, besides a few of the officers, capable of doing any duty upon deck.[14]

In one month, forty-three men died of scurvy on the flagship alone; twice that number the following month. On the *Tryal*, Lieutenant Philip Saumarez blamed scurvy on 'a mysterious *je ne sais quoi* to be found only in fresh fruit and vegetables'.[15] Anson forlornly relied on sulphuric acid to ward off scurvy, and his flagship surgeon equally hopelessly favoured 'any food of a glutinous nature, such as salt fish, bread, and several sorts of grain.'[16]

Revd Walter's descriptions of the outbreaks of scurvy, which James Lind was later to approve of as 'justly exploding some opinions which usually pass current about its nature and cause', are descriptive of the whole range of secondary symptoms which so often coexisted, or gave rise to confusion, with other diseases:

> . . . it is not easy to complete the long roll of the various concomitants of this disease. For it often produced putrid fevers, pleurisies, the jaundice, and violent rheumatic pains. And sometimes it occasioned an obstinate costiveness [constipation]; which was generally attended with a difficulty of breathing; and this was esteemed the most deadly of all the scorbutic symptoms.[17]
>
> But a most extraordinary circumstance, and what would be scarcely credible upon any single evidence, is, that the scars of wounds which had been for many years healed, were forced open again by this virulent distemper. Of this there was a remarkable instance in one of the invalids on board the *Centurion*, who had been wounded above fifty years before at the Battle of the Boyne: for though he was cured soon after, and had continued well for a great number of years past; yet on his being attacked by the scurvy, his wounds, in the progress of his disease, broke out afresh, and appeared as if they had never been healed.[18]

Pascoe Thomas shows in his account that the expedition was not prepared for the virulence of the scurvy:

> Since our passing Cape Horn, our Surgeon, Henry Ettrick (who was a very good practical surgeon, but in the theory part vain and pragmatical, making science to conflict in a flow of words with little or no meaning) had been very busy in digesting a Theory of Scurvies.

But this passage, in a very hot climate, where the symptoms were not only more dreadful, but the mortality much more quick and fatal, put our scheming doctor to a sad nonplus; he could not account for this. All this obliged him to own that the grand centre was certainly the long continuance at sea and that no cure but the shore would ever take place.[19]

The flagship having survived Cape Horn, a disaster occurred that was typical of the uncertainty brought about by the inability to calculate longitude correctly; and there was an irony. In 1736 the clockmaker John Harrison had carried his first huge experimental marine timekeeper, H-1, aboard ship in his first successful sea trial during a passage to Lisbon. The ship had been *Centurion*. Now, six years later, *Centurion* and Anson were in trouble, with no Harrison sea-clock on board. For fifty-eight days they battled against violent storms, with scurvy claiming half a dozen men each day. Anson headed west until he thought he had travelled 200 miles beyond Tierra del Fuego. He then headed north, towards the island of Socorro (now known as Isla Guamblin) where the fleet intended to regroup, having become dispersed. He expected to sight land to starboard, but it appeared dead ahead. It was in fact the western tip of Tierra del Fuego – he had been virtually static for weeks, unwittingly battling against fierce currents. Anson had no choice but to make what he hoped were intelligent guesses. *Centurion* reached Socorro, but after two weeks, no other ship appeared, and Anson decided to make for the next rendezvous, Juan Fernandez, the island of the real Alexander Selkirk and the fictional Robinson Crusoe. Scurvy was attacking again:

> . . . it was no uncommon thing for those who could do some kind of duty, and walk the deck, to drop down dead in an instant.[20]

Anson again headed west, then north as before. He knew and could calculate the latitude of Juan Fernandez, but when he reached the correct latitude, he decided to sail west to reach the island. After four days, he decided he had been wrong, turned the ship around and headed east. Two days later, he reached the coast of Spanish Chile. His original guess had been correct, and at the point of reversing his course he had been almost within sight of the island; now he had no alternative but to reverse course yet again. His lack of longitude had forced him to zig-zag for two weeks in vicious sea conditions while scurvy claimed an extra eighty lives.

What was left of the fleet eventually met up again at Juan Fernandez. Only *Centurion*, *Tryal* and the small supply-ship *Anna* had survived the Horn; *Wager* had been completely wrecked; *Severn* and *Pearl* failed to navigate the Cape and had returned to Rio, suffering scurvy, dysentery and other deficiency diseases. *Wager*'s crew (or at least those who had escaped scurvy) made it ashore, where some of them mutinied. One man was shot dead by the desperately sick and deranged captain, some deserted, and after numerous adventures, several groups returned to England by various convoluted routes. Sir James Watt, late director-general of the Naval Medical Service, has stated that in rounding Cape Horn over 750 men died, mostly of scurvy and other deficiency diseases.[21]

Gloucester arrived at Juan Fernandez after another three weeks with two-thirds of her crew dead from scurvy; it took her sick, weak crew six days from being within sight to making anchor. *Centurion* had hardly a man fit to work; *Tryal* had two officers and three men fit. A dozen men died while actually being carried ashore. The Revd Walter recorded that 'for the first ten or twelve days we buried rarely less than six each day; and many of those who survived recovered by slow and insensible degrees.'[22]

The remaining ships stayed at anchor for three months, repairing, refitting and recovering health, thanks to fresh water, vegetables (radishes, scurvy grass and celery) and goat meat available on the island. A Spanish ship, the *Monte Carmelo*, was taken as prize and added as a fourth to the depleted fleet. When they departed from Juan Fernandez in September 1741, they had been away from home for a year; three ships had been lost, an appalling sixty-seven per cent of the men had died, mostly from scurvy, and not a shot had been fired. There was no means of communication between the fleet and England. The Admiralty did not know what had happened, and could not have helped in any case. Anson's small, beleaguered squadron was on its own. They had almost another three years ahead of them before they would see home shores.

* * *

Already, James Lind was busy coming to grips with preliminary thoughts about scurvy, having had modest experience of its effects while on patrol in the English Channel. His first conclusion, which was echoed by the experience of the Revd Walter, was that the quality of the air (in particular its moisture) was a major predisposing factor in the contracting of scurvy:

> We often observed our Channel cruisers quickly overrun with scurvy; while their consorts, fitted out at the same port, and consequently with the same state of provisions and water, who soon left them, stretching into the main ocean upon a voyage to the Indies, or upon a much longer cruise off the Canaries or Cadiz, kept pretty free from it. For my own part, I never could remark any alteration upon our scorbutic patients, while we continued for many days close in upon the French shore, with the wind or air coming from thence, or when, at a greater distance from any land, we kept the middle of the Channel: and yet, in either of those stations, difference of weather had a remarkable influence upon scorbutic ailments.[23]

Lind's thinking was to be further confused by Anson's subsequent brushes with his deadly medical enemy. After leaving Juan Fernandez, the squadron headed for the South American coast, where they took four more prize ships. They attacked and set the town of Payta ablaze, taking some prisoners, valuable plunder, wine, brandy and fresh provisions, and sinking six vessels in the bay. Although their plan to capture the governor and demand a ransom was not carried out, this was a remarkable assault by a severely depleted fleet. *Centurion*, *Gloucester* and three prize ships headed for the Panamanian port of Quibo for supplies, in advance of seeking out the Manila treasure galleon off Acapulco. The prizes were disposed of and the two ships left Acapulco, heading across the vastness of the Pacific for China. They left in May, which turned out to be a mistake, since the ships were to encounter long becalmed periods, accompanied by blistering heat. Soon after leaving, both ships suffered broken mainmasts and within a month, the first deaths from a second violent eruption of scurvy had occurred.

The outbreak at Cape Horn had occurred in cold, foul weather, with no fresh provisions, and a crew of already sick and weak sailors crammed tightly together. This time, there were two warm, well-ventilated ships, a much smaller crew and, although no vegetables, at least sufficient fresh meat and water. With several men dying each day, Pascoe Thomas recorded the desperation that resulted in the use of the dreaded Pill and Drop. Perhaps those who suffered a quick death were lucky:

> The Commodore, on this great mortality, having by him some quantity of Ward's pills and drops, in order to experience whether they would be of any use, first tried them on himself; and then gave a quantity of them to the surgeon, to give to such of the sick people as were willing to take them. The surgeon would not recommend them to any person, but several took them; though I know of none who believed that they were of any service to them. They worked on most people who took them very violently, both by vomit and stool; after which, as several of themselves have told me, they would seem to be a little easier (though weaker) for perhaps a day or two, but then they always relapsed, and became worse than before. And this together with the inefficacy of all our surgeons could do in the case, sufficiently showed the vanity of attempting the cure of this distemper at sea.[24]

It was an extraordinary but revealing conclusion from an intelligent person that man was vain to imagine he could find a cure for scurvy. Thomas nevertheless proceeded to berate those who favoured Cockburn's theory that scurvy was due to idleness. He insisted that sailors had for too long suffered not only from the vile disease itself, but from the prejudice and hardship heaped upon them:

> I shall endeavour to remove a very great prejudice and hardship from which the unhappy persons who labour under this affliction have too long severely and most unjustly suffered; which is, that none but the idle and indolent are thought ever sick of this disease; and this so generally received, though vilely mistaken opinion, has caused many poor sufferers to endure more from their commanding officers than from the distemper itself; being drubbed, kicked and cuffed to do their duty when utterly incapable of it, and often when ready to expire; with the good-natured epithets of idle, lazy, skulking dog, or rascal liberally bestowed on them into the bargain, when perhaps they can scarcely hear it. The most laborious, active, stirring persons are often seized with this disease; and the continuation of their labour, instead of curing, only helps to kill them the sooner.[25]

He spared nobody from his attack, pointing out acidly that Cockburn's approach had been adopted and promoted 'by persons of approved veracity.'

To the ravages of scurvy was added the disaster of having to abandon *Gloucester* due to severe leaking and accumulated damage to rigging. On board, only sixteen men and eleven boys were fit, the others were sick or dead. In an increasing squall, the pathetic, sick crew was transferred to the flagship, and *Gloucester* set ablaze and scuttled. She took hours to burn, and finally blew up as the flames reached the munitions. The crippled *Centurion*, with ten men dying every day, was now the sole remaining vessel of the eight-ship fleet that had left

Spithead twenty months earlier. Lieutenant Philip Saumarez of the *Centurion* later recorded the critical event in his journal:

> We had a passage of three months and a half to the Ladrone Islands, which is generally made in two: that it was a vulgar opinion among our people that we had sailed so far as to pass by all the land in the world! Length of time and badness of weather rendered both our ships leaky. This, joined to our mortality, the scurvy raging amongst us as much as ever, we were obliged to destroy the *Gloucester*, which was ready to founder, and receive the men on board, which were all sick and dying. It's impossible to represent the melancholy circumstances wherein we were involved previous to our arrival at these islands.[26]

There was only a surgeon's mate left on board *Centurion* to tend the sick, but even he had to take his due turn at manning the pumps. Pascoe Thomas noted the miserable conditions:

> ... the Ship, considerably lumber'd with Prize Goods, and the small Room we had left throng'd with the Sick, whose Numbers were now very much increas'd with those from the *Gloucester*; the Dirt, Nauseousness, and Stench almost every where intolerable.[27]

Centurion finally reached Tinian, one of the Ladrone or Mariana Islands, and only with great difficulty did the few healthy men left make anchor. One hundred and twenty-eight of the most sick were taken ashore and installed in a store house which was converted to a hospital. Although there were fresh vegetables, exotic fruit, water and livestock on the uninhabited island, thirty of the sick died and the remainder took weeks to recover. Accounts depict Anson cutting oranges and squeezing the juice directly into the mouths of the worst afflicted. Not only scurvy was to blame, however; vitamin B deficiency resulted in extensive dementia. During the extended period on Tinian, something happened which has the ring of a scene from a Keystone Cops film: the flagship broke moorings and disappeared, leaving Anson and most of the crew ashore. They attempted, without any tools or equipment, to prepare for sea a Spanish vessel they had taken as prize at Tinian, with the aim of making for China. However, three weeks later, *Centurion*'s skeleton crew was successfully able to return the ship to the anchorage.

Eventually, Anson made it to Macao, and after wintering there, set out to make a last attempt to capture the Spanish treasure galleon. After cruising for a month around the island of Samar in the Philippines the *Nuestra Señora de Cavadonga*, with 42 guns and a crew of almost 600, was sighted. After an action lasting only an hour and a half, the treasure ship was Anson's, and he appointed Philip Saumarez as her captain. The plunder amounted to $1.3 million in cash, 35,682 oz of silver and assorted merchandise. Two of Anson's men were killed and eighty-four wounded. The prize ship was sold in Canton – after the crew of the *Centurion* was involved in saving part of the port from destruction by fire. The flagship was provisioned, and she left Canton, bound for home, on 15 December 1743. She reached Spithead after a wholly uneventful voyage, on 15 June 1744 just under four years after departure.

Of the original complement of the expedition, only 188 returned with Anson; some others had returned from *Severn*, *Pearl* and *Wager*, which had failed to navigate Cape Horn. Of just under 2,000 who sailed in 1740, 1,400 had died – 4 killed by enemy action, a few from injury, but most from scurvy and vitamin A and B deficiencies. The personal and social consequences of such carnage must have been staggering, but any righteous anger and distress was overwhelmed by the noisy, national celebration of a great hero and a unique treasure-hunting voyage across the world. Thirty-two wagonloads of treasure were paraded from Portsmouth, through the streets of London to the Tower. The total value has been put at almost £1½ million – at 1744 values this is a sum of truly colossal magnitude. The previously unknown Anson became a national celebrity, and the politicians and gentlemen of the Admiralty were happy to bask in any reflected glory. After all, any great military campaign had to expect a large death toll. Only a couple of years earlier, 10,000 out of a total of 14,000 troops had died of disease in the Caribbean. Even in the Channel Fleet, one ten-week period produced 2,400 cases of scurvy. There was nothing new.

The matter of prize money raised its ugly head. Ordinary sailors who had received an advance instalment were soon observed drinking and fighting it away on the streets of Portsmouth and London. The position of the officers became mired in legal actions lasting several years. Most of the dispute seems to have centred on the rights, or otherwise, of officers transferred to the flagship after their own vessels' destruction. Of those who returned with Anson, many suffered continuing health problems, including 'deep scurvey', some eventually succumbing to premature death. Many senior officers pleaded with the Admiralty in later years to be released from service early as a result of their state of health after having been with Anson to China and back. Anson himself became fabulously wealthy following the voyage. He had been born and brought up at Shugborough Hall in Staffordshire, and was now able to buy the opulent Moor Park in Hertfordshire.

It seems that nothing was learned by the Admiralty about the depredations brought about by scurvy, or about measures to prevent or treat the disease. It was as if there had been no problem in the first place. Pascoe Thomas's remark about the vanity of even considering a cure seems to have had the quality of prescience. Dr Richard Mead, Physician to George II and one of those who advised the Admiralty on health matters before departure, interviewed Anson on his return. Mead was by no means wholly obstinate in his views about scurvy, but it is dispiriting to read in the opening remarks of his book that 'it is therefore very plain that this malady is a kind of corruption of the blood.' His conclusions on scurvy, which appear in his *Discourse on the Scurvy* originally published in 1749, agreed with the doubtful Dr Cockburn that the main predisposing factor was putrid or malignant sea air. Mead was so convinced of this connection that his *Discourse* was published as an addendum to a report by Samuel Sutton for a system of 'Extracting Foul Air out of Ships'. Mead also agreed with the rather anodyne, conservative conclusion of the College of Physicians that 'wine-vinegar' should be issued to crews. If ever there was a time for a new approach to scurvy this was it; wine-vinegar was not the answer.

Mead ironically repeats a story that had been told to him by Admiral Sir Charles Wager. Sadly, he appears not to have taken any account of its practical example in relation to scurvy. Apparently, while at Leghorn in Italy, the Admiral had bought several cases of oranges and lemons:

> Recollecting, from what he had often heard, how effectual these fruits were in the cure of this distemper, he ordered a chest of each to be brought up on deck, and opened every day. The men, besides eating what they would, mixed the juice in their beer. It was also their constant diversion to pelt one another with the rinds; so that the deck was always strewed and wet with the fragrant liquor. The happy effect was that he brought his sailors home in good health.[28]

It seems astounding today that Mead had not recognised the value of Wager's experience. He admitted in his *Discourse* that Anson had found citrus fruits '[had] the most extraordinary benefit,' yet still he ignored the point. He even goes on to note:

> ... it is very commonly known that, in our East India ships returning home, the men are very much affected this way, and that upon their very approach to the island of St Helena, they are strangely relieved by the fresh odoriferous air; and perfectly recovered, after some days, by eating the fruits we have mentioned, and living chiefly on the vegetables, which kind nature has supplied that place with in profuse plenty.[29]

'A LEARNED MAN'

Two years before Mead's *Discourse* Dr John Huxham, a fever expert from Plymouth who had sailed with the Channel Fleet, published anonymously that fresh fruit 'do surprising things in the cure, and what will cure will also prevent.' He recommended that all ships should be ordered to carry cider, lemon juice mixed with rum, fresh lemons and oranges wrapped in flannel to preserve them.[30] His ideas were more fully detailed in essays published in 1750 and 1766, by which time he was unaccountably blaming lemon juice for what was called 'Derbyshire colic' and no longer recommended it in treating scurvy. Nevertheless, had the well-intentioned but spectacularly heedless Mead been alert to his own potent examples of the efficacy of citrus fruit, he might have made recommendations in the aftermath of Anson's voyage which could have been of real significance. As it was, nothing changed.

James Lind, on patrol in the English Channel, was appalled by the experiences of Anson's circumnavigation. He could not immediately read many of the surgeons' journals and individual reports, which were not published for some years, and the Revd Walter's authorised account for Anson only appeared in 1748. However, he tried to relate what information he did acquire to his own initial experiences in the Channel. He concluded that the moisture of sea air was a contributory factor, and he was particularly interested in the different conditions that had applied in the two major outbreaks during Anson's voyage:

> ... the great Lord Anson cruised for four months, waiting for the Acapulco ship, in the Pacific ocean; during which time, we are told, his crews continued in perfect health: when, at another time, after leaving the coast of Mexico, in less than seven weeks at sea, the scurvy became highly epidemic, notwithstanding plenty of fresh provisions and sweet water on board. And when it raged with such uncommon malignancy in passing Cape Horn, it destroyed above one half of his crew, in less time than he kept the seas in perfect health, in the before mentioned cruise.[31]

Lind was moving from his intellectual interest in scurvy to considering a novel practical experiment. He was on the verge of taking up the problem of scurvy in a manner which no-one had attempted before. He would be scientific, systematic and observant. Sir Richard Hawkins' 'learned man' was taking up the challenge. The Royal Navy was about to enter a period of great success and development, partly aided by political support in the shape of the First Earl of Chatham, otherwise known as William Pitt the Elder. Chatham believed in England's superior role in Europe, to be achieved by the pursuit of trade, bolstered by the aggressive protection of the Royal Navy. As Paymaster General and Secretary for War with the powers of Prime Minister in all but name, Chatham presided over the strengthening of the Royal Navy and its operations, appointing George Anson First Lord of the Admiralty. Anson was to be a strategic and administrative genius. In the new Royal Navy that was coming, there was a clear opportunity for the lessons that desperately needed to be learned about the medical implications of naval affairs to be addressed. James Lind was ideally placed to take advantage of that opportunity.

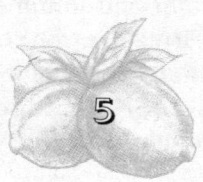

'I Shall Confirm All by Experience and Facts'

During 1746 and 1747, James Lind was the surgeon on board HMS *Salisbury*, a newly built fourth-rate ship of fifty guns on one of the deathless harassment patrols in the English Channel. The War of the Austrian Succession was still under way. The *Salisbury* was constructed by the shipbuilders Ewer of Bursledon, at Hamble near Portsmouth; the keel was laid in May 1744 and she was launched in January 1746; she weighed 976 tons, and had a complement of 350 men. This was the fourth Royal Navy ship of that name, and there were to be four others after this one was condemned in the East Indies in 1761. The *Salisbury*'s captain during Lind's period was Lieutenant George Edgcumbe (a protégé of Admiral Haddock) whom Lind described as being a man of generous liberality. While still serving in *Salisbury* in 1746, Edgcumbe became MP for Fowey. From an old family with landed Cornish connections (one of his ancestors was referred to as 'the good old knight of the castle'), Edgcumbe took part in many dramatic sea battles, and was later to become an admiral, and the first Earl of Mount-Edgcumbe.

Lind regarded the medical circumstances of Anson's circumnavigation as a scandal but praised the 'lively and elegant picture' of scurvy given by the Revd Walter, who had recorded the voyage for Anson:

> This disease, so frequently attending all long voyages, and so particularly destructive to us, is surely the most singular and unaccountable of any that affects the human body. For its

symptoms are inconstant and innumerable, and its progress and effects extremely irregular; for scarcely any two persons have the same complaints; and where there hath been found some conformity in the symptoms, the order of their appearance has been totally different.[1]

Lind verified that the best descriptions of the disease came from those voyages, but bemoaned the fact that 'no physician conversant with this disease at sea had undertaken to throw light upon the subject.' Even after the Anson disaster, there was no sign that either the Admiralty or the Sick and Hurt Board was interested in tackling the issue, despite the chaos that scurvy caused to naval operations. During his time aboard *Salisbury* his responsibility for the practical treatment of scurvy led him into a more intellectual consideration of the disease and its history. Although scurvy gained infamy when the Navy began to embark on very long voyages, it made severe inroads into the operation of the Channel Fleet, which was prevented by scurvy from sustaining squadrons at sea for longer than six weeks or so. Lind was clearly exasperated in his initial researches by the realisation that despite the scores of supposed remedies tried and recommended over the years, there was no contemporary consensus as to what might be the best answer. Custom dictated that the favourite remedy of whichever society doctor was in fashion (or attracted the appropriate patronage) suited the day. Lind realised from the outset that, despite the confused situation, he was likely to break with what passed for established medical opinion.

For almost two centuries it seemed to have been quite casually recognised in naval circles that citrus fruits might prevent scurvy. Yet no authoritative decision was made to use them for that purpose, although they were fairly readily available, or even better to conduct proper research on the subject. Dutch merchant and whaling ships in particular were known to suffer little from the disease, and this was widely put down to their use of sauerkraut. Yet again, no-one seemed willing to examine the supposed efficacy, or study the implications. Perhaps there were simply too many potential remedies, some with the supposed benefit of traditional usage and others with their influential promoters. Even the evangelist and founder of Methodism, John Wesley, published a volume in 1745 entitled *Primitive Physic* which promoted the use of popular remedies for a vast range of diseases. He included a dozen remedies for scurvy, including nettle juice, goosegrass juice, pulped orange, orange juice and milk, lemon juice and sugar, and a mixture of cress, mustard and scurvy grass.[2] Items such as mustard became very common aboard ship, and it was usually grown fresh on deck. Its use at sea with all forms of meat gave rise to a popular retort by shore-bound gourmets, 'Mustard with mutton! Naval officer, I presume?'

In broad terms, as far as the Admiralty was concerned, there were probably three reasons for the continued inertia; short-sightedness, financial strictures, and the fact that acquisition and preservation of potential remedies was difficult if not impossible. Fresh fruit and vegetables, wherever obtained, simply could not be preserved at sea for any length of time. That fact alone seems to have been enough to discourage any interest in investigating their real worth. The rationale seemed to be that if lemons worked it was due to their acidity, therefore 'oil of vitriol' (sulphuric acid) or vinegar would be just as good. However, as Lind said of each of these two remedies, 'bringing this to the test of experience, we find the contrary'.[3] He felt that there were two reasons for the lack of success in preventing scurvy. Every attempted treatment was applied too late in the course of the disease; and most physicians adopted treatments that did not take adequate account of conditions prevailing at sea – in particular, the use of salt in the preservation of meat. The only points of agreement among most surgeons were that exposure to cold, damp, fatigue and spiritual depression were all significant preconditions. No doubt such preconditions could, however, as easily be applied to many other sea diseases.

In April 1747, Admiral Steuart at the Admiralty received a report from the surgeon John Hammond of HMS *St George*.

Steuart seems to have had regard for Hammond, and had at some point asked him to address the problem of scurvy. Hammond says that he had made detailed observations during three cruises on a 90-gun ship, and reported that nineteen in every twenty deaths at sea were from scurvy. He particularly blamed victualling, especially salt provisions; bad, moist salt air, and the drinking of 'stinking water.' Taking a sideswipe at the views of the highly influential William Cockburn, Hammond described it as a 'vulgar error' to claim that scurvy sought out the lazy and slothful, and deprecated the insistence on 'driving scorbutic men about by way of exercise.' He had little good to say of most of the medicines tried against scurvy, and especially condemned as poisons those based on mercury and antimony:

> If anything can be of service here it must be something endowed with balsamic and saponaceous qualities, introduced by a dietetic course into the constitution. Our spruce beer at Newfoundland has all those properties; accordingly we seldom meet with any scurvies on those voyages. But as it is impossible to have these in our long western cruises I am well assured that their intentions may in a great measure be answered by allowing a certain quantity of good sound cider to every ship in such a proportion as each man (supposing one-fourth of the company always down) might have at least a quart a day.[4]

Hammond further approved of wine, good ventilation and the provision of hospital ships. He ended his letter with a plea to the Admiral for trials to be organised on the efficacy of tar water, which he had been unable to complete due to a shortage of water. He had made many entirely sensible observations and inferences, with which James Lind would have found little argument, but was somehow unable to analyse the results and implications in any meaningful way.

As a result of his practical observations with the Channel Fleet, Lind himself was among those inclined to believe that cold, moist sea air was the most important precondition:

'I SHALL CONFIRM ALL BY EXPERIENCE AND FACTS'

> It appears that the strong predisposing causes to this calamity at sea are not constant, but casual, upon that element. For though it should be granted, that the sea-air gives always a tendency to the scorbutic diathesis, yet the evil proves often highly epidemic and fatal in very short voyages, or upon a very short continuance at sea, to crews of ships who, at other times, have continued out much longer, cruising in the same place, and in parallel circumstances of water and provisions, and yet have kept entirely free from it.[5]

Lind was careful to plan a comparison of his own direct experiences with those of others, and while he did not attribute scurvy to weather conditions, he was initially adamant that 'the principal and main predisposing cause to it, is a manifest and obvious quality of the air, *viz.* its moisture.'[6] He went on to state – as had others before him, including Richard Mead and even William Cockburn – that secondary disposing causes were 'preceding sickness, lack of exercise and melancholy humour.'[7] The most notable outcome of his preliminary thinking was that, despite his suspicion of other factors, the variables he planned for his experiment were all dietary. However, it is important to state that Lind never rated diet at the top of his list of preconditions. Indeed, he stated that he did not accept the idea that:

> . . . the constitution of the human body is such that life and health cannot be preserved long without the use of green herbage, vegetables, and fruits; and that a long abstinence from these is alone the cause of the disease.[8]

It seems clear that Lind had a predisposition towards the efficacy of citrus fruit. He wrote that there had hardly ever been an instance in which an affected ship had been short of vinegar, tar-water, salt water or sulphuric acid. On the other hand, he pointed out that there was not a single instance of a ship ravaged with scurvy which had been adequately supplied with oranges or lemons properly administered:

> Some will perhaps say, that these fruits have been used in the scurvy without success; as appears from the experience of physicians who prescribe them every day in that disease at land. And here we may again observe the fatal consequence of confounding this malady with others. Legions of distempers very different from the real and genuine scurvy, have been classed under its name: and because the most approved antiscorbutics fail to remove such diseases, hence we are told by authors that it is the masterpiece of art to cure it.[9]

He concluded that such claims were contradicted by the experiences of the East India Company and others, and pointed out that nothing could be more absurd than rejecting the efficacy of citrus fruits against scurvy because they failed to cure quite different diseases:

> Some new preservative might here have been recommended; several indeed might have been proposed, and with great shew of the probability of their success; and their novelty might have procured them a favourable reception in the world. But these fruits have this peculiar advantage above any thing that can be proposed for trial, that their experienced virtues have stood the test of near 200 years.[10]

Lind quoted the experience of one of his fellow surgeons, Mr Murray, who had spent time at the naval hospital in Jamaica, and had recently been surgeon on the *Canterbury* and *Norwich*. While Murray also favoured the theory of 'moist air' as a precondition, he had found citrus fruit a success:

> As to oranges and lemons, I have always found them, when properly and sufficiently used, an infallible cure in every stage and species of the disease, if there was any degree of natural strength but left; and where a diarrhoea, lientery, or dysentery, were not joined to the other scorbutic symptoms. Of which we had a most convincing proof, when we arrived at the

Danish island of St Thomas; where fifty patients belonging to the *Canterbury*, and seventy to the *Norwich*, in all the different stages of this distemper, were cured, in little more than twelve days, by limes alone; where little or no other refreshments could be obtained.[11]

Murray unusually mentioned the use of limes against scurvy, and it is important to remember that the lime was a discrete fruit, different from the more commonly mentioned oranges and lemons. The role of the lime enters this story significantly at a later stage.

One of Lind's other preliminary considerations related to clothing. He was to make important recommendations on naval hygiene in later years, and was largely responsible for the adoption of changes of clean uniform as a means of combating disease. On scurvy, he insisted that:

No person sensible of the bad effects of sleeping in wet apartments, or in damp bed-cloaths, and almost in the open air, without any thing sufficiently dry or warm to put on, will be surprised at the havock the scurvy made in Lord Anson's crew in passing Cape Horn, if their situation in such uncommon and tempestuous weather be properly considered.[12]

Lind's decision to investigate scurvy was taken with the pioneering objective that would satisfy the definition of Hawkins' 'learned man':

... lastly, I shall propose nothing dictated merely from theory; but shall confirm all by experience and facts, the surest and most unerring guides.[13]

What he proposed was to conduct clinical trials at sea aboard *Salisbury* in a series of experiments that has been recognised as the first documented example of a controlled clinical trial.[14] This was not a technique he adopted from the textbook, since it did not exist in the textbook. His intuition and overriding desire to make statements based on scientific observation were what convinced him that he might find an answer. He seems to have had a prophetic insight into undreamed of techniques.[15]

Today, most people are aware of the concept and practice of clinical trials, as they have arisen largely from pharmaceutical testing in modern times. Refined statistical analysis has become an important partner of such trials, which can involve periods of time from hours to years and subject numbers from half a dozen to many thousands. There are sophisticated methods of subject selection and ethical controls; there are 'double-blind' trials involving control groups who unwittingly receive placebo treatment; and researchers who are neutral to the design and purpose of the trial. In fact, the issue of the analysis of probabilities in epidemiological statistics has become fiendishly complex, and arcane professional arguments rage over competing models. For example, whereas it might be thought that subjectivity was a quality resolutely to be avoided, there are many who advocate the modification of 'subjective prior opinion' only in clearly defined circumstances.

Lind was a stranger in this particular unexplored forest and his proposed trials were unsophisticated. Today, the idea of taking a sample of only twelve patients would be ridiculed, but Lind's practical efforts were nothing short of revolutionary at the time. His carefully observed, controlled experiment in determining remedy has been contrasted with the more overconfident and thus disastrous efforts of another extraordinary physician in treating yellow fever during the same century.

Benjamin Rush was born in Philadelphia as Lind was conducting his trials aboard *Salisbury*. He trained in medicine at Edinburgh University, under Cullen and Black, and became one of the most prominent physicians in the USA. He was a man of intriguing contradictions. On the one hand he was a signatory of the Declaration of Independence, an enlightened enemy of slavery and capital punishment, an advocate of the emancipation of women and better care of the mentally ill. Yet this same imaginative man was an entrenched promoter of the medieval practices of blood-letting, or phlebotomy, based on an analysis of 'the state of the blood'. He was a heroic figure during the great epidemic of yellow fever that killed 5,000 people in the summer of 1793 in Philadelphia, but was heavily censured for his simplistic, untested reliance on blood-letting.[16] In practice, and as a teacher, Rush was a dogmatic theorist who strove to prove the existence of a unitary explanation for disease, one which allowed the possibility that all diseases were actually different forms of the same. His cures were often more feared than the diseases. An undoubtedly great and influential physician, the comparison with the philosophy and methodology of Lind could hardly be greater.

Lind's purpose was clear from the outset, and he insisted that he would not be swayed by theory alone. He stated that, having reached conclusions as to the most efficacious remedy:

> I shall then endeavour to give it the most convenient portable form, and shew the method of preserving its virtues entire for years, so that it may be carried to the most distant parts of the world in small bulk, and at any time be prepared by the sailors themselves.[17]

Lind must have canvassed his intentions within certain medical circles, since he received letters and diaries from other naval and Army surgeons offering contributions to the debate. Some of these, such as that of Surgeon Murray, he obviously found to be highly relevant, and he later included copious extracts in the course of discussing various treatments in his *Treatise*. A journal detailing scurvy and fever attacks aboard the *Dragon* in the Mediterranean from July 1743 until May 1745 was submitted by his friend, 'the ingenious Mr Ives', who was physician to the East India Company Fleet. Lind had information from Army surgeons such as James Grainger, surgeon to Lieutenant-General Pultney's regiment, who detailed the ravages of scurvy in 1751 at Fort William, on the west coast of Scotland. The same surgeon also reported on a high incidence of fatal scurvy among lead miners at Strontian, a village on the shore of Loch Sunart in Morvern.[18]

Lind's description of his practical experiment is short and clear:

> On the 20th of May 1747, I took twelve patients in the scurvy, on board the *Salisbury* at sea. Their cases were as similar as I could have them. They all in general had putrid gums, the spots and lassitude, with weakness of their knees. They lay together in one place, being a proper apartment for the sick in the fore-hold; and had one diet common to all, *viz.* water-gruel sweetened with sugar in the morning; fresh mutton-broth often times for dinner; at other times puddings, boiled biscuit with sugar, etc; and for supper, barley and raisins, rice and currants, sago and wine, or the like. Two of these were ordered each a quart of cyder a day. Two others took twenty-five gutts [drops] of *elixir vitriol* three times a day, upon an empty stomach; using a gargle strongly acidulated with it for their mouths. Two others took two spoonfuls of vinegar three times a day, upon an empty stomach; having their gruels and their other food well acidulated with it, as also the gargle for their mouth. Two of the worst patients, with the tendons in the ham rigid, (a symptom none of the rest had), were put under a course of sea-water. Of this they drank half a pint every day, and sometimes more or less as it operated, by way of gentle physic. Two others had each two oranges and one lemon given them every day. These they eat with greediness, at different times, upon an empty stomach. They continued but six days under this course, having consumed the quantity that could be spared. The two remaining patients, took the bigness of a nutmeg three times a day, of an electuary [medicinal paste] recommended by an hospital-surgeon, made of garlic, mustard-seed, *rad. raphan.* [horseradish] Balsam of Peru, and gum myrrh; using for common drink, barley-water well acidulated with tamarinds; by a decoction of which, with the addition of *cremor tartar*, they were gently purged three or four times during the course.[19]

Several other men were kept as what might be described as 'negative controls'; they were given a pain-killing paste, laxatives and cough syrup. After six days, one of the men who took citrus fruit was fit for duty, although still showing spots and spongy gums; by the use of the acid gargle he was completely healthy before returning to Plymouth on 16 June. The second man to take citrus fruit was 'the best recovered of any in his condition' and was appointed to nurse the others. This was a significant result, particularly given the fact that the citrus supplement was only available for six days as against the two weeks for the alternatives. Lind said of the citrus fruit that 'all that could be spared' had been used in the experiment, which suggests that he was not permitted to use all the fruit on board *Salisbury* at the time solely for his experiment.

Lind found that the next best dietary supplement appeared to be cider. Improvement seems to have been much less marked than for citrus, but it did produce 'a fairer way of recovery than the others at the end of the fortnight.' Lind included in his *Treatise* a letter recommending the use of cider from a fellow surgeon (the ingenious Edward Ives) who had given scorbutic patients a quart of cider per day together with three quarters of a pint of sea water twice a week. The incidence of scurvy had dropped dramatically, rising again only when the cider was finished.

Lind was scathing about the efficacy of the ubiquitous 'elixir vitriol'. He admitted that the mouths of those who used the gargle were in a better condition than those who had used vinegar, 'but perceived otherwise no good effects from its internal use upon the other symptoms.' Of the other patients:

> There was no remarkable alteration upon those who took the electuary and tamarind decoction, the sea-water, or vinegar, upon comparing their condition.[20]

The two men who had been given sea water alone fared no better than the 'controls' who supped the cough mixture. This possibly surprised Lind, who may have been ambivalent about sea water. He admits to having experienced its use against scurvy and notes that the Royal College of Physicians favoured a manufactured salt water rather than crude sea water. He goes on to say of salt and some of the other popular remedies, 'experience has abundantly shown that they have not been sufficient to prevent this disease, much less to cure it.'[21]

What Lind devised, observed and began to describe clearly now appears to us as common sense. That is a measure of the significance of his achievement. On the basis of his admittedly limited experiments, Lind was firmly of the view that oranges and lemons were the best remedies for use against scurvy at sea, but decided that he would seek the views of others before he finalised his opinions. Initially, he had intended his work on scurvy to amount to a modest paper on the topic for the Society of Naval Surgeons, which had been formed only the year before in the wake of the medical disaster of Anson's circumnavigation.[22] However, he now also decided that a full historical review of the literature on scurvy was necessary. A straightforward journal article was no longer appropriate. That decision was to lead to major changes to Lind's life. There would be infinitely greater effects on the fighting strength of the Navy and on the country's prosperity. To take his work on to the next stage he decided to leave the Royal Navy.

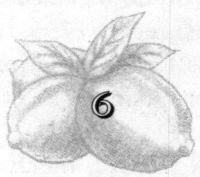

'The Province Has Been Mine'

IN 1748, when Lind left the Navy, a peace treaty had just been signed at Aix-la-Chapelle. The end of the European war would have resulted in a considerable reduction in manning throughout the Navy. It is possible that he was able to take advantage of an administrative status that allowed him to step down from active duty of his own volition, while receiving a modest pension allowance – essentially joining 'the reserves'. He had decided to complete the formal studies for a university medical degree and that decision, coupled with his desire to concentrate on a study of scurvy, may have hastened his departure. There appears to have been no overriding dissatisfaction, on either side, with his experience of the Navy, nor any interest on his part in taking an appointment at a shore hospital.

Given his considerable practical experience, his medical studies were not onerous. His main duty was to complete a doctoral thesis in Latin. Curiously, in view of what was the supposed relationship to scurvy, he chose as his subject venereal lesions, and his thesis entitled 'De morbis venereis localibus' was duly accepted. Guthrie and Meiklejohn, writing in their bicentenary edition of Lind's *Treatise* say of Lind's thesis that it was probably completed in a hurry and is a trivial piece of work that was never published in English. However, it served the purpose of gaining Lind his medical degree and the vital licence from the Royal College of Physicians of Edinburgh to practice 'within the City of Ed. & Libertys yrof without any tryal or Examination' as he was 'a Graduat Doctor of Medicine in the

University of Edin.' In 1750 he was elected a Fellow of the Royal College, became its Treasurer in 1756, and earned his living in private practice. This was Lind's situation in Edinburgh medical circles as he began the formidable task of analysing the historical work on scurvy.

There was a great deal to read, much of it in Latin. Lind was prepared to be critical. He made a detailed analysis of the contributions of over 60 writers on scurvy, together with comments on a further 140 – an extraordinary effort in itself. He sought out the contributions of medical quality and derided those of folklore. He observed that Pliny had described an outbreak of scurvy in the Roman Army under Caesar Germanicus. But he had no truck with what he described as Pliny's 'fabulous credulity'. He abhorred the intolerable 'vanity and presumption' of the early seventeenth-century Dutch physician Eugalenus, who wrote that scurvy was 'a Proteus-like mischief, lurking under various and surprising appearances', and who insisted that the disease was 'sent by divine permission, as a chastisement for the sins of the world'.

Lind would have none of this medieval mumbo-jumbo. Nor had he any time for the later theoretical subdivisions of scurvy – hot or cold, land or sea, acid or alkali. He did however endorse a distinction between what he called 'adventitious' scurvy (as suffered by seamen and due to external conditions) and 'constitutional' scurvy, which was contracted by those with particular combinations of pre-existing physical tendencies. He knew that many physicians classed all sorts of skin diseases under the term 'scurvy' and derided what he called this 'very improper denomination'.[1] He rigorously contended that scurvy deserved its own, discrete classification, 'with the same accuracy that botanical writers have observed in describing different plants.' The term 'scorbutic' had become the preferred term for any disease that ignorant or lazy physicians could not identify. Lind condemned the seventeenth-century Professor, Thomas Willis of Oxford University, who declared that any medical condition 'which cannot properly be referred to any disease, may justly be called scorbutic'.

Like a botanist, Lind knew the value of radical pruning. Many writers had relied too heavily on reproducing the opinions and errors of their predecessors, especially Eugalenus, whom they followed 'most religiously and minutely'.

'The English Hippocrates', Thomas Sydenham, was a friend and follower of both the chemist Robert Boyle and the philosopher John Locke, both of whom were noted empiricists who stressed the importance of observation. That characteristic alone connected those three with James Lind. In 1685, Sydenham gave considerable credit to scurvy grass as an antiscorbutic, and in some recipes he combined the herb with oranges and white wine. (Sydenham first distinguished the symptoms of venereal disease, which many considered had features in common with scurvy; some writers spoke with authority on both diseases, and Lind himself was expert.) Robert Boyle also made many contributions to the debate on scurvy, and offered one remedy in particular that he had used himself:

> Take English Barley, and having wash'd it, boil it in a sufficient quantity of fresh Spring-water till it be just ready to burst: Then pour off the clear upon the yellow part of the Rhinds of Lemons, freshly cut off from the white part, and put them into a Bottle, which being carefully stopt, the Liquor is to be kept so for Use, which is, that the Patient make it his constant Drink.[2]

A military surgeon who had much to say about scurvy was the eccentric Dr John Colbatch of Worcester, who was knighted in 1716. He had extensive military experience, and wrote widely recommending his secret powders and the importance of diet. He was apparently obsessed with the possibility of scurvy intervening in most other ailments, and with trying to effect miraculous cures using his secret methods. However, he was equally fanatical on the efficacy of citrus fruit:

> Why should we fly to Acids chymically prepared, when, as I said before, Nature has provided Oranges, Lemons, Citrons,

Limes, and a great many more not necessary to mention, which for the most part answer our intentions, if skilfully given by an experienced hand?[3]

He also used citrus fruit against open wounds, viper stings, smallpox, gout and arthritis:

If they are at any time very thirsty, they may drink Lemmonade; and if what they eat does not digest well, they may about an hour after dinner eat the Pulp of a Lemon, cut into slices, with some double-refined Sugar, it greatly helping Digestion, and strengthening the Stomach.[4]

He helpfully gave out his recipe for lemonade, which he regarded as 'the most grateful liquor in the World':

Take of clear Spring-Water one quart; then pare off the outward thin Rine of two Lemmons, and put into it; afterwards squeeze in the Juice of the Lemmons, and then sweeten it with about two Ounces of fine Sugar.[5]

For some reason, Lind did not consider in his study the use of citrus fruit by John Woodall, nor his great 1639 work *The Chirurgeon's Mate*. However, he did pay homage to the observations ('the best ever made on this disease') that had been recently published in 1737 by Dr Kramer, physician to the Hungarian Imperial Army:

The scurvy is the most loathsome disease in nature; for which no cure is to be found in your medicine-chest, nor in the best-furnished apothecary's shop. Pharmacy gives no relief, surgery as little. Beware of bleeding; shun mercury as a poison; you may rub the gums, you may grease the rigid tendons in the ham, to little purpose. But if you can get green vegetables; if you can prepare a sufficient quantity of the fresh noble antiscorbutic juices; if you have oranges, lemons, or citrons; or their pulp and juice preserved with sugar in casks, so that you can make a lemonade, or rather give to the quantity of three or four ounces of their juice in whey, you will, without other assistance, cure this dreadful evil.[6]

Kramer, giving practical example to Lind's concerns, complained that thousands of German soldiers had perished from scurvy because no-one recognised the true disease as distinct from the theoretical but spurious and indefinite subdivisions that were current.

Lind resolved to be a determined pioneer of detached scientific observation, recording and logical interpretation, and declared that 'it was necessary to remove a great deal of rubbish.' This rejection of much of what had been written about scurvy in history was no show of arrogance on his part; by all accounts he was a very modest man and a kindly and considerate physician. A description of Lind's character, as revealed in his writing, was published in the journal *The Practitioner* in 1896:

> ... a man of truth-loving and humane spirit, perhaps with something of the canny Scot in his respect for rank and authority, but independent in his judgement and fearless in expressing his opinions. He always appears anxious to give full credit to the workers who had preceded him, and he keeps himself in the background, except when necessary, to refer to his own experiences. He was evidently a man of extensive learning, but without pedantry; his style, without literary pretence, is simple and lucid.[7]

The first edition of Lind's *A Treatise of the Scurvy, in Three Parts, Containing an inquiry into the Nature, Causes, and Cure, of that Disease, Together with a Critical and Chronological View of what has been published on the subject* was published in 1753 by Kincaid & Donaldson of Edinburgh. The publishing company, which existed in several forms over perhaps 150 years, was the royal printer and stationer in Scotland, and published medical and academic works, including those of the philosopher David Hume.

Lind was a civilian in private medical practice; there was no automatic means by which his work would have been accepted, or even recognised, by the Admiralty. It is not clear in precisely what way his work was offered to The Sick and Hurt Board or to other parts of the hierarchy, although correspondence exists within Admiralty records that makes clear that it was. As we shall see, his proposals were subjected to a rather partial, biased scrutiny by those who were the current favourites in naval medical advisory circles. What he did – and it was to have great bearing on his later life – was to dedicate the work to Lord Anson, who had been made First Lord of the Admiralty two years earlier and whose interest in Lind's work is likely to have been both genuine and informed:

> To
> The Right Honourable
> GEORGE LORD ANSON
> Etc, Etc, Etc,
> Who, as a just reward for the great and signal
> services done to the BRITISH NATION, does
> now preside over her NAVAL AFFAIRS,
> The following Treatise is INSCRIBED,
> With the greatest respect, by his
> LORDSHIP'S *Most devoted, and*
> *Most obedient humble servant,*
> JAMES LIND

In his preface, Lind offered in acknowledgement of his critique of some of the earlier writers on scurvy that:

> Where I have been necessarily led, in this disagreeable part of the work, to criticise the sentiments of eminent and learned authors, I have not done it with a malignant view of deprecating their labours, or their names; but from regard to truth, and to the good of mankind. I hope such motives will,

to the candid, and to the most judicious, be a sufficient apology for the liberties I have assumed.[8]

Lind's extensive synopsis and chronology of earlier publications on scurvy, together with his own critical commentary, is a work of considerable scholarship in its own right; most of these early works would have been in Latin. One academic, K.J. Carpenter, who has compared Lind's digest with many of the original publications, has described Lind's summaries as accurate and objective.[9]

Lind began his 'Theory of the Disease' by declaring his belief (abandoned in a later edition) in an ancient hypothesis that the pores of the skin were the vital means by which the body excreted 'putrescent noxious humours'. The blood could be freed of these substances mainly via urine and perspiration. He believed that a cold, wet climate could result in such a mechanism becoming inefficient:

> ... by the uninterrupted circulation of its fluids, their violent attrition, and mutual actions on each other, and their containing vessels, the whole mass of humours is apt to degenerate from its sweet, mild, and healthful condition, into various degrees of acrimony and corruption. Parts of the solids themselves, continually abraded by the repeated force of the circulating fluids, are again returned into their channels. Hence the necessity of throwing out of the body, by different outlets, these acrimonious and putrescent juices.[10]

To modern eyes, this all might seem rather too similar to the medieval nonsense that he claimed to reject, but it was part of a rational approach in a period when there was a distinctly mechanical understanding of physical functions. Today 'conditioned deficiencies' are recognised for a number of vitamins and minerals, and some illnesses can reduce the concentration of vitamin C in the blood. Scurvy might therefore be precipitated by infection.

Lind proceeded to discuss other features relating to the actions of moist air. What he called 'the elasticity of the air' in assisting lung and digestive functions, and the production of blood could both be inhibited by atmospheric conditions. Lind's ideas on moist air affecting the 'spring and elasticity' of air in ships at sea were rather similar to those of Dr Richard Mead, whose own 'Discourse on the Scurvy' of 1749 was also prompted by Anson's disastrous voyage. Mead was a prodigious promoter of the ship ventilation system of Samuel Sutton. Lind also had strong views on the virtues of good ventilation below decks, and made recommendations of his own elsewhere in relation to naval hygiene, but was unconvinced of any special association with scurvy. Ventilation of ships was a matter that was getting some attention. Aside from Sutton, the chemist and botanist Dr Stephen Hales, 'the father of plant physiology',[11] perfected a hand-operated mechanical pump. In 1756 Hales ventilators were ordered to be fitted in all ships over twenty guns, and Hales pumps were also available for use in hospitals. (Hales was an enormously gifted clergyman, philanthropist and inventor whose biographers have suggested that of all his technological work, his efforts to improve water distillation attained the highest merit.)[12] The only concession Lind made to the Mead/Sutton view of ventilation was that warm, dry air might be beneficial:

> ... the noxious qualities of the moist air at sea were greatly heightened by being confined in so close a place as a ship, without a succession, or fresh supply of it. But as that inconvenience is sufficiently guarded against by the excellent invention of Sutton's machine, which extracts all such foul and putrid air, and this will prevent many infectious malignant fevers from thence; so there seems nothing wanting to make it likewise an excellent preservative against the scurvy, but that it should correct the moisture of the sea-air, and dry or warm it betwixt decks when needful.[13]

Although at odds with much else of his thinking, Lind also partly agreed with some of the views of the controversial William Cockburn. He concluded that physical inactivity (Cockburn characteristically preferred the more abusive 'indolence') was a predisposing factor, as was a discontented nature – both of these states being no doubt equally likely to exacerbate almost any medical condition.

One of Lind's first topics in relation to the causes of scurvy was that perennial companion of the sailor – salt, which had for a long time been blamed for all manner of maladies and injuries, and in particular a supposed form of scurvy ('muriatic') entirely attributable to excess salt. Lind pointed out that he had not intended to reach any particular conclusion about salt, and set out open-minded as to whether it might either be a component cause of scurvy or – by its antiseptic attributes – a partial remedy. He concluded categorically that salt in the form of salt water was not a direct cause. He was less sure about the innocence of salted meat and fish, which were usually so heavily tainted as to be impossible to decontaminate.

Lind made a number of simple everyday recommendations to which individuals could try to adhere as a matter of good habit. He advised the use of clear open fires; the burning of myrtle wax candles or similar aromatics; the wearing of dry, clean clothes, and dryness and cleanliness of the body:

> We often observe many asthmatic persons affected with a moist wind, and in a damp season hardly able to breathe; but upon throwing a little benzoin, or the like aromatic gum, on a red-hot iron, by which their chamber is well perfumed, they are sensible of relief, and the air replete with these aromatic particles. So here . . . I would recommend putting a red-hot loggerhead in a bucket of tar, which should be moved about, so that all the ship, once or twice a day, may be filled with this wholesome antiseptic vapour.[14]

Thinking of the 'putrescent, noxious humours' he recommended the chewing of raw garlic or onion to promote perspiration; plenty of mustard and onions to be used with food; and at bedtime, water-gruel and vinegar should have added lemon juice. He was not much in favour of the use of spirits, but when used, they should be acidulated with oranges or lemons; fermented liquors such as cider, beer and wine were all useful. All of these examples were dealt with at some length, as were the issues of the provision of fresh water (extremely difficult) and dried victuals (almost always corrupted by mould and vermin).

Lind favoured the regular use of a variety of fresh green vegetables, especially for their ability to become acidic through fermentation. However, he was not so zealous as to suggest, as some had done, that the lack of such vegetables alone was a cause of scurvy:

> . . . if this were truly the case, we must have had the scurvy very accurately described by the ancients; whose chief study seems to have been the art of war; and whose manner of besieging towns was generally by a blockade, till they had forced a surrender by famine. Now, as they held out many months, sometimes years, without a supply of vegetables; we should, no doubt, have heard of many dying of the scurvy, long before the magazines of dry provisions were exhausted.[15]

Green vegetables were the most popular suggested preventative in cases of 'land' scurvy, but Lind pointed out that there were many countries, such as Scotland and Newfoundland, where for half the year green vegetables were not readily available, yet there was no unusual incidence of scurvy. Although vegetables were less common at sea for reasons of lack of preservation, he detailed further examples from his own sea experiences to support his contention that fresh vegetables alone did not prevent scurvy. The concept of the 'accessory food factor' had not yet been developed, and Lind did not consider that both green vegetables and citrus fruit conveyed the same factor.

Following his clinical trial on *Salisbury* Lind was in no doubt as to the cure for scurvy, although he was equally sure that there was nothing new in what he had discovered. He clearly indicated the 200-year history of the casual use of citrus fruit at sea. However, he was still convinced of the inseparable connection of a whole series of conditions that prevailed in the lives of sailors. He was more interested in encouraging that 'holistic' concept, and in nurturing improvements, than in attempting to identify the mysterious factor in citrus fruit that was so potent.

Lind had promised that, if he found the cure, he would devise a method of 'preserving their virtues entire for years in a convenient and small bulk.' This he did, and he described his method for producing what he called the 'rob' of lemons and oranges:

> Let the squeezed juice of these fruits be well cleared from the pulp, and depurated by standing for some time; then poured off from the gross sediment; or, to have it still purer, it may be filtrated. Let it then be put into any clean open earthen vessel, well glazed; which should be wider at the top than bottom, so that there may be the largest surface above to favour the evaporation. For this purpose a china bason or punchbowl is proper; or a common earthen bason used for washing, if well glazed, will be sufficient, as it is generally made in the form required. Into this pour the purified juice; and put it into a pan of water, upon a clear fire. Let the water come almost to boil, and continue nearly in a state of boiling (with the bason containing the juice in the middle of it) for several hours, until the juice is found to be of the consistence of oil when warm, or of a syrup when cold. It is then to be corked up in a bottle for use.[16]

Lind noted that two dozen good oranges weighing over five pounds would produce over one and a half pounds of depurated juice, which in turn would yield five ounces of the extract. Thus the juice of twelve dozen oranges or lemons could be contained in a quart bottle and preserved for several years. As he was writing, he said that he had by his side lemon juice bottled four years earlier. When mixed with water or punch, no-one could tell that it had not been freshly squeezed juice. Lind was very enthusiastic about the use of such juice in acidulating other liquids, including spirits:

> When made in a proper place and season, it will come very cheap; and our navy may be supplied with it at a much easier rate than anything as yet proposed. It will be found extremely wholesome on all occasions, but especially to correct bad brandy, and other noxious spirits, often drank by sailors in immoderate quantity. Rum in the West Indies, arrack or brandy, when served them by way of allowance, should always be first mixed up with the extract. This will not only make them more palatable, but what is a matter of much greater moment, will convert these poisonous pernicious draughts into a sovereign remedy, and a preservative against a scorbutic habit, the bane of seafaring people.[17]

Lind made a major error in his method of preservation, an error which no-one would appreciate for 150 years. In heating the juice, he was destroying the vitamin C, and therefore the only antiscorbutic constituent. Within a few years of Lind's recommendations, other techniques would involve the use of olive oil, or of 15 per cent rum and sugar in an effort to preserve the juice. However, these adulterations also reduced the efficacy. In a later edition of his *Treatise* Lind was even more specific about the boiling, recommending a period of at least twelve to fourteen hours. He also changed his mind about the type of boiling vessel; he advised against a glazed vessel to avoid the hazard of lead being dissolved from the glaze.

In discussing the currently accepted remedies for scurvy, Lind insisted that 'there are but few medicines carried out in a sea-chest which are here of service.'[18] Worse, he wrote that many commonly used minerals such as steel, antimony and mercury were positively dangerous. There were only two components of the usual medical chest that he was able to recommend –

Peruvian Bark infused in wine, and the squill or sea-onion. The latter he initially regarded as encouraging the discharge of his 'putrescent, noxious humours'. Both onions and wine, while containing no vitamin C, had an antioxidant effect and thereby aided the conservation of the vitamin.

It is important to note that in his *Treatise* Lind recommended oranges and lemons (*citrus limonum*) or their juice, and not limes (*citrus acida*); the latter had played no part in his *Salisbury* trials and he did not discuss them. His only comment on limes was in a footnote to the effect that lime juice brought from the West Indies was usually mixed with rum or covered with oil, and in either case was generally musty.[19] His other general recommendations to ships' commanders were based on some of the remedies used for centuries, to which he gave credence: onions, green vegetables stored dry in salt, cabbages 'pickled in the Dutch style' (sauerkraut), and fermented drinks such as spruce beer and cider. He favoured the dry bottling of fruit such as gooseberries 'gathered two-thirds ripe on a dry day'; and he suggested that cider was a good medium in which to ferment fruit such as gooseberries, blackberries, currants, elderberries and Seville oranges. In making his recommendations, he was careful to advise that a scorbutic patient who had not been able to eat fresh fruit or vegetables for a long time, 'should be treated like one almost starved to death.' If they were allowed to eat voraciously, they were liable to die of dysentery.

It might be useful here to show the comparative content of ascorbic acid in some of the common remedies for scurvy. Lind and his contemporaries knew none of this; and it is important again to remember that many of the items in the table could not have been (or were not in practice) adequately preserved for use at sea. Also, a substance with a lesser ascorbic acid content, such as the potato, could in practice have been more available on a daily basis (and therefore been more useful) than more potent items. The table gives approximate ascorbic acid in milligrammes per 100 grammes (or 100 millilitres for liquids):

LIMEYS

	mg/100g
Apple cider, fresh	5
Banana	0–31
Barley seed, fresh sprouted	30–100
Blackcurrants	180
Cabbage, fresh	45–60
Cloudberries	80
Cranberries	10
Gooseberries, fresh	65
Gooseberries, preserved	0
Lemon juice, fresh	45
Lime juice, fresh	30
Malt, dried powdered	10
Onions, fresh	10
Onions, pickled	0
Orange juice, fresh	48
Parsley	140
Potato	20
'Rob' of oranges, fresh but consumed diluted	240
'Rob' of oranges, (stored 1 month), consumed diluted	60
Rosehip syrup	200
Sauerkraut (stored 1 month)	10–15
Scurvy grass, leaves and buds	200
Spruce, pine needles	65–200
Spruce, leaves and shoots	30–270
Spruce, fresh infusion	14–100
Spruce, fermented infusion	<0.5
Sweet potato	23
Watercress	43
Wine	<0.5
Wort (fermented malt)	0.1
Miscellaneous foods, including sugar, molasses, fresh bread, rice, vinegar, coffee and 'portable soup'	Negligible or zero [20]

Following the publication of his *Treatise* in 1753, Lind remained in private practice in Edinburgh for another five years, during which time he remained continuously busy with research and writing. He was Treasurer of the Royal College of Physicians of Edinburgh, and a member of the Philosophical and Medical Society of Edinburgh (later the Royal Society of Edinburgh). In 1754 he published an article suggesting the possibility of lead poisoning arising from the action of lemon juice on the lead glaze of earthenware vessels. He recalled several fatal incidents and noted that the Swedish authorities had recently prohibited the use of copper vessels:

> I knew a dozen people who narrowly escaped with life after drinking moderately of wine that had been pumped out of a cask with a copper pump, which had stood in it for some time.[21]

He quoted from a letter he had received from 'a gentleman in London' who had conducted research on this problem. The unknown gentleman was obviously intending to produce lemon juice commercially:

> . . . intending to make the extract of lemons, he squeezed the juice of a thousand lemons into a large, glazed, coarse earthen vessel, and allowed it to stand for two days; he then poured off an English gallon of the clear juice into another glazed flat earthen vessel, and put it in a pot of boiling water to evaporate. During the evaporation, a great quantity of sediment appeared among it; which, upon examination, he found to be the salt or sugar of lead, to the quantity of several ounces. He then poured off the remaining part of the juice out of the first earthen vessel, which had not been put upon the fire, and was surprised to find the sides and bottom of it also loaded with a large proportion of the same sort of salt.[22]

Lind was clearly concerned about the potential ill effects upon 'persons less judicious, and ignorant of the effects of this deceitful poison' and conducted a series of tests on various kinds of pottery. He advised against the use of all common brown or black pottery, and very particularly warned against delftware. He recommended porcelain or genuine Chinese china (as opposed to the European copies), or Staffordshire flintware.

Lind's *Treatise* was reprinted in 1757, and there was a major revision published in 1772, which will be referred to in a later chapter. The book was also translated into various editions in French, German and Italian. Also in 1757, Lind published yet another classic and important work on naval medicine, *An Essay on Preserving the Health of Seamen in the Royal Navy*. This would form the basis of a whole series of new principles of naval hygiene, and was printed in three editions. Ten years later came his *Essay on Diseases Incidental to Europeans in Hot Climates*, another significant work which had six editions in Britain and one in the USA in 1811.

The proposals contained in Lind's *Treatise* made their way through the Admiralty to the Commissioners of the Sick and Hurt. They wrote in March 1754 to the Admiralty Secretary suggesting that the College of Physicians be consulted on the matter, 'ere we ventured upon what seemed to us a thing of great consequence.' The issue was consequently placed before Dr Schomberg, Dr James and Mr Hill (surgeon at Woolwich Dockyard) for scrutiny. Unfortunately, Dr James was one of those charlatans with vested interests who made a vast income from his secret powders – 'the aspirin of the eighteenth century'. (Lind was later asked by the Admiralty to give an opinion of James's powders, and was unenthusiastic: 'this medicine, until made public, is not likely to be of great benefit to mankind.'[23] Lind recommended instead the continued use of Peruvian Bark, which suggestion reduced the opportunity for the continued sales of James's violently diuretic powders.)

Schomberg was short and sweet:

> These proposals are ingeniously founded on reason and observation and I am of opinion that they are likely to be of public use whenever carried into execution.[24]

James was obtuse and complained of the shortage of time in which to offer comment; he pointed out however that he had gone out of his way to obtain a copy of Lind's *Treatise*. While he was in agreement with Lind on the general points relating to salt and digestion, on other issues he managed to sound positive while surrounding his remarks with reservations:

> I think the extract of rob of lemon would make a most excellent preservative against that scurvy proceeding from putrefactions which the sailors are subjected to when diluted with punch or wine and water, but I highly disapprove of British Spirits, which I know from experience to be more pernicious than either rum or brandy.
> What Mr Lind says of the Bark I think very reasonable and likely to succeed. And no doubt what he says of fresh air and clean linen is of great importance to the preservation of health and the dissipation of contagion.[25]

Dr James took the opportunity to take a sideswipe at the 'filthy and pernicious custom' of chewing tobacco, to which he obviously had an obsessive antagonism, noting that, 'as a narcotick it palls the appetite, impairs digestion, and renders the use of drams almost unavoidable.'

Surgeon Hill was acid, and insisted at every opportunity that Lind's proposals were not practicable. He also revealed himself to be a supporter of the various mechanical ventilation systems, and of the conservative treatments of his colleagues in the higher echelons of the college:

> ... it was [Dr Mead's] opinion that if vinegar was allowed to eat with their salt provisions, that would greatly prevent the bad effects of their salt beef, and on our report to their Lordships a certain quantity was and is still allowed to every mess, which has been found to have a very good effect in greatly preventing that distemper rising to the height it used to do before ...

> Dr Mead, Dr Monro and if I mistake not Dr Cockburn were another time consulted on this distemper when it was agreed that Elixir of Vitriol made according to Dr Mead's prescription if given plentifully in barley water, to be drank at least a quart or two in 24 hours, and also for lotions to wash their mouths with when they become foul and stinking by the distemper. Though this method did not always cure, yet it kept the distemper under till the ships arrived in port and the men could be sent on shore where they soon recover'd. This method had been found very efficacious in all sorts of scurvys. Mr Lind further observes to their Lordships that Captain Palaseer kept his ship's company in health by giving them beef and pork but once a week. I wish the captain had told him what he gave them in lieu, but presume it must have been oatmeal and pease which are better than salt provisions. Mr Lind's method of treating sea distempers in long voyages at sea I am afraid are not quite practicable though they seem very rational; at present it will take up more time to digest and proportion quantities, for each ship cannot so soon be done as proposed.[26]

Hill went on to recommend what was clearly his own favoured method – a system of mechanical ventilation, 'which will keep a ship's company better in health than all the methods ever yet proposed'. The situation was left that, at some unspecified time, trials of Lind's proposals might be made on voyages to Guinea and the West Indies.

It would be interesting to discover (and I have not yet done so) what, if anything, Tobias Smollett had to say about Lind's work. Smollett was not only a novelist, but founder of, and editor and contributor to a number of critical journals. He made considerable use of his medical training, controversially editing the famous 'man-midwife' Dr William Smellie's *Midwifery* and campaigning against the accepted, narrow-minded but long-established tradition that men had no place in such sensitive areas of medicine as obstetrics and midwifery. That particular issue was viciously schismatic, and it was not the only such medical controversy in which Smollett became involved. He wrote an essay, 'On the External use of Water', in support of the surgeon Alexander Cleland, attacking the vested medical interests at Bath Spa. For a number of years Smollett wrote critical reviews (mostly anonymous) of medical works, such as John Pringle's 'Observations on the Diseases of the Army in Camp and Garrison', published in 1752. Among others, he wrote reviews of works dealing with venereal disease, dentistry, phlebotomy, and aneurism.[27] Some example of Smollett's opinion of Lind's *Treatise* may yet be identified. Even more to be enjoyed (had Smollett sustained his earlier interest in heckling the medical old guard) would be an account from Smollett's sarcastic pen of Lind's treatment at the hands of that establishment.

There were criticisms of the *Treatise* from some, like Surgeon Hill, who had their own axes to grind. Others doubted the scientific rigour of Lind's presentation and complained of the ease with which he gave weight to what some critics saw as relatively untested assumptions. A French naval surgeon wrote in 1867:

> It is astonishing that Lind, that rigorous and severe spirit, who in matters of therapeutics will recognise no authority but experience, should have accepted too readily, as the basis of his arguments, ideas that are far removed from any kind of scientific precision.[28]

Lind's presentation of the text was also seen as difficult, since he discusses the same detailed matters in different ways under various headings. In later years, some also suggested that Lind either did not appear to recognise the full import of what he recommended, or that he did not express himself sufficiently forcefully. In his later edition, he favoured the use of cream of tartar, and recommended greater general hygiene and the fumigation of ships. This later led to suggestions that he had lost sight of his main recommendations. That allegation was highlighted when one of his disciples, Nathaniel Hulme, appeared more active than Lind in promoting the production of lemon juice, and in setting out detailed ideas for the victualling of ships. Lind has been criticised in recent years, perhaps rather mischievously and certainly with hindsight, for having made judgements based more on enthusiasm and faith than experimental science.[29] But sins of omission identified 250 years after the event have little potency. Not even his critics have been able to deny that Lind had an unusual ability to observe and record carefully, and to draw accurate conclusions from his observations.

In 1758 James Lind was made a surprise offer that he probably could not refuse. Ten years after leaving the Royal Navy, he was offered the appointment of Physician-in-Charge of the largest naval hospital in the world. He might have been forgiven for thinking that his *Treatise* had struck a chord with the Admiralty, and that major changes were to be made to the lives of all who sailed the oceans. However the problem, then as now, was that politicians did not understand the nature of scientific evidence. In practice, as far as scurvy was concerned, nothing much happened. Inertia and neglect were to surround the whole subject. A host of works published by other naval surgeons would cloud the issue, and the disproportionate influence of Captain James Cook was to be a major frustration to Lind and the cause of substantial delay in the proper treatment of scurvy. Lind was about to encounter a time of great professional disappointment, during which he pointedly observed, 'The province has been mine to deliver precepts; the power is in others to execute.'[30]

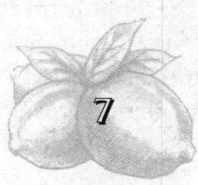

7

'But the Power is in Others'

IN the summer of 1758, James Lind was appointed to be Physician-in-Charge of the Royal Naval Hospital at Haslar, Portsmouth, which had opened four years earlier, in succession to Dr Cuthbert the first physician. Lind would retain the post with distinction for the next quarter of a century. This was the largest naval hospital in the world, and Lind had been a civilian for ten years; perhaps he had reason to hope that his efforts against scurvy had not been in vain. This prominent naval posting was one that fell within the realm where candidates would normally be expected to display considerable political or social influence in order to be considered. Although Lind did not court favouritism, the appointment seems to have come out of the blue, and it is probable that he was directly recommended for the post by Lord Anson. It is most unlikely that Anson, of all people, did not know of his work on scurvy and the later important volume on naval hygiene. The Admiralty Secretary's Register records:

> Whereas we have thought fit to establish a Physician to the Sick and Hurt seamen at Haslar, and to support Dr James Lind of whom we have received good testimony to that employment; these are, therefore, to direct and require you to cause him, the said Dr James Lind, to be entered Physician of the said Hospital accordingly; to hold the said place, and be allowed the salary of two hundred pounds a year, for his care and trouble therein until further order.[1]

The board confirming the appointment, headed by Admiral Forbes, would normally have included Lord Anson, who was apparently not present on that occasion. The relatively handsome salary was accompanied by living quarters, dining allowance, and the opportunity to engage in research and private practice.

There had been a 700-bed privately owned hospital, called the Fortune Hospital, at Gosport since 1713. Its owner had a contract with the Commissioners of the Board for the Sick and Hurt.[2] However, Haslar Hospital was authorised by George II in September 1744, along with similar institutions at Plymouth and Chatham. Although the naval hospital at Greenwich had been in use since the 1690s, the tradition was that sick sailors were expected to be cared for at the expense of any convenient seaport. But as the Navy expanded and voyages became extended, it was clear that changes were required. Consideration had been given to the conversion of Porchester Castle, but this was rejected and a 95-acre site on a peninsula at the western entrance to Portsmouth Harbour was acquired in 1745. The design was by John Turner and Theodore Jacobsen, who had designed the London Foundling Hospital in Bloomsbury in 1739 (of which Dr Richard Mead was a governor). The plan at Haslar was for a quadrangular establishment approximately 560 feet square covering 7 acres, and accommodating 1,500 patients. Each of the Palladian, three-storey blocks was to consist of a double row of buildings, similar in style to the hospital at Greenwich, separated by about 34 feet. The building of this, the biggest brick building in Europe, began in 1746 and it was a true product of Hampshire. Red bricks were made of local clay, white facing stone came from the Isle of Wight and timber was cut from the New Forest. All the workmen on the site were given official protection from the roaming press gangs. The foundations contained massive arched cellars, and there were staff residences, a cemetery, asylum, mortuary, brewhouse and church within the site. The original design was modified to leave one side of the planned quadrangle open, and the first block was opened in October 1753. The final blocks were opened eight years later, with the total cost reaching £100,000. In its original form, small boats could approach the main entrance, as a visiting American naval surgeon described:

> There is a water-carriage, by means of a small creek or canal, from Spithead-roads, up to the door of the receiving-room, for the easy and tranquil conveyance of wounded and sick seamen.[3]

Since the incidence of disease in the Navy increased while the hospital was under construction, the building was modified to accommodate approximately 2,000 patients. Eventually the open side of the quadrangle was walled as a preventive measure against desertion by patients, who tended to regard the institution as more of a prison than a hospital.

James Lind was to take charge of a substantial enterprise. Four months after taking up his appointment, he wrote a descriptive letter to Sir Alexander Dick, President of the Royal College of Physicians of Edinburgh:

> The hospital is under the direction of the Physician and Council – the latter consisting of the Physician, who presides, two Surgeons, the Agent, and Steward, and lately two members are added to the Council, *viz.* Dr Welch, Physician to Forton Hospital (which receives the Marines only, about half a mile distant from us) and the Surgeon of that hospital. But this Council must act entirely on orders from the Board of Sick and Hurt.
>
> We are remarkably clean. No patient is admitted into the hospital until he is stripped of all his clothes and well washed with warm water and soap in tubs always kept ready for the purpose; he is allowed the hospital dress during the time he continues in hospital, or until his clothes are returned to him quite clean, and he is regularly shifted and kept quite nice, clean and sweet at the Government's expense. None of his clothes, bedding, etc., is ever permitted to be brought into the hospital: we have large outhouses for their reception.

In cases of fever the patients' clothes are directly fumigated with brimstone in the smoke house and baked in an oven sprinkled with vinegar. The fever wards are cut off from all communication with the rest, and nothing but hospital dresses are used in them. We have sometimes 90 women nurses at a time; their pay is £12 per annum. In our wash houses we have seldom less than 24 women constantly employed. All these are under sober and discreet Matrons.[4]

Lind was a naval surgeon who was now obliged to take on the unaccustomed role of administrator of a huge hospital, and to become concerned, however reluctantly, with the inevitable politics involving the hospital's council and the Admiralty Board of the Sick and Hurt in London. In theory, power was devolved from the board to the physician and council. In practice, the political relationships were fractious, and became more so after the Commissioners of the Sick and Hurt Board appointed one of their number to sit on the hospital's council. One of Lind's earliest achievements was to devise the hospital's first comprehensive regulations, which included a clear system of preventing dangerous mistakes in the dispensing of medicines. In addition to the general administration and higher-level politics, he also, inevitably, had to deal with endless trivial disputes involving staff, such as one row over an assistant dispenser calling a nurse a 'saucy slut'.

In his first two years, Lind recorded 5,734 patients, of whom 1,146 were suffering from scurvy. There is little doubt he was following his own counsel as far as treatment was concerned, but there were no indications whatsoever that his methods were to be adopted on a wider scale. If the influence of Anson had indeed resulted in his appointment to Haslar, it appeared that it was to go no further. As we shall see, the power of patronage in practice worked against Lind rather than in his favour. He continued to conduct research on scurvy, and to prepare a second edition of his substantial *Essay on the most effectual means of preserving the health of Seamen in the Royal Navy*. At the same time, he was beginning work on a major research into tropical diseases which would culminate in a hugely influential book.

Scurvy was still taking its toll at sea. In 1754 Lind's friend Edward Ives had been surgeon aboard Admiral Watson's flagship on a voyage to India protecting an East India Company expedition. By the time they reached Bombay, 1,214 men out of a fleet complement of 1,800 were in hospital with various diseases; in two years, there were over 6,000 hospital cases and 328 deaths. 'When Mr Watson's squadron entered the Bengal river, a most melancholy scene was exhibited by the scurvy'. Ironically, the *Salisbury*, on which Lind had conducted his trials, was part of the squadron. Ives, honouring his 'ingenious friend' was giving sailors on his own ship orange and lemon juice which he had himself bought on the outward journey, with the result that there were few scorbutics: 'I now ordered it to be daily given to the seamen in their common liquors.'[5] This was the only instance later quoted by Gilbert Blane of 'any effectual means ever taken for a general supply of this antiscorbutic specific'.[6]

In 1758 Admiral Lord Anson was deeply concerned about the potential effects of scurvy in the Western Squadron blockading the French off Brest; the following spring the Admiralty adopted one of James Lind's major recommendations. It was ordered that the squadron should be victualled at sea by the use of special transports carrying fruit, vegetables and live animals sent out from England especially for the purpose. This was a far-reaching new technique which has remained a standard practice since, and the beneficial effects were rapidly obvious. Anson's senior commander, Sir Edward Hawke, won the important battle at Quiberon Bay, and of the total of 14,000 men in the fleet, less than 20 were sick. The irony was that while none of the fighting fleet had scurvy, the store-ships carrying the provisions were ravaged by the disease, forbidden as they were from making use of the anti-scorbutics. More than any other decision, replenishment at sea ensured that naval squadrons could remain at sea for much longer periods without recourse to port for revictualling or for putting sick sailors ashore in hospital. James

Lind had foreseen the health benefit years earlier, and had the satisfaction of noting:

> It was hardly ever known before, that ships could cruise in the Bay of Biscay, much above three or four months at a time without having their men afflicted with the scurvy. An exemption from which was entirely owing to this fleet having been well supplied with fresh meat and greens. It is an observation, I think, worthy of record, that fourteen thousand persons, pent up in ships, should continue, for six or seven months, to enjoy a better state of health upon the watery element than it can well be imagined so great a number of people would enjoy, on the most healthful spot of ground in the world.[7]

But long voyages could not benefit from replenishment at sea. From 1764 to 1766 Commodore Byron led a circumnavigation. On Friday 17 June 1765 the crews celebrated the fact that their two ships had made an arduous seven-week passage through the Strait of Magellan:

> I sent the boat with an officer to look for an anchoring-place, who to our great regret and disappointment returned with an account that he had been all round the island, and that no bottom could be found within less than a cable's length of the shore, which was surrounded close to the beach with a steep coral rock. The scurvy by this time had made dreadful havock among us, many of my best men being now confined to their hammocks; the poor wretches who were able to crawl upon the deck, stood gazing at this little paradise which Nature had forbidden them to enter, with sensations which cannot easily be conceived; they saw cocoa-nuts in great abundance, the milk of which is perhaps the most powerful antiscorbutic in the world; they had reason to suppose that there were limes, bananas, and other fruits which are generally found between the tropics; and to increase their mortification they saw the

shells of many turtle scattered about the shore. These refreshments, indeed, for want of which they were languishing to death, were as effectually beyond their reach as if there had been half the circumference of the world between them.[8]

The expedition was saved, temporarily at least, by consuming the coconut milk on which they had laid such confidence:

> By the 21st, all our cocoa-nuts being expended, our people began to fall down again with scurvy. The effect of these nuts alone, in checking the disease, is astonishing; many whole limbs were become as black as ink, who could not move without the assistance of two men, and who besides total debility, suffered excruciating pain were in a few days, by eating these nuts, so far recovered as to do their duty, and could even go aloft as well as they did before the distemper seized them.[9]

By 31 July, when Byron made Tinian, where Anson had anchored twenty years before, 'not a single man [was] wholly free from the scurvy, and many in the last stage of it.'[10] Scurvy was indisputably a mysterious foe. Sometimes the occurrence was easy to understand; at other times its virulence was inexplicable. There were advocates of a latent form, in which the body harboured the disease before any symptoms were evident. An account has been quoted in support of this idea which relates a visit to Anson by several senior captains just returned from a long voyage. Anson's wife complained in a letter that their presence in the cabin had been so offensive, due to their state of health, that it had been hardly bearable, even after they had gone.[11] However, this hardly supports the latency idea, since their bad state of health had been clearly visible. If foul breath was the problem, then they were simply displaying an early, classic symptom of scurvy.

One of the main reasons for the lack of progress on scurvy was probably that there was a rush of essays and papers of conflicting opinion being produced by physicians. Had there been any interest in the matter among the higher reaches of the Admiralty, they would probably have been unable or unwilling to quantify the conflicting evidence. The fashionable Dr Richard Mead still actively promoted ideas of corruption of the blood. However Mead was no fool, and much of what he had to say about scurvy found no argument from Lind. He also promoted improved ventilation, and the idea that specially produced brine was preferable to sea water for both the salting of provisions and for medicinal drinking:

> The trials already made of Mr Lowndes's salt made from brine, prove it to be much preferable, for salting provisions, both flesh and fish, to that made from sea-water, even to the bay-salt. Some experiments of its use I have made myself; and our College, being consulted by the Lords of the Admiralty, gave their opinion in its favour. I cannot but say, that I am sorry to see some of our physicians, of late years, so fond of prescribing the drinking of sea-water to their patients, particularly in scrofulous distempers. I am well assured, that it has sometimes brought on scorbutic symptoms, besides other mischiefs.[12]

Charles Bisset was another Edinburgh-trained surgeon who had served in the West Indies. In his treatise of 1755 he blamed salt provisions and heat, and recommended vegetables, wine, rum punch, spirits and in particular, rice. A later essay of 1766 on 'land scurvy' recommended tamarinds and Seville oranges taken in hot rum punch, but confusingly and disastrously, it also favoured the use of mercury, sulphur, antimony and sea water.[13]

In 1762 a London surgeon, John Leake, was promoting 'The Lisbon Diet-Drink for the cure of Venereal Disease and Scurvy'. This nostrum, whose constituents he did not reveal, was apparently so called after a German who was employed as Physician to the Queen Dowager of Portugal. Although the causative agents of the disease were unknown, Leake's script was an example of the kind of professional insincerity that would have angered James Lind:

> Though I shall only mention the most evident Properties by which it expels the Venereal Poison or Scorbutic Acrimony, yet I am far from limiting its Powers of Action solely to those secretions which it principally tends to promote; since Medicines often operate by Qualities too abstruse to be discovered by the Senses.[14]

Leake blandly referred to scurvy as 'a Complication of Disorders' and was clearly a promoter of the concept of the bad state of the blood. He was also against flesh-meats, salt and the drinking of 'corrupted, stagnating Water.'

The promotion of remedies for scurvy appealed to a number of doctors who otherwise specialised in venereal diseases. One such was John Profily, who in 1748 introduced his pronouncements with one of those claims to humanitarian good that were so common:

> ... the common Class of mankind are kept still in the dark, and the unfortunate Sufferers in this Distemper having no notion of the Nature, Cause or proper Remedies, are still imposed upon by Quacks and ignorant Pretenders.[15]

Profily, whose lengthy account of the symptoms of scurvy merits a special acknowledgement, condemned pickles, vinegar and 'High Sauces' along with 'unwholesome waters, corrupted, stagnating, blackish, thick, heavy Malt Drink, and Bad Wines'. He recommended a decoction made with scurvy grass, cresses and strawberry leaves; or the use of milk with a decoction of guaiacum wood (which produced a green resin often used in medical potions); *in extremis* he suggested the use of brimstone (sulphur) taken every morning with vegetables.

In 1757, a Scarborough doctor named John Travis produced the startling theory that what was being diagnosed in the Navy as scurvy was actually copper poisoning. The Navy generally used copper boilers for cooking purposes, and the merchant fleets – where scurvy was less prevalent – preferred cast iron. Travis proposed that long cooking times in copper pots led to a reaction with salt to produce copper acetate. He claimed that this copper salt was ingested with the food and produced the toxic effects that were diagnosed as scurvy. This theory was largely ignored at the time, but it has more recently been acknowledged that small amounts of copper salts destroy ascorbic acid. Experiments were conducted in the 1970s in which a typical shipboard cabbage soup was prepared in both copper and iron vessels (as Lind said, 'a soup of boiled cabbage and onions will cure an adventitious scurvy'). The percentages of vitamin C remaining after 10, 20, 30 and 40 minutes boiling in the copper pot were 90, 40, 30 and 25 respectively. Those for the iron pot were 98, 80, 84 and 56.[16] Copper is known as a source of the free radicals that interrupt the utilisation of vitamin C, and it is therefore true that boiling in copper pots would have destroyed the relatively low levels of vitamin C in vegetables in the eighteenth-century Navy.[17] Travis had been simultaneously right and wrong. (Copper cooking pots are however likely to receive a boost. Recent research suggests that the use of copper vessels kills the virulent E-coli 0157 within four hours, whereas the more commonly used stainless steel will sustain the live virus for over a month.)[18]

Another naval surgeon of the time who began well, but became confused, was Nathaniel Hulme. In 1768 he supported James Lind and recommended that 'orange and lemon juice and sugar should be so mixed with spirits and water as to become the common drink of sailors when at sea.' Hulme insisted that scurvy was due to bad diet, and had nothing to do with moist air. For some time, a number of surgeons adhered to Hulme's promotion of Lind's ideas and his own methods of preserving lemon juice. Inexplicably however, in a revised version of his published theory ten years later, Hulme made no mention of citrus fruit, preferring instead a 'fixed air' remedy consisting of alternate draughts of spirit of vitriol and potassium carbonate to produce, in effect, a fizzy drink. He was now wholeheartedly in favour of 'fixed air' and devised his own simple apparatus to replace the much more complicated equipment used by Priestley and others.[19] (The theory was that 'fixed air', or carbon dioxide, in water acted to prevent the putrefaction of human tissue by disease.) The muddled thinking that overtook Nathaniel Hulme seemed destined to swamp the truth.

Infinitely more confusion, controversy and intrigue was brought to the topic by a young Irish doctor, who formed his own obsession with the treatment of scurvy and promoted it mercilessly, supported by several people of influence. His self-promotion was successful in attracting the interest and authority of the Admiralty, and in gaining him the celebrity reputation he so clearly sought. David MacBride was born in Ballymoney, County Antrim in 1726, became apprenticed to a local doctor and joined the Royal Navy during the War of the Austrian Succession, which ended in 1748. He then attended lectures in Edinburgh by Alexander Monro, and in London by William Hunter and William Smellie. MacBride practised in Dublin before graduating from Glasgow University and publishing his first medical work. MacBride agreed suspiciously closely with 'the ingenious Dr Lind's excellent Treatise' that the principal predisposing cause of scurvy was moisture in the air, with salt diet, bad water and foul air as secondary causes. He agreed with Lind that the fermentative quality of fresh vegetables was beneficial, but set out to raise that particular possibility to greater significance.

> If it be true what was published in 1762, taken as is supposed from returns made to the House of Commons, that of 185,000 men raised for sea service during the late war, above 130,000 perished by diseases, and that two-thirds of this number may be safely charged to the account of diseases which take their rise from putrefaction; surely every motive of policy and humanity should excite men to endeavour at finding out somewhat to check this fatal and destructive diathesis; for if seamen could be preserved from it, few other kinds of diseases would endanger them.[20]

MacBride's ideas had begun with the work of Joseph Priestley, and support came from, among others, Sir John Pringle, the influential Surgeon-in-Chief of the Army (who had himself conducted similar fermentation experiments, upon which MacBride extemporised) and John Hunter the great comparative anatomist. MacBride was also championed by Henry Tom, a Commissioner of the Sick and Hurt Board, 'whose zeal in the prosecution of this affair, and in endeavouring to get the proposal carried into execution, demands a public acknowledgement'.[21] The practical experiments were devoted to discovering the most appropriate means of delivering the carbon dioxide. MacBride's development of this idea, together with the powerful backing which it received, resulted in the Admiralty instructing that his methods be tried on two circumnavigations, before being adopted by James Cook on his famous South Sea voyages. MacBride himself had never treated a single case of scurvy. This was a level of official support and sanction that had never been offered to Lind.

Controversy has raged over MacBride's theories, and the manner of his promotion. Anthony Lorenz referred in 1953 to MacBride's 'verbiage' and to his 'dabbling' in the scurvy issue.[22] In 1979 the recently retired medical director-general of the Navy, Surgeon-Admiral Sir James Watt, said that the ravages of scurvy in the eighteenth century were due to 'the extraordinary arrogance and persistence of David MacBride' in obtaining backing for his own theories at the expense of those of Lind.[23] MacBride almost certainly plagiarised James Lind and undoubtedly promoted his own mistaken theories with the assistance of the sponsorship of Commissioner Henry Tom, John Montagu, 4th Earl of Sandwich and First Lord of the Admiralty, and Admiral Sir Hugh Palliser. Montagu (the 'inventor' of the sandwich) was notoriously corrupt in his employment of political power and the exercise of patronage. He was extremely adroit at manipulating people, but was widely accused of ineptitude during the American War of Independence. The Montagu 'clique' at the Admiralty had in the previous century been patrons of Samuel Pepys, and was later responsible for the promotion of MacBride's brother John to the rank of admiral.

With patronage being so endemic, and originating at such a high level, it is difficult to know how to distinguish its effects from those of corruption and conspiracy. It seems inevitable that the effects of preferential patronage in favour of one person would have the effect of conspiracy without the necessity of a deliberately malevolent action against another. In that sense at least, Lind was clearly the victim of a conspiracy arranged by MacBride's supporters, including James Cook, who was also a beneficiary of the patronage of Montagu and Sir Hugh Palliser.[24] Lind's *Treatise* was superior in every respect to that of any other writer on the subject; he had also based his opinions on practical research that was truly unique. To have ignored it was negligent. To have done so while placing such overwhelming support behind the insubstantial MacBride seems very deliberate. The fact that MacBride plagiarised Lind's substantial theories on maintaining health at sea, on which he had done no work of his own, simply increases the sense of conspiracy.

MacBride claimed that common malt could be used to replicate the fermentation of vegetables, thereby producing an efficacious 'fixed air' effect against scurvy. Malt could be carried aboard ship in all climates for lengthy periods without detriment. It could be easily used to produce a drinkable wort infusion, available for distribution as and when required. However, MacBride's form of malt did not have the benefit of being produced from freshly germinated grain. More to the point, and unfortunately unknown to MacBride, malt wort contained no vitamin C whatsoever. That is not to say that, in his time, the idea was not worth developing. There was, after all, no understanding of what the magic component in food might be. However, he could be quite provocative in his declarations when promoting himself at the expense of others, as in this case advocating fresh vegetables for their fermentative quality:

> Notwithstanding the many impudent assertions every day published in the common newspapers, which among other much-boasted remedies, promise not a few as peculiarly

specific against scurvy, yet it may be laid down as a position, not easily to be controverted, that the *genuine putrid scurvy* has never been known to yield to any other medicines than to such as are composed of fresh vegetables and provided they be fresh, and of such a nature as will allow them to be taken freely, it is almost no matter what they are. The acid and the alcalescent, the mild and the acrid, the sweet and the bitter, all of them cure the scurvy.[25]

He recommended boiling up a panada (a pulpy stew) with ship's biscuit or dried fruit; three measures of boiling water to one of ground malt, left to stand for four hours. Patients were to make at least two meals a day of this 'palatable mess', and to drink a quart of a fresh infusion every twenty-four hours. He warned that the most likely effect 'will be to open the belly' – the contemporary euphemism for the violent purging of the bowels. He noted that spruce beer was a powerful antiscorbutic, but claimed the effect was produced by the molasses that was usually added to make it ferment. He added slyly, 'honey, on the same principle, must be a good antiscorbutic, and as such may be recommended to officers and others who can carry it conveniently.' MacBride, organising his supporters in Dublin and London, noted that they:

> . . . being persuaded of the reasonableness of the scheme, engaged very warmly in the promotion of it; so that, in consequence of this application, permission was readily obtained from the Board of Admiralty for having the wort fairly tried in the naval hospitals at Portsmouth and Plymouth.[26]

These trials of 1762 appear not to have been concluded. MacBride's demands at Plymouth required the withdrawal of normal meat and vegetable rations before a group of scorbutic sailors were given malt. After one man died, the others refused further treatment and demanded the return of vegetables and meat.[27] The Admiralty Board wrote to the Sick and Hurt Board on 1 July with the order 'not to proceed any farther in making experiments of the Regimen lately proposed to eradicate the Scurvy, its effects having upon trial [been] found to be fatal.'[28]

Lind placed 130 men on a treatment of wort at Haslar, but it was found only to be a nourishing drink with no curative properties. The general hostility of naval surgeons to MacBride resulted in no report on the test being sent to the Sick and Hurt Board. In any case, the signing of a peace treaty put an end to any chance of conducting experiments. MacBride later persuaded the East India Company to conduct trials. He also obtained a glowing testimony for the use of malt wort from the voyage of HMS *Jason* to the Falkland Islands in 1765 – his brother being the captain. However, Captain John MacBride somewhat ruined the effect for his brother by simultaneously supplying the same scorbutic sailors with oranges and apples. The following year, Samuel Wallis and Philip Carteret sailed with two ships on a three-year circumnavigation. They were instructed to take MacBride's wort with them. Carteret reported that vegetables, especially coconut tops, were excellent restoratives from scurvy, and urged that naval surgeons do more studies on vegetables. Portable Soup and Salop (a thickening powder made from orchid roots) were also taken in quantity. Apparently Carteret found the wort of no use at all against scurvy, although it had some value as basic nourishment.[29]

While MacBride was trying to consolidate his position with the hierarchy at the Admiralty, James Lind was revising his *Treatise*. His extended researches at Haslar (where he saw 'three or four hundred scorbutic patients a day' sent from the various fleets) had failed to confirm his earlier belief in the idea that scorbutic patients were in a state of putrefaction – a discovery that incidentally also undercut MacBride's ideas. As he reviewed his work, Lind was not optimistic that he had done enough:

> I can carry my researches no further. . . . A Work, indeed, more perfect, and remedies more absolutely certain might have been expected. Though a few partial facts and

observations may, for a little, flatter with hopes of greater success, yet more enlarged experience must ever evince the fallacy of all positive assertions in the healing art.[30]

Despite a weary pessimism, he was still convinced of the major causes of scurvy (although he continued to rate confinement over diet):

> Many diseases have been well known and accurately described for above a thousand years, yet for which of them have we an infallible remedy? What medicine can counteract the continued influences of improper diet, air and confinement, the last of which in particular I may judge to be a principal cause of the great obstinacy and frequent mortality of the scurvy in long voyages at sea?[31]

Lind, ever the man of practical observation, insisted that the answer would not come from any shore-bound theorist:

> It is indeed not probable that a remedy for the scurvy will ever be discovered from a preconceived hypothesis, or by speculative men in the closet, who never saw the disease, or who have seen, at most, only a few cases of it.[32]

Another disappointment for Lind was that doubt surrounded the efficacy of his 'rob' of orange or lemon juice. In the summer of 1766, The Lords of the Admiralty had ordered the 'rob' of lemons and oranges to be prepared and tested at Haslar, and the Sick and Hurt Board responded negatively the following year:

> . . . it was thought proper to reduce one gallon of the simple juice till only one and a half pint of the rob was remaining, which is in the proportion of 3 to 16 . . . the juice of 1637 lemons when evaporated in the above proportion yielded 22 pints and a half of the rob and nearly the like number of oranges yielded 17 pints.

> ... at the prime cost of the lemons and oranges without carriage or any expense in making, the charge of one quart of the rob of lemon is twelve shillings and one quart of the rob of oranges ten shillings and seven pence.
>
> ... we before observed to their Lordships that we did not think the rob of lemons and oranges would be efficacious in preventing the scurvy, and we now find by the experiment which has been made that it would be almost impracticable to supply the navy in general therewith to be issued with that intention on account of the great quantities which would be required.[33]

Trials of the 'rob' were recommended to be conducted, but not before Lind's revision was to be published. However, there is no doubt that boiling destroys vitamin C, and controversy has continued in recent years over the suggestion that Lind's preparations of the 'rob' were so lacking in vitamin C that they could not provide even the minimum dose required for protection against scurvy. Likewise, some of his other antiscorbutic recommendations (other fruit, fermented liquors, onions, etc.) have been condemned as lacking sufficient vitamin C.[34] They may, however, have had an antioxidant effect which could conserve low levels of the vitamin.

In his revision, Lind reiterated his belief in his principal original finding:

> To what has already been said of the virtues of oranges and lemons in this disease, I have now to add that in seemingly the most desperate cases, the most quick and sensible relief was obtained from lemon juice; by which I have relieved many hundred patients, labouring under almost intolerable pain and affliction from this disease, when no other remedy seemed to avail.[35]

There was still no particular recommendation of limes. He finally endorsed the usefulness of sauerkraut, onions, wine and sugar, fresh vegetables, scurvy grass, coconut juice, orange peel, chamomile flowers, infusions of fir or pine tips, and Peruvian bark. He began to develop the idea that what is now recognised as 'emotional stress' was a predisposing cause of scurvy, and recommended simple entertainment such as a fiddler or singer to reduce the effects of homesickness or monotony. Perhaps surprisingly however, given his abandonment of the theory of fermentation and putrefaction, he also restated his agreement with the use of the infusion of malt.

In the 1760s a new vegetable appeared, with claimed antiscorbutic properties. Samuel Bowen, an ex-employee of the East India Company, first brought soya beans from China to London at the end of 1763 before settling in Savannah, Georgia. Bowen claimed:

The Chinese use these vetches for the following purposes – From them they prepare an excellent kind of vermicelli, esteemed by some preferable to the Italian: nothing keeps better at sea, not being subject to be destroyed by the weevil. In Canton, and other cities of China, they are used for salad, and also boiled like greens, or stewed in soup.[36]

Bowen declared that in soup, the new beans were an excellent antiscorbutic; that fact had been his principal reason for introducing them to the USA, where they were first planted by Henry Yonge, the Surveyor-General of Georgia. Bowen stated 'it would be a most valuable remedy to prevent or cure the scurvy amongst the seamen on board his majesty's ships.'[37] Bowen went on to substantial success producing soy sauce and related products for export to Britain. (Experiments in Britain at the end of the First World War were to show that 'germinated pulses' – in particular haricot beans – were as potent as raw lemon juice in the treatment of scurvy, and they were recommended for use by the Army.)[38]

David MacBride, meanwhile, was having success in gaining the support of the Admiralty. Their lordships were considering the trials of malt wort on board HMS *Endeavour*, which, in 1768, was to voyage to the South Seas under Captain James Cook. Thus another character entered the mischievous web that trapped and blocked James Lind's work on scurvy. Cook was an explorer, cartographer, navigator and sea captain of enormous stature. Cook had been a shop assistant before going to sea with traders from Whitby. In the Royal Navy, he was a humane captain, had a scientific curiosity, and gained a reputation as a man who laid great store on his sailors being provided with the best of hygiene and victuals. He is often portrayed as the man who, more than any other, was responsible for defeating scurvy. Oliver Wendell Holmes, the great American physician and writer, is sometimes credited with incorrectly perpetuating the irony that it was a sailor (Cook) who taught the medical profession how to defeat scurvy. However, James Cook added confusion rather than clarity to the scurvy issue. His willingness to promote MacBride's remedy was largely responsible for the delay in the implementation of Lind's recommendations. Cook's influence on the Montagu clique would have been disproportionately powerful compared to that of Lind.

In June 1768 the Admiralty ordered the Commissioners of the Sick and Hurt Board that trials of the rob of lemons should be conducted aboard *Endeavour*:

> ... we think that the *Endeavour* bark, now fitting out at Deptford, will afford a good opportunity for the said trial; you are hereby required and directed to cause a proper quantity of the said rob to be put on board her for that purpose, giving her surgeon such instructions as you shall judge necessary in respect to the issuing thereof and letting us know upon her return the success of the experiment.[39]

At the urging of the Royal Society, Cook had been commissioned to sail with *Endeavour* to the South Pacific to observe and record the transit of Venus in 1769 and to conduct general exploration duties. There were two naturalists, an astronomer and two artists assigned to the voyage. This was to be the first of three such extended expeditions. He was ordered to try a variety of antiscorbutic remedies, including sauerkraut and rob of oranges and lemons. However, MacBride sidestepped the Sick and Hurt Board and lobbied the Secretary of the Admiralty directly, who wrote to Cook as the vessel was being provisioned at Galleons Reach in the Thames:

> Whereas there is great reason to believe from what Dr McBride has recommended in his book entitled 'Experimental Essays on the Scurvy and other subjects' and his pamphlet entitled 'An Historical account of the new method of treating the scurvy at sea' (of which you will herewith receive copies) and from the opinion of other persons acquainted with scorbutic disorders, that malt made into wort may be of great benefit to seamen in scorbutic and other putrid diseases, and whereas we think fit experiments should be made of the good effects of it in your present voyage, and have with that view directed the Commissioners of the Victualling to put a quantity on board the bark you command.[40]

Cook was instructed to store the wort in the Bread Room, and to prepare and administer it according to specific instructions enclosed with his orders, with the surgeon keeping detailed notes and observations. This decision came as Dr John Clerk, surgeon on an East India Company ship, reported on his own attempted use of malt wort, which he had initially adopted with enthusiasm, 'but had the mortification of observing the distemper to increase daily'. When he administered two spoonfuls of lemon juice, scurvy disappeared.[41]

Cook had direct personal experience of severe scurvy on an earlier voyage to Nova Scotia, but there was no intention on his part, or that of his ship's surgeon, to conduct any proper trial of the several authorised treatments aboard *Endeavour*. On other occasions he had been well supplied with antiscorbutics (he favoured sauerkraut) and punished his crew for refusal to use them. Cook had the strength of character, and the status with the

Admiralty, that enabled him to get what he wanted; a well-fitted ship, the pick of the best crew (no pressed men for Cook), and first-class provisions, described in one account as 'lavish for the period'[42]. Sir James Watt pointed out that normal sea rations provided about 4,450 calories, which he described as 'ample for energy requirements, but nutritionally disastrous'. While enjoying a relaxed schedule, *Endeavour* was not expected to be out of sight of land for more than three months at any one time, and was unlikely to encounter scurvy in its severest manifestation.

Some years later the naval surgeon Frederick Thomson referred, in his *Essay on the Scurvy*, to the kind of conditions on Cook's *Endeavour* that were clearly the envy of everyone who was unable to command the same Admiralty largesse:

> Other material advantages attended Captain Cook's crew, some of which were, their being all chosen men; seamen in the prime of life; inured to a sea life, therefore less liable to the diseases incident to seamen; and being less numerous in proportion to the size of the ship; consequently less crowded than in ships of war; they were of course less prone to diseases arising from crowding people together; and what added to this advantage was, the ship being more lofty, in proportion to her size, than men of war, they could keep their hatchways and scuttles open longer; and would be less liable to have the sea break in on their decks. When to the above circumstances we add the frequent large supplies of fresh vegetables of different kinds; of animal food, fish etc, which they procured at the different islands and other places where they anchored; that they were never more than 117 days at any one time without such a supply; and even during that time they were not entirely without fresh diet, and good preservatives; that the greatest part of the time they were at sea, they were either in a warm or a temperate climate; without excessive fatigue, or want of rest, having nothing but the common duties of the ship to do; no chasing, nor being called 'all hands to quarters' night after night.[43]

Although scurvy arose, there were no deaths from it during the three-year voyage. However, the ship experienced appalling medical problems, and a third of the crew of ninety-eight died from malaria and dysentery. Cook explained his success against scurvy principally by his use of MacBride's wort, and to a lesser extent to his persuasive techniques in getting his conservatively minded crew to eat sauerkraut. But John Clerk, the East India Company surgeon, observed that, 'he aided the wort with so many excellent preventatives, such as saurkraut, rob of lemon and oranges, as it is improper to place the preservation of his crew to that article.'[44] The use of a wide range of antiscorbutics was confirmed by William Perry the ship's assistant surgeon (the surgeon himself having died of fever). Perry's letter is dripping with obsequiousness, and begins thus:

> The sanguine and well-grounded expectations of the certain efficacy of the wort possesses to cure the sea-scurvy and the very great probability of that distemper raging at some time or other in the course of a long voyage induced, I apprehend, the Rt. Hon. the Lords Commissioners of the Admiralty to send out a quantity of malt in the *Endeavour*, as well to determine and fix its character in that respect as through an humane and tender care for the preservation of her crew. It may at first appear strange that I reckon this last motive secondary to the first, but a recollection of the ample and various assistance the same provident minds had afforded for that purpose, will remove this seeming absurdity.[45]

Perry, despite admitting the successful use of lemon rob, declared boldly:

> ... from what I have seen the wort perform, from its mode of operation, from Mr MacBride's reasoning, I shall not hesitate a moment to declare my opinion; that the malt is the best medicine I know, the inspissated [condensed] Orange & Lemon juices not even excepted.[46]

However, Perry was extraordinarily contradictory, and stated that since they used so many other antiscorbutics, they had had little opportunity for a trial of the wort, and that, 'It is impossible for me to say what was most conducive to our preservation from Scurvy, so many being the preservatives used.' These preservatives included sauerkraut, mustard, vinegar, wheat, rob of lemon and orange, saloup, portable soup, sugar, molasses and vegetables. The crew had also been prevented from eating salted beef and pork. He rather ingratiatingly apologised for not having made more use of the wort:

> What opportunities have occurred of using it have constantly been embraced; that more have not happened is, if a fault, the fault of the humanity of the Lords of the Admiralty and the care of the captain of the ship.[47]

James Cook himself was less enthusiastic about MacBride's wort than his assistant surgeon claimed to be, and depicted a pretty prosaic use of the wort:

> To Mr Perry's remarks I have only to add that in February 1770 we found the malt so indifferent (notwithstanding it was perfectly dry and sweet) that the surgeon could make little or no use of it in the common way; having at this time a good deal remaining and in order that we might reap some benefit from it, I ordered as strong a wort to be made of it as possible and in it boiled ground wheat for the people's breakfasts.[48]

Sailing aboard *Endeavour* as botanist was Joseph (later Sir Joseph) Banks, a brilliant, wealthy, 25-year-old Fellow of the Royal Society. He subsequently published his own account of the scurvy incidents. He recorded an attack of scurvy at Tierra del Fuego that was beaten by a diet of soup made from locally grown scurvy grass and wild celery. Banks himself was afflicted, and wrote that he also ate sauerkraut and, as a pleasant substitute, drank a pint of wort each evening to no good effect. 'I then flew to the lemon juice, which had been put up for me according to Dr Hulme's method.'[49] He had been supplied with citrus juice prepared by Lind's disciple Nathaniel Hulme; two gallons of lemon rob; seven gallons of orange juice with brandy, and five quarts of lemon juice with brandy:

> Every kind of liquor which I used was made sour with the lemon juice, so that I took nearly six ounces a day of it; the effect of this was surprising, in less than a week my gums became as firm as ever, and at this time I am troubled with nothing but a few pimples on my face, which have not deterred me from leaving off the juice entirely.[50]

According to Banks, successful treatment with the rob of lemons cured other cases of scurvy, despite the ambiguous claims for malt wort by the assistant surgeon. Nathaniel Hulme had written to Banks before the voyage, carefully describing the rob and giving instructions for its use:

> When you come to make use of the juice which is in the casks, do not open the bung-hole, but draw it off at the end of the cask by means of a wooden cock, and make a vent-hole with a peg in it at the top of the cask; and always observe this method when you draw off the juice.[51]

Hulme warned against even the smell of 'stinking water' and recommended the brewing of beer as a daily drink:

> I would recommend to you to carry out a quantity of molasses, and two or three pounds of the best Chio and Strasburg turpentine, in order to brew beer with. So small a quantity of molasses as two gallons, or two gallons and a half, are said to be sufficient for making an hogshead of tolerably good beer.[52]

Endeavour returned in the summer of 1771 with the issue of the proper treatment of scurvy more confused than ever, and

'BUT THE POWER IS IN OTHERS'

MacBride's remedy achieving an overrated status in the lexicon. It is easy to understand the tone of depressed resignation that Lind used in the third edition of his *Treatise*, which was about to be published. There had also been a dramatic incident in London which probably increased Lind's despondency. William Stark was a brilliant young physician who had studied in Glasgow, Edinburgh and Leyden, and who was working in London. He was a protégé of both John Hunter and Sir John Pringle, and a friend of Benjamin Franklin, who was living in London at the time. It has been suggested that Franklin, who had a particular interest in diet, may have encouraged the young Stark in his course of action. He determined to prove the details of the course of scurvy by personal experiment, and to show that simple diets such as those discussed with Franklin and Pringle, were compatible with good health.

> I confess it will afford me singular pleasure if I can prove by experiment, that a pleasant and varied diet is equally conducive to health, with a more strict and simple one; at the same time I shall endeavour to keep my mind unbiased in my search after truth, and if a simple diet seems the most healthy I shall not hesitate to declare it.[53]

Beginning in June 1769, Stark devised twenty-four dietary experiments over several months, all carefully recorded, and took a particular interest in the nutritional values of animal fats and of lean meat. Initially, he confined himself to a diet of bread, water and sugar with a little olive oil. This diet he compared with one containing milk and a little meat. He had originally intended, in a discrete phase of his experiment, to study the effects of fruit and green vegetables, but for some unknown reason, cancelled this procedure. Instead he later ate honey and Cheshire cheese. Thus his fate was sealed. Eventually, as was common at sea, he succumbed to one or more unidentified infections and became progressively more ill. It is a dreadful comment on Sir John Pringle and his blind devotion to the opinions of MacBride and Cook that all he suggested to his young friend was to omit salt from his diet. Even *in extremis* he did not attempt to save his protégé's life by suggesting the use of Lind's orange or lemon juice, of which he was, without a doubt, fully aware. After eight months of detailed note-taking on his consumption and condition, a colleague arrived to 'bleed the patient' but Stark died of deliberately induced scurvy on Friday 23 February 1770.[54]

James Cook set out on his great easterly circumnavigation in HMS *Resolution* and HMS *Adventure* in July 1772. The aims were to search for the supposed 'southern continent' (Australia), to explore the Antarctic and to conduct research for the Board of Longitude on four marine chronometers – an exact copy of the famous, compact H4 of John Harrison, and three others by John Arnold. Joseph Priestly, who had recently sent papers and drawings to the Admiralty describing his apparatus for impregnating water with 'fixed air', was considered by Joseph Banks for the post of astronomer. However, his employment was blocked by the academics who held sway over such appointments. Another candidate was the younger James Lind of Edinburgh. As Cook noted in his Journal:

> The Parliament voted Four thousand pounds towards carrying on Discoveries to the South Pole, this sum was intinded for Dr Lynd of Edinburgh as an incouragement for him to embark with us, but what the discoveries were, the Parliament meant he was to make, and for which they made so liberal a Vote, I know not.[55]

There was clearly considerable disagreement over the scientific personnel, and Banks finally complained that there was not enough space for him. Cook's view was derisive:

> ... not only Mr Banks and his whole suite but Dr Lind gave up the Voyage and their Baggage etc were got out of the Sloop and sent to London, after which no more complaints were heard for want of room etc.[56]

'BUT THE POWER IS IN OTHERS'

Cook was able to obtain even better levels of victualling than he achieved for his first voyage. An early demand was for the preferred antiscorbutics – David MacBride's malt wort, sauerkraut and 3,000 pounds of portable soup. When Cook queried supplies of the rob of oranges and lemons, he was told by the Victualling Board that there was none in stock. However, eventually a miserly supply of twenty-four pints was obtained, with sixteen pints for the second vessel. In any case, it seems that Cook's surgeon preferred elixir of vitriol and the even more useless Dr James's Powder. Priestley's soda water and the new 'carrot marmalade' (a syrup of evaporated carrot juice devised by a Berlin aristocrat) were both to be given trials as antiscorbutics.

Cook's extraordinary second voyage lasted three years, and consists of a wonderful series of hazards, adventures and encounters with new places, people and events. The popular characterisation of Cook as the man who conquered scurvy – an accolade which he happily accepted – is due to the fact that on his return, he was able truthfully to report that on such a lengthy and arduous voyage, not a single man had died from scurvy. He declared:

> After such a long continuance at sea in a high southern latitude, it is but reasonable to think that many of the people must be ill of the scurvy. The contrary, however, happened. Sweetwort had been given to such as were scorbutic. This had so far the desired effect, that they had only one man on board that could be called very ill of this disease, occasioned chiefly by a bad habit of body and a complication of other disorders.[57]

This indeed seemed a remarkable outcome; however scurvy had attacked the expedition on several occasions, sometimes with a vengeance, and from the recorded statements and events it seems clear that attempts to deal with it were of a rather haphazard nature, using all the available treatments. Sir James Watt noted that *Resolution* had excellent surgeons, but that they did not possess Lind's experimental methods:

This led to a blunderbuss approach to antiscorbutic treatment which confused the issue by failing to differentiate true antiscorbutics from the empirical remedies of longstanding tradition.[58]

Much can probably be attributed to the fact that, as ever, Cook's ships and crews were very well provided for; they must have had every expectation that, whatever disease encroached, they would be better able to withstand and recover from it than any previous expedition. Despite these conditions, Cook has been blamed for allowing his men too much access to alcohol, which contributed directly to several deaths, and indirectly to other medical complications.

Cook insisted that his own crew gathered fresh vegetables at every available opportunity, and noted that he did not have to order them once they saw the restorative effects. The crew of the second ship was less inclined to follow suit, and throughout the voyage there was more scurvy on board *Adventure*. In reports to the Admiralty and the Royal Society, Cook rated both sauerkraut and portable soup very highly, and was careful – and somewhat ambiguous – in his praise of the wort:

> We had a large quantity of malt, of which was made sweet-wort, and given to those who had manifest symptoms of scurvy, and to such also as were judged to be most liable to that disorder from one pint to three quarts in the twenty-four hours. This is without doubt one of the best antiscorbutic medicines yet discovered; and if used in time will, with proper attention to other things, I am persuaded, prevent the scurvy from making any great progress for a considerable while. But I am not altogether of opinion that it will cure it at sea. We have been a long time without any, without feeling the want of it, which might be owing to other articles.[59]

Cook's surgeon was equally happy to praise the effects of the wort, but also suggested that it was successful if 'aided by' other

'BUT THE POWER IS IN OTHERS'

remedies. Neither man made much mention of citrus juice or the rob, which Cook said was for use only under the care of the surgeon, who, 'made use of it in many cases with great success.'[60] In Cook's final report, he made one comment that would undoubtedly have pleased James Lind; 'the introduction of the most salutary articles, either as provision or medicines, will generally prove unsuccessful, unless supported by certain rules of living.'[61] He then proceeded to expound on the virtues of humane watch-keeping hours, cleanliness, dry clothes, ventilation and fresh drinking water.

Cook's report to the Royal Society resulted in his being awarded the Society's Sir Godfrey Copley Gold Medal for his care and attention to life at sea, and for keeping his expeditions free from scurvy. Cook was preparing his third (and fatally last) great voyage, and did not attend the official presentation to his wife in the summer of 1776, at which the society's president, Sir John Pringle, extolled the virtues of MacBride's wort and called up the name of Cook in support. Pringle said of the rob of citrus fruit that the ship's surgeon thought that it was 'of so little advantage that, judging it not advisable to lose more time, he set about the cure with the wort only, whereof the efficacy he was certain.'[62] Cook wrote a damning letter to Pringle on 7 July following the award, in which he indicated an obvious prejudice in favour of the wort. It also gave a clear indication from this undoubtedly great and influential naval hero that there was no future in considering the rob of citrus any further:

> I entirely agree with you that the dearness of the rob of lemon and oranges will hinder them from being furnished in large quantities. But I do not think this is so necessary; for though they may assist other things, I have no great opinion of them alone. Nor have I a higher opinion of vinegar.[63]

Despite the contradictions in Cook's use of different remedies, his letter was like the turning of the knife in a wound. However, Lind did not attempt to counter the rebuttal of his recommendations, or any associated hint of conspiracy that may have existed. Either he could not, or was disinclined; perhaps both. If Anson had indeed been Lind's patron at the time of his appointment to Haslar in 1758, then that patronage came to an end four years later with his death in 1762, when Lind was assuredly on his own again. Cook's willingness to accept deserved public approbation was one thing; but also to wear the mantle of 'the man who defeated scurvy' together with his condemnation of any further consideration of citrus juice were distinct setbacks to the Physician-in-Charge at Haslar.

In the third edition of his *Treatise* Lind had said:

> It would indeed be happy for mankind, if in all the various calamities and distresses, to which they are subject, the means of relief were so well ascertained, as they are in this painful disease (scurvy), an ignorance of the nature of which has long been productive of fatal consequences.[64]

The fatal consequences were to continue. Despite Lind's lifetime spent improving the health and hygiene of sailors, and despite the outbreak of new hostilities in the Americas, when both scurvy and typhus raged dramatically, the Admiralty's advisers increased pressure against citrus juice. In addition, there was to be a new attack on Lind in another pioneering area of his work – the provision of fresh water. Again, James Cook would be party to the blind refusal to give Lind's efforts credence.

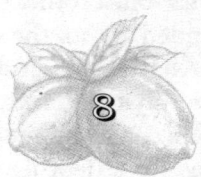

'My Attendance was Never Again Asked'

THE Royal Navy was a complicated beast of state that acquired an equally unwieldy series of administrative controls. The earliest formal hierarchy was headed by an all-powerful 'great officer of state' known as the Lord High Admiral; he was above a vice-admiral and a rear-admiral, all three above the eight principal officers comprising the Navy Board. These commissioners were lieutenant of the admiralty, treasurer of marine causes, comptroller, surveyor, clerk of the king's ships, master of ordnance for the king's ships, and two assistants. The commissioners of the Navy controlled all the big issues; expenditure at sea and ashore, ship construction and repair, dockyards, stores, ordnance, and so on. The Navy Board was probably the largest department of government, and the biggest industrial employer.

Eighteenth-century society in general was one in which patronage flourished. The Navy and the Board of Admiralty were similar to other branches of the body politic in that respect. Today there is a general abhorrence of systems based on prejudiced, personal motive rather than liberal public interest. Yet it is true that while the mid-eighteenth-century Admiralty Board was composed almost entirely of men placed in position by patronage, they were names which are universally attached to some of the greatest naval victories. One story illustrates how patronage could be entirely accidental and also highly successful; a captain injured in a carriage accident took refuge in a vicarage. Subsequently, the vicar's thirteen-year-old son went to sea under the captain's protection, soon to be followed by his fifteen-year-old brother. They were Samuel and Alexander Hood, and ended up as the naval heroes Viscount Hood, Lord of the Admiralty, and Viscount Bridport, commander-in-chief of the Channel Fleet.[1]

More commonly, a young man might be assisted in entering the Navy as a *quid pro quo* for a debt paid off or for some other favour within family or business. Having become an officer, it would be necessary to find a patron, under whose influence further promotion could be sought. In the mid-eighteenth century, regulations allowed officers to have an extraordinary number of 'servants' on board ship at sea. A captain could have 4 servants per 100 of the complement; a rear-admiral could have 15, up to Admiral of the Fleet, who was allowed 50 servants, of whom 16 were paid for by the Navy. 'Servant' might literally mean a retainer similar to those found in the household of a wealthy gentleman – 'tailors, barbers, footmen and fiddlers followed their patron.'[2] Often, a captain would use his 'allowance' of servants to introduce a young man into naval service, where he could be coached and prepared for a position as an officer in due course.

Patronage, and all the devious rule-bending that went with it, also operated in the awards of contracts, and in the support given to outsiders who came to the Admiralty with business or scientific propositions of one sort or another. As one quote from the second half of the eighteenth century put it:

> Reports are gone about of the immense profusion of the public Treasury; of the enormous emoluments of some places; of large sums not accounted for; of a vast expense in favouring contractors . . . and providing for a useless set of men.[3]

A colourful pair of letters indicates one particular swindle that was being worked which typified small-scale attempts to defraud the system. In November 1794 an anonymous 'Friend to The Government' made allegations concerning the production of portable soup:

'MY ATTENDANCE WAS NEVER AGAIN ASKED'

It is well known a certain officer at the Soup House has a deal of fat to dispose of which is <u>hid</u> after you sell what you advertise, beside his salary won't afford him to keep his Horse and Chaise and drink the <u>best wine</u> which he boasts of, as also to buy annuities every year – but fat for that, if you look sharp you will detect him.[4]

Enquiries were clearly made, for the following month there appears a desperate letter from George Clode, landlord of The White Hart at Windsor:

I beg you will be pleased to observe that I am an innkeeper at Windsor, and know nothing of the trade of fat, neither have I received any fat, or even had any offered to me to dispose of. I hope you will be pleased to give some reasons for the clause of this letter to me, as nothing else can conciliate the minds of my wife and eight children.[5]

Patronage did not only involve the illicit expenditure of money; preferential treatment, or sponsorship, was rife. The eighteenth-century Navy employed many private contractors and was engaged in supporting important expeditions in the fields of cartography, marine chronometry, natural history and astronomy. In such circumstances, it is easy to see what a dangerous minefield it might be for an innocent party, who could easily become a victim of shifting alliances. The more or less reputable, such as David MacBride, were able to progress their theories or contractual relationships against all others if they were able to attract powerful support. The worst effects were to be seen where the complexity of the situation encouraged sloth in decision-making. In the face of two centuries of conflicting evidence and hearsay on remedies for scurvy, it may have been easy, if wholly inexcusable, for the Admiralty to rely on the kind of partisan lobbying that enabled a 'society doctor' such as Joshua Ward to have his fraudulent pills authorised.

Since the late 1750s, James Lind had been giving thought to the problem of providing potable water aboard ship. Perhaps the most vital everyday factor in any long sea voyage, and one constantly referred to by naval surgeons, was water. Good, clean water was vital not only for drinking, but for the boiling of provisions, and for cleanliness. Even in hot climates, the daily ration per man for all purposes was about three pints – often less during the frequent intervals of shortage. Water was a real health issue, and scurvy and other diseases were advanced not only by lack of good water, but by the consumption of sea water either in desperation or by mistaken ideology. The role of sea water in preventing scurvy was a live issue, with dispute raging over its efficacy as a direct remedy; sea water and salt were also heavily ingested in a variety of preserved provisions, provoking further controversy. Fresh water stored in barrels in ships' holds did not last long in good condition, yet it was carried for months and formed the only realistic supply in most circumstances. Surgeon Leonard Gillespie wrote of the water on board the sloop *Racehorse* on patrol in the North Sea:

> The water we have at this time is Thames water filled six months ago at Deptford in new unseasoned casks. The astringent principle of the oak and the iron rubbed off the cooper's tools have impregnated it so as to form a dilute sort of ink. Putrefaction has made it fetid and stinking. It would appear to be impregnated with inflammable or hepatic air, first from the taste, second smell, third discoloration of silver immersed into it.[6]

Wooden casks were especially notorious for producing noxious water, but after 1815, iron casks or tanks were gradually introduced. For ships departing from England and hoping to avoid the worst of the Thames water, there were sweet wells at Bembridge on the Isle of Wight, which reputedly delivered the best water destined for long storage.[7] But the chances of acquiring fresh water in the course of a long voyage were extremely unreliable, and water obtained from a dubious source could turn out to be a prime cause of disease. In any case, the practicalities of obtaining water and ferrying it aboard ship were so time-consuming as to make the prospect impossible in many inhospitable or dangerous places. Small volumes of rainwater could be regularly saved on deck when possible, but the amounts gained by this method were usually negligible or still poisonous:

> ... it is all rainwater, and covered close up, which, for want of air, breeds poisonous animalculae, and becomes foul and putrid.[8]

A means of turning sea water into fresh drinking water on board ship during long voyages was a long-cherished dream of sailors. Various means had been attempted since the earliest circumnavigations. Richard Hawkins had some unknown system off the coast of South America as long ago as 1593:

> Although our fresh water had fayled us many dayes by reason of our long Navigation, without touching any land, and the excessive drinking of the sicke and diseased (which could not be excused) yet with an invention I had in my Shippe, I easily drew out of the water of the Sea, sufficient quantitie of fresh water to sustaine my people, with little expence of fewell; for with foure Billets I stilled a Hogshead of water, and therewith dressed the meat for the sicke and whole. The water so distilled, we found to be wholesome and nourishing.[9]

A variety of purification methods were in use in the mid-eighteenth century; they usually involved the addition of a number of substances to bad water in the hope of purging or neutralising the worst poisons. Many of these substances themselves acted as adulterants, and produced severely tainted water that was often nauseous. Vinegar and cream of tartar were popular additions; troops in Canada added powdered ginger;

again in Canada, burnt ship's biscuit was added to bad water on the St Lawrence River in 1759 (four pounds of biscuit to the hogshead). In Senegal, where water had been found to be very bad indeed, lime was used; this was a method that could not be used at sea since the process sometimes lasted for weeks and involved much boiling. One method of obtaining fresh water on shore was to bury a cask drilled with small holes in a pit dug ten to fifteen yards from the sea; this method provided the basis of primitive filtration systems for use by watering parties.

The ability to distil sea water on board ship was clearly a much sought-after benefit, and the Admiralty in its usual half-hearted fashion encouraged work on solving the problem, without any clear concept of analysing the results. James Lind had been attempting to perfect a shipboard distillation process that made use of the heat of the sun. Initial trials failed, but he persevered with more conventional methods:

> Let us suppose a ship at sea to be in distress for want of water, having eight men on board, and that the pot for boiling their provisions can contain five gallons and an half, being twelve inches in diameter; by the following simple contrivance, with only a tea-kettle, a musket, and a cask, one gallon of fresh water may be procured every three hours, which is a pint for each man.[10]

The musket barrel was inserted into the spout of the kettle inverted over a hole in the pot cover. The musket barrel passed through holes on opposing sides of the cask and was caulked to stop leakage. Cold sea water was retained in the barrel, acting as a condenser. With heat applied to the pot, steam rose through the kettle and musket barrel, and was condensed as it passed through the water-filled cask, trickling out as pure water from the end of the barrel. This was a crude trial, but it satisfied Lind's requirement for a system that was simple, could be set up in a crisis without special equipment, and did not rely on the addition of chemicals that would taint the water.

Lind decided to make further experiments, and in his usual fashion gave critical attention to the attempts that had been made by others. He researched the progress of distillation since Francis Bacon in the early seventeenth century. There was Sir Theophilus Oglethorpe's patent of 1683 for 'An Engine for rendering salt and brackish water sweet'; Dr Stephen Hales' powdered chalk system of 1739; and that of Joshua Appleby of Durham in 1754 which used *lapis infernalis* (silver nitrate) and calcined bones. Lind made a critique of all the earlier proposals, and pointed out of the Appleby scheme:

> The attention of all Europe being at that time drawn towards this discovery, which was then esteemed the most fortunate of the age, various substitutes were proposed, instead of the noxious ingredients used in Mr Appleby's process. For this purpose, Dr Butler recommends capital soap leys, Dr Alston limestone, and Dr Hales powdered chalk.
>
> The manner in which I fortunately discovered that all those ingredients were unnecessary, and that a simple distillation rendered sea-water perfectly fresh and wholesome, may be seen in my letter to the Royal Society.[11]

Lind had succeeded in developing a system that was simple, with no spurious adulterants and was capable, even in its experimental form, of delivering sufficient quantities of fresh water for practical use at sea. A paper outlining his proposals was read before the Royal Society in London in May 1762, and the notes of the meeting state that:

> The still employed by Dr Lynd was of tin, without a worm containing about two quarts. When this still ran slow, the sea-water boiling gently, the water which came over was found free from salt than the common rain water which usually falls near the Sea-side, with a sea breeze. The distilled water appeared to be equal in taste and purity to rain water distilled from the said vessel. Dr Lynd is not without hopes of being

able to distil sea-water by an accumulation of the solar rays; though an attempt of that kind with an 10-inch speculum belonging to Mr Robertson did not succeed at Portsmouth.[12]

Robertson was the late master of the Royal Academy at Portsmouth; another witness to Lind's experiments was Captain Richard Hughes, the Royal Navy commissioner at Portsmouth. Lind also published a more detailed, less experimental method in a second edition of his *Essay on the most effectual means of preserving the health of Seamen in the Royal Navy*. This was published in March 1763 at the instruction of the Lords Commissioners of the Admiralty, whom Lind, not unnaturally, assumed were honouring him 'on account of the important discovery I had then made of rendering sea-water perfectly fresh and wholesome by a simple distillation.'[13] In support of his distillation system, he included an extract from a letter sent to him from Cuba in September 1762:

Before the surrender of this place, our distress for want of water became inexpressible; I would have given with pleasure half a guinea for a pint of such distilled sea-water as I have frequently drank at your table. Numbers of our men died, from a real want of water, and many more from drinking water which was unwholesome and poisonous.[14]

Nothing was heard from the Admiralty. But news arrived from Paris in July 1764, when Doctor Poissonnière laid claim to what he described as an 'improvement' in the construction of a still for use at sea. Poissonnière was a naval physician who was to receive a pension from the French government for the 'discovery' of what was in effect Lind's process. Lind remarked with some sarcasm in the 1779 edition of his *Essay on the Most Effectual means of Preserving the Health of Seamen* that his process had no sooner attracted public attention than it suffered the common fate of having its discovery claimed by others. He pointed out that it was fully two years after his own experiments before Poissonnière made his own 'discovery' at Brest and Toulon. An account exists of the remarks of the captain of the frigate *Epouée* in 1768 who, on arriving at Brest, extolled the virtues of Poissonnière's method. However, he added the comment that, 'the method was first practised by our countryman Dr Lind, from whom the French physician has taken the process.'[15] It is ironic that the good doctor Poissonnière became one of Lind's fervent disciples on the question of scurvy. In 1767 he published a book on diseases of seamen in which he offered ample homage to Lind, and in which he recommended punch containing a high proportion of lemon juice and sugar; he also advocated the use of oranges in the late stages of scurvy.[16]

Lind stoically proceeded with the task of perfecting his own design. He concentrated on devising the best means of connecting the still heads to the normal arrangement of ships' boilers so that whenever the boilers were fired, water could immediately be distilled irrespective of other demands on the boilers. He worked out that 200 gallons of fresh water could be obtained in 12 hours from a still of 32 inches diameter. He claimed that a 60-gun ship of 400 men could obtain half a gallon per day per man at the expense of 3 chaldrons of coal (a chaldron is a defunct measure equal to the contents of a 288-gallon container).

In 1766, Surgeon Frederick Thomson recorded his impressions of a successful use of distillation:

> For some weeks we had used no other water; On banyan days we generally distilled from the spare copper; and on other days, after the dinners were dressed, and the coppers cleaned, filled with sea-water etc, we began to distil; which was continued until four or five o' clock in the morning, and in that time we commonly obtained 80 or 90 gallons, sometimes more, of good pure water. We had but one apparatus on board; but when a ship is supplied with one for each copper, there can never be any danger of scarcity of water, while the fuel lasts.[17]

LIMEYS

In 1768 Lind was successful in arranging an official trial at sea on board HMS *Dolphin* under Captain Wallis during a three-year circumnavigation. In the vicinity of Cape Town in February 1768, the captain and surgeon were delighted to have the opportunity of showing off their distillation system to the officers of a nearby East Indiaman:

> At five o' clock in the morning, we put 56 gallons of salt water into the still, at seven it began to run, and in about five hours and a quarter afforded us six and thirty gallons of fresh water, at an expense of nine pounds of wood and 69 pounds of coals. Thirteen gallons and two quarts remained in the still, and that which came off had no ill taste, nor as we had often experienced, any hurtful quality. I thought the shewing this experiment of the more consequence, as the being able to allow plenty of water not only for drink, but for boiling any kind of provision, and even for making tea and coffee, especially during long voyages, and in hot climates, conduces greatly to health, and is the means of saving many lives. I never once put my people to an allowance of water during this whole voyage, always using the still when we were reduced to five and forty tons, and preserving the rain water with the utmost diligence.[18]

The following year, an emergency took place on HMS *Dorsetshire* on a passage from Gibraltar to Port Mahon. The ship carried a regiment of troops, and in a crisis, the kettle-and-musket still was rigged up; this produced nineteen quarts of fresh water from twenty-two quarts of sea water in four hours. Lind still hoped for a wholehearted response to his distillation proposals from the Admiralty (that had ordered the publication of his method), but instead of support he saw their Lordships effectively hand his work on a plate to someone else. This was Charles Irving, a junior surgeon on the ironically named HMS *Arrogant*, who in 1771 invited Lind to a demonstration of his 'new and hitherto not practised' method of distillation at sea. This claim was made in the same year that a second edition was

'MY ATTENDANCE WAS NEVER AGAIN ASKED'

published of Lind's *Essay on Diseases Incidental to Europeans in Hot Climates*, containing an even more detailed description of the distillation scheme. Irving's proposal was essentially Lind's own system, with a few modifications of his own which have been described as 'inferior'. Irving, completely ignoring the *Dolphin* trials and the previously published details, later had the nerve to say of Lind's work:

> He distilled sea-water without the addition of any ingredients; but as the experiment he made was performed in a vessel containing only two quarts, with a glass receiver, in his study, nothing conclusive can be drawn from it for the use of shipping. Indeed experiments of the like kind had been made by the chemists in their laboratories, for at least a century before.[19]

With considerable insolence, Irving asked Lind to countersign a document enabling him to claim a reward for his 'invention'. Lind initially refused, but the Admiralty convened an official board to consider and evaluate Irving's scheme; Lind was, no doubt reluctantly, appointed to this committee, which was simply 'required' to endorse Irving.[20] Lind took a pragmatic, unselfish view and relented;

> ... desirous that in any form so important a discovery as the freshening of sea-water by distillation might be introduced into general use; this, Mr Irving said, he had reason to believe he could effect if he obtained the certificate; and to me it appeared a matter of indifference whether the distillation was performed by means of a still head and refrigiratory, as I had proposed, or by a long tin tube wet with mops, as set forth in the certificate: in that particular alone Mr Irving's method having differed from what I had before published.[21]

It is hard to imagine the feelings that must have tormented Lind when he was unable to do anything other than stand aside and watch as Irving was awarded the very substantial reward of £5,000 for his invention. Inevitably encouraged by the Admiralty, the House of Commons passed the appropriate vote on 11 March 1772. It is extraordinary that the Admiralty, having publicly supported Lind's proposals, should now have turned on him in such a manner. Remarking on Irving's 'pretentions' [sic], Lind remarked philosophically of the Admiralty committee, 'my attendance was never again asked'.

That year, the Admiralty directed that all warships were to be fitted with a still and related apparatus.[22] It is not clear whose system (if any one in particular) was preferred, but in any case, various trials seem still to have taken place. Despite the Admiralty's sponsorship, and his substantial financial reward, Irving's distillation system seems never to have been universally adopted. He took his equipment on board HMS *Racehorse* under Constantine John Phipps, later Lord Mulgrave, seeking a passage to the East Indies via the North Pole (when one young midshipman aboard was Horatio Nelson). Phipps recorded a detailed diary of this momentous Arctic exploration:

> 20th June 1773:
> We began this day to make use of Dr Irving's apparatus for distilling fresh water from the sea; repeated trials gave us the most satisfactory proof of its utility; the water produced from it was perfectly free from salt, and wholesome, being used for boiling the ship's provisions; which convenience alone would be a desirable object in all voyages, independent of the benefit of so useful a resource in case of distress for water. The quantity produced every day varied from accidental circumstances, but was generally from 34 to 40 gallons, without any great addition of fuel. Twice indeed the quantity produced was only 23 gallons on each distillation; this amounts to more than a quart for each man, which, though not a plentiful allowance, is much more than what is necessary for subsistence. In cases of real necessity I have no reason to doubt that a much greater quantity might be produced without inconvenient expense of fuel.[23]

'MY ATTENDANCE WAS NEVER AGAIN ASKED'

James Cook also took Irving's inefficient apparatus on board *Resolution* and *Adventure*. It was apparently hardly used, and Cook himself had a poor opinion of it, 'a useful invention, but only calculated to provide enough to preserve life without health.'[24] Cook placed a high value on the provision of fresh water. Even where there were none of the recommended antiscorbutics available, he was convinced 'that with plenty of fresh water, and a close attention to cleanliness, a ship's company will seldom be much afflicted with scurvy.'[25] Whatever Cook's views on the importance of fresh water, he was not induced to use Lind's distillation system either. Given Cook's status and influence, this refusal was as unfortunate as his repudiation of citrus fruit against scurvy. In 1979 Sir James Watt suggested that Cook deserved even heavier criticism for his failure to use Lind's water distillation apparatus than for the blinkered attitude that favoured malt over lemon juice.[26]

Lind's distillation system continued to attract interest and approval from individual voyages. One Irish captain experienced a severe water shortage en route for India and constructed an emergency version of Lind's kettle and musket which in three hours produced 'ten quarts of fresh water, exceedingly clear and well tasted.' Lind was given an account of this incident by Mr Davis, surgeon aboard HMS *Dolphin*, who stated that he 'tasted the distilled water, which was the purest and best water he ever remembers to have tasted.'[27] The Admiralty appears to have made little attempt to reach any conclusion on the issue of distillation, and individuals continued from time to time to take up the matter as if for the first time. In 1786 Charles Fletcher published in his book *Health for Seamen* an account of a system devised by a surgeon's mate named Smyth. He had sufficient nous to allow himself a reference to Lind's ill-treatment:

> Mr Smyth was thirty years a Surgeon's Mate in the navy, when he pointed out this ingenious improvement to the Lords of the Admiralty, who ordered that it might be used on board the *Intrepid*, in which ship I had the opportunity of seeing it at

Madras; it was supplied with water from the forecastle by means of the fire-engine, and perfectly answered the purpose for which it was intended. Whether he got anything for the above, I know not; but I should think it rather probable that he did not; as Doctor Lind, acknowledged inventor of this important discovery, was not considered.[28]

As the petitions for consideration of 'new' ideas rolled in to their lordships, the production of fresh water would be referred to as a matter of national importance, yet it seemed destined to remain largely unresolved. In September 1797 Henry Dundas (Viscount Melville) was in communication with Joseph Black, the chemist who succeeded William Cullen as Professor of Medicine and Chemistry at Edinburgh University. Black assured him that one paper submitted was 'a Farrago' which attempted to suggest that filtration was a new idea. Black noted that 'he encumbers his filtrating process (which he names precipitation) with much useless trumpery.'[29] Black submitted some notes of his own on the water problem, which he attributed to two causes; initial impurity of the water, and secondary impurity caused by the wooden storage casks. He was particularly scathing of River Thames water:

> It contains dissolved animal and vegetable matter in sufficient quantity to dispose it to undergo a putrid fermentation, which begins not long after it is put into the casks, and I believe it would undergo this fermentation much in the same manner although it were carried to sea in glass vessels.[30]

Black recommended coating the interior of water casks with GUM LAC, or Lacca – commonly sold as SHELL LAC – in order to prevent the wood affecting the water quality. He also suggested the use of pure sulphur, but blandly noted 'its propensity to take fire.' A later letter of 1804 from another hopeful to Melville, then First Lord, was typical of several in its appeal to the vital importance of the subject matter:

'MY ATTENDANCE WAS NEVER AGAIN ASKED'

As every object of national importance is known to engage your lordship's attention, I presume to submit to you a method of making salt water fresh and which can be effected without any incumberance [sic] to the ship or any other expense to His Majesty's Navy than the original cost of the apparatus which for a ship of the line would not exceed £35.[31]

It is not known if the writer, Richard Younger, was encouraged to proceed with his plans. The previous year he had registered a patent (No. 2,740 of 1803) for 'Extracting worts from malt, barley and other grains and substances', so it is possible that he was petitioning their lordships on a number of issues related to shipboard life.

The problem of providing distilled fresh water at sea was not solved for some years, and the problems of foul water continued, despite numerous attempts to promote a variety of shipboard systems. One 1837 writer was unreserved:

[No-one] who had not felt it can imagine the distress that was often endured within the tropics, from the intense thirst thus excited and the only means of quenching it – water so putrid and offensive, often so thick and green from vegetable decomposition, and emitting so strongly the factor of rotten eggs, as to disgust at once the sense of smell and of taste.[32]

Three years later, Edward Cree was assistant surgeon on the troopship HMS *Rattlesnake* in the East China Sea, and was still able to record the weary, philosophical acceptance of putrid water:

Fri. 25th: Poor Tracey, Assistant Surgeon of *Melville*, a great friend of mine, died this morning after an illness of four days of dysentery. He was a general favourite. He died in the temporary hospital ship *Victoria*. Death is making great havoc in the force, which is very sickly. I don't wonder at it considering the water we are drinking, stagnant from the paddy-fields, all well mixed with liquid manure. It stinks and is white and flatulent, but there is no other to be got in the neighbourhood.³³

Distillation became a much greater possibility after the advent of steam power, and an apparatus developed by Dr Normanby that was capable of delivering one gallon of fresh water from six gallons of salt water was becoming widely installed in ships by 1880.³⁴

* * *

During his years at Haslar, Lind was inevitably part of the special role of the Navy in the spectacular expansion of the British Empire to include Canada, India and Australia. Haslar under James Lind dealt with the diseases and injuries that colonial exploitation generated; it also saw the effects of the War of American Independence and the start of the French Revolution. Lind's considerable reputation enabled him to devote effort to new editions of his three great works on scurvy, naval hygiene and tropical medicine. His work on hygiene was translated into French, German and Dutch, and the one on tropical medicine achieved five editions during his lifetime. In Europe, in particular, his work was highly regarded. Together, the three books constitute what Sir James Watt described as 'a compendium of naval preventive medicine argued from sound principles'.³⁵

Apart from his recommendations on scurvy (which were still not accepted by the Admiralty) Lind has been credited with conquering typhus and other sea diseases. He instituted better ventilation, regular bathing, physical exercise, clean clothing and uniforms. On its own, the introduction of regular changes of clean clothing for all sailors was a simple improvement with far-reaching implications. His work also led to the introduction of depot ships for the proper regulation of quarantine; supply ships to ensure the victualling of squadrons at sea, and hospital ships. In 1953, Surgeon Vice-Admiral Sir Sheldon Dudley, late Medical Director-General of the Royal Navy, celebrated the fact that Lind was responsible for the banishment from the Navy of both scurvy and typhus:

> I myself am unable to add anything to Lind's clinical observations because, thanks to him, in the forty years I followed Lind's vocation of preserving the health of sailors, I never saw a seaman suffering from scurvy or typhus.[36]

Given Lind's enormous contribution to naval medicine, it is certainly puzzling to consider that he – and more especially his work – was treated with such indifference by the Admiralty and that he was given so little recognition. There is no evidence that he was at all bitter about this situation, or felt himself to be personally humiliated. He was sufficiently realistic to understand that his recommendations would have to await the arrival of someone else to bring them into effect. A conspiracy theorist might claim that there seemed to be a will to airbrush Lind out of the picture entirely. In William Laird Clowes's seven-volume *History of the Royal Navy from the Earliest Times to 1900* Lind is referred to, in passing, as 'one Dr Lynn'[37] and that is a minor reference to water distillation rather than scurvy or any other of his principal medical fields of achievement. He undoubtedly suffered the worst effects of patronage. John Montagu, Earl of Sandwich, may not have conspired directly against James Lind, but his ill-considered patronage of David MacBride had the same effect. Not only did Lind's own work fail to achieve merited recognition under such a malign system, but, ironically, the efforts of both David MacBride and Charles Irving came to nothing.

Lind's apparent willingness to remain silent in the face of official neglect is a puzzle – whether that neglect was bred of conspiracy or simply lack of regard for his prodigious work. This neglect has attracted comments ranging from 'a national disgrace' and 'one of the most tragic in the history of medicine' to 'criminal and disastrous'. Others have questioned whether it is an adequate explanation that his supposed inability to acquire the appropriate social connections could really have remained an obstacle for half a century. By all accounts, he apparently abhorred publicity and self-promotion, and was a man whose nature was one of absorption in his own administrative and academic works rather than in bureaucratic squabbles. He seems not to have been the kind of man who would have been happy to parade through the corridors of power seeking out patronage. For all that, in an age when such patronage was so dominant, it may be a fair criticism of Lind that he did not recognise a greater responsibility to ensure that his work received wider knowledge and understanding.

In February 1772 Lind's son John was appointed assistant surgeon at Haslar, and was promoted to assistant physician (effectively, deputy to his father) in July 1778, at an annual salary of £200. Scurvy was continuing to take a heavy toll within the Navy, and the controversy over treatment did not abate. In 1780 the Channel Fleet blockading France returned to Portsmouth with 2,400 men suffering from scurvy, of whom 1,500 ended up in Haslar.[38] The following year, 3,000 were stricken with scurvy in the West Indies Fleet under Rodney, and the military situation was saved only by the French Fleet suffering to an even greater extent.[39]

James Lind decided to retire in 1783 at the age of sixty-seven, and the Commissioners of the Board of the Sick and Hurt accepted his resignation with regret and the unusual award of an annual pension of £200 – equal to his annual salary. However, the commissioners wanted to ensure that this was seen as a highly unusual agreement.

> We think that this allowance equal to his full pay, if their Lordships are pleased to grant it, should not serve as a precedent in favour of any future physician.[40]

Lind's son John succeeded him at the same salary, but without the benefit of his own vacated position of assistant physician being filled.

However, the battle against scurvy was about to take a new

'MY ATTENDANCE WAS NEVER AGAIN ASKED'

turn. Sailing with Rodney in the West Indies as his personal physician was the 31-year-old Gilbert Blane, a graduate of Edinburgh and Glasgow Universities. Blane was already well-connected in London society, and apart from his medical abilities, his social, political and royal connections were to give him unusual influence. Even before Lind retired, Blane took the unusual step of writing directly to the Admiralty about his experience of scurvy in the West Indies. After a few months in London, Blane returned with Rodney to the West Indies, where with Surgeon Thomas Trotter he actively treated scurvy with fresh lemons, limes and oranges. Two new and powerful champions of Lind's methods were moving themselves into the limelight.

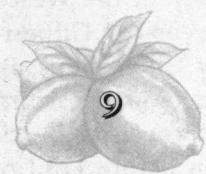

'Policy as Well as Humanity Concur'

GILBERT Blane was born on 29 August 1749 into a comfortably off family at Blanefield, a tiny hamlet near Kirkoswald in Ayrshire, about 2 miles from the imposing Culzean Castle, overlooking the Firth of Clyde. A brother made a vast fortune with the East India Company, and bought extensive land in Kentucky, Pennsylvania, Virginia and Washington DC. In addition, family estates were owned at Foliejon Park in Berkshire. Gilbert entered the faculty of arts at Edinburgh University at the age of fourteen, originally intending to study theology. After five years, he entered the faculty of medicine, finally taking his MD degree at Glasgow University in 1778.

Blane's entry into the Navy was, to say the least, unusual. Suffice to say that he was the beneficiary of patronage of a high level right from the beginning. After he graduated, he left Scotland for London, carrying letters of introduction from his mentor, Dr William Cullen, to one of his ex-pupils, Dr William Hunter, the renowned Scottish anatomist and obstetrician. This led, in 1779, to Blane being appointed private physician to Admiral George Rodney, who was widely regarded as a brilliant naval commander after momentous victories at Cape Finisterre, Le Havre and the West Indies. Rodney was something of a hypochondriac, but he suffered very real and severe gout. Blane sailed with Rodney to the West Indies, where he encountered the ravages of scurvy at first hand. He was present in a strictly private capacity as Rodney's doctor, but had so impressed the Admiral with his behaviour in battle conditions that when

Rodney was appointed Commander of the Windward and Leeward Islands station in late 1779, he commissioned Blane Physician to the Fleet. This appointment, involving a most blatant example of patronage, has been described as 'a piece of jobbery which had the most beneficial consequences.'[1] The third of the quartet of great naval surgeons (Lind and Blane being the first two), Robert Robertson, was already a young surgeon in the fleet, and noted the new promotion with some cynicism:

> A Dr Blane, who never was in the Navy before, is taken under Lord Rodney's protection and was, he said, ordered to superintend the hospital while the fleet was at Gibraltar.[2]

Blane later said of his own appointment that he was determined, as much as possible, to take advantage of the opportunities that had been opened to him:

> ... in order to satisfy my own mind as a matter of duty, as well as to find out, if possible, the means of bettering the condition of a class of men, who are the bulwark of the state, but whose lot is hardship and disease above that of all others.[3]

One of the first points that Blane made at that time, in a direct echo of James Lind, was that he was concerned about *prevention* and not just cure. He made another nod to Lind and his observational techniques by confirming that, 'the only true method of cultivating any practical art is to collect and compare a great number of facts.'[4]

The West Indies Fleet had headed for Gibraltar to convoy supplies for the reinforcement of Gibraltar and Minorca. Blane was appalled by the medical condition of the fleet, which even in these waters had a mortality rate of one in seven. He also discovered that naval surgeons were despised by their captains. In response, Blane wrote and printed, at his own expense, a volume outlining the medical responsibilities of officers, which he had distributed to the fleet captains.[5] He called for the immediate improvement of ventilation, the use of lemon juice, and reduced access to cheap rum.⁶

In January 1780, the fleet sailed for the West Indies, where over the following two years Blane achieved a reputation for his bravery in battles against the French Fleet under the Comte de Grasse. The main naval stations were the Leeward and Windward Islands; Port Royal, Barbados; and English Harbour, Antigua – a place characterised by James Lind as 'remarkable for its unhealthiness.' Blane was not content to be the administrator who occasionally toured the hospitals and wrote reports home. His habit at sea was to make himself visible to the seamen on deck during battle. He carried supplies of tourniquets immediately ready to staunch blood loss, rather than manhandle the wounded to the cramped medical station below decks. Clowes in *History of the Navy* recorded Blane's opinion of the French Fleet:

> Gilbert Blane, who though Physician to the Fleet, obtained permission to be on deck throughout the action, wrote ten days later, 'I can aver from my own observation that the French fire slackens as we approach, and is totally silent when we are close alongside.'⁷

In various fleets, senior surgeons and commanders were at last beginning to complain at the highest levels about the continuing effects of scurvy. It is shocking to consider that thirty years had passed since Lind demonstrated clearly the course of action required to defeat the disease. Thousands of sailors had perished, thousands more had become incapacitated, and the military and economic objects of the country had been constantly imperilled by an incompetent response to the perennial problems of death, disability and the resulting inability to maintain ships at sea. Now, senior commanders were stating unequivocally that not just single ships but entire squadrons at war would simply be removed into port from patrol due to the disastrous effects of scurvy.

'POLICY AS WELL AS HUMANITY CONCUR'

In early August 1780, Rear-Admiral Richard Kempenfelt was aboard HMS *Victory* under the elderly and sick Admiral Geary at sea off Ushant, France's most westerly point, where the English Channel met the Bay of Biscay. Kempenfelt, a progressive in the field of naval hygiene and a disciple of Lind, was to win a brilliant victory against the French at Ushant the following year. He wrote to Admiral Charles Middleton (later Lord Barham, and First Lord of the Admiralty):

> The scurvy now shows itself in most of the ships of the fleet; in some very severe; and according to the nature of that disorder, increases fast, so that there is a necessity for the fleet's going into port. Torbay, which has many advantages to recommend it, it is judged will not answer upon this occasion. How to dispose of the sick?[8]

He eventually put the sick ashore at Spithead, a decision he said was unavoidable due to the fact that 2,400 men were suffering from scurvy. The situation was so bad that he insisted the proper way to have dealt with it was to split the fleet, sending the five worst affected ships to Portsmouth, the eight healthiest to Torbay, and the rest to Spithead. However, Admiral Geary had refused to split his fleet. Kempenfelt insisted to Middleton that proper means of both dealing with the sick, and reprovisioning the fleet, would have to be found, all in the face of an admiral whose faculties were in question:

> Four line-of-battle ships and a frigate, which lately joined us at sea, are brought in to add to our embarrassment at Spithead. Had they been cruising for short intervals, putting in from time to time at Torbay, they would have been in the way to have annoyed the enemy and protected our trade, to have kept themselves healthy and have formed their raw men by practice.[9]

Admiral Hawke, who had suffered so badly in his blockade at Quiberon Bay, wrote of Geary's experience:

I do not wonder at the men being sickly after so long a cruise. Six weeks is long enough in all conscience. Any time after that must be very hurtful to the men, and occasion their falling down very fast. I wish the Admiralty would see what was done in former times. It would make them act with more propriety.[10]

But when it came to the point, Kempenfelt minced no words in stating his opinion of his admiral's abilities:

In fine, if the Admiralty will not appoint a suitable person to command the fleet, you must expect nothing but bad conduct, and, in consequence, bad success; the present person is brave, generous, and may perhaps have been a good officer; but he is wholly debilitated in his faculties, his memory and judgement lost, wavering and indetermined in everything.[11]

A few days later, Kempenfelt was ordered back to sea again by Geary with most of the fleet's crew still very sick. Frustrated and angry, he wrote from *Victory*:

The positive order for sailing when half our people are scorbutic – probably the whole somewhat tainted – however necessary, disconcerts us greatly. The fatigue is too much for Mr Geary; I have just left him in bed, ashore, much indisposed. This increases our embarrassment and must produce delay.[12]

Two weeks later, Kempenfelt's complaints were acted upon, at least as far as Geary was concerned; the admiral resigned and was replaced by Vice-Admiral Darby.

From HMS *Sandwich* at New York, as part of the West Indies Fleet, Captain Young also wrote to the Admiralty, in September 1780, complaining about the quantity and quality of provisions, and the inevitable advance of scurvy:

James Lind in a stipple engraving after the now lost painting of 1783 by Sir George Chalmers. (*Wellcome Trust*)

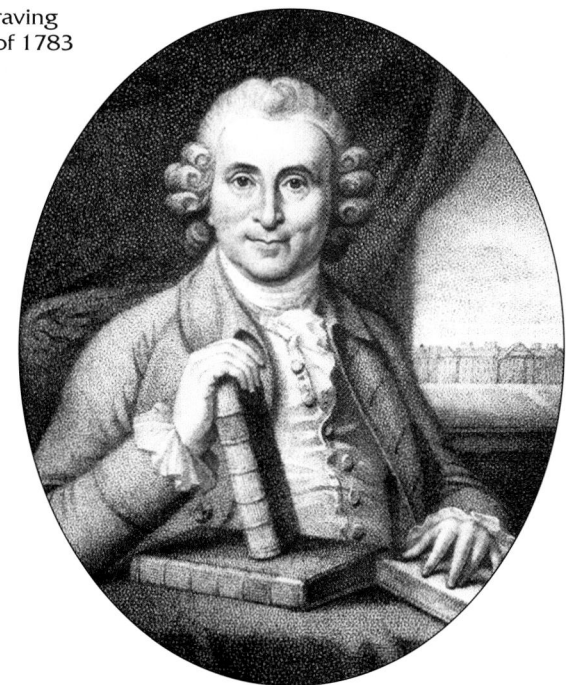

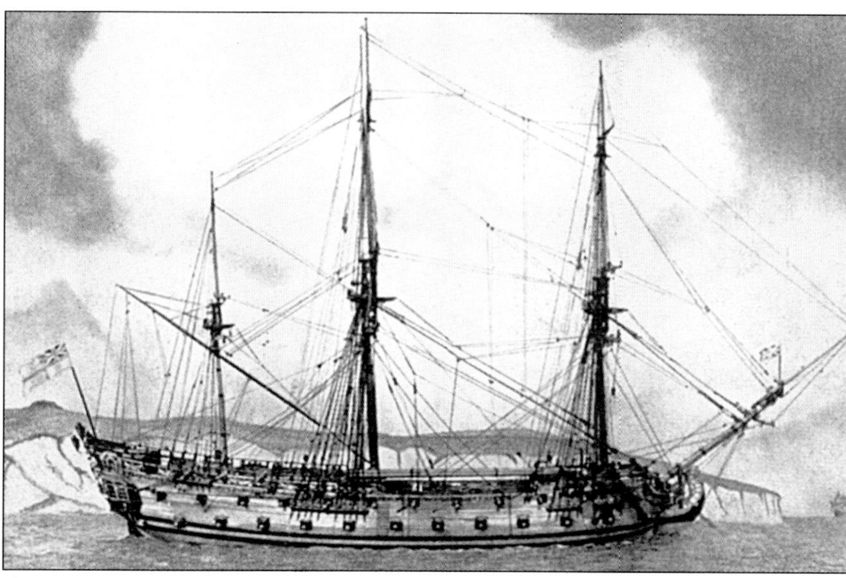

Model of HMS *Salisbury*. (*Edinburgh University Press*)

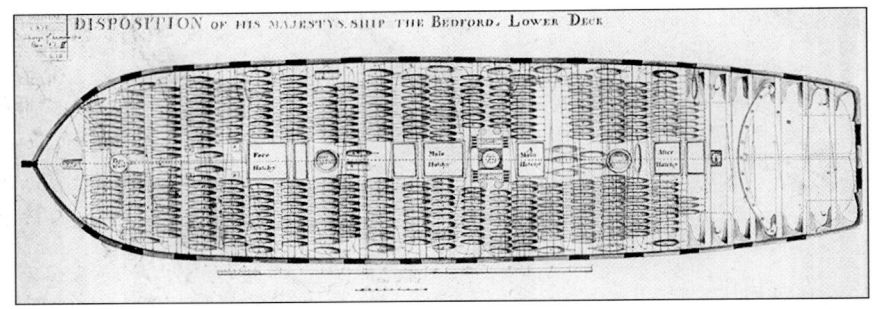

Typical disposition of hammocks, 14 inches apart, on a mid-eighteenth-century 70-gun ship. (*Copyright: National Maritime Museum, London*)

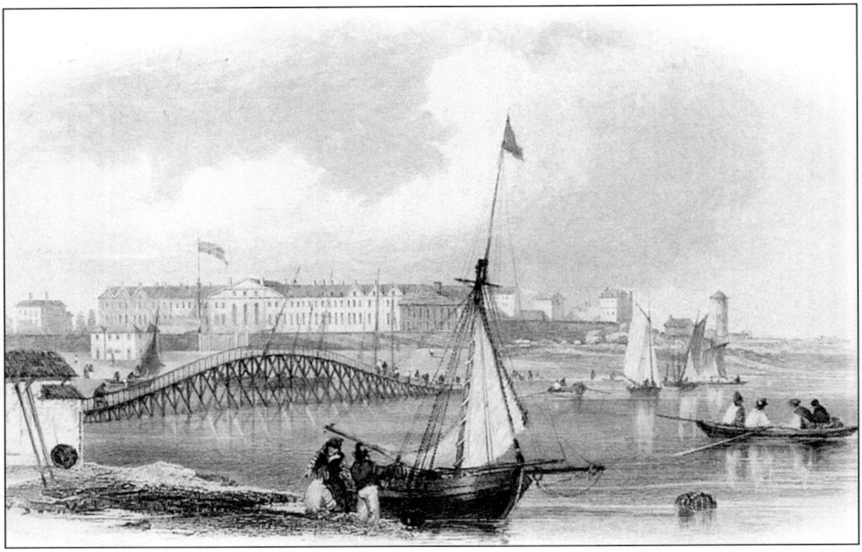

Haslar Hospital, Portsmouth (*c.* 1790), the largest naval hospital in the world, where Lind was Physician-in-Charge.
(*Copyright: National Maritime Museum, London*)

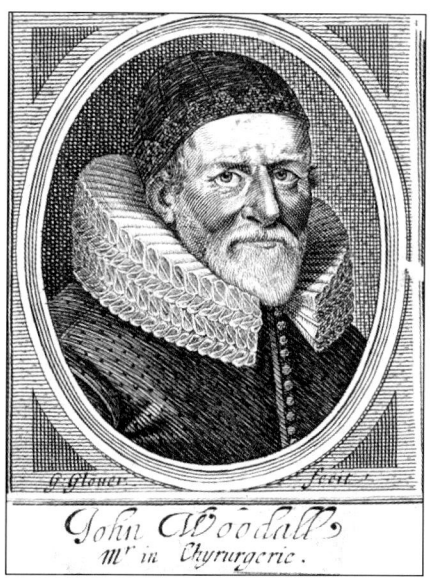

Dr John Woodall (1556?–1643), first Surgeon-General of the British East India Company. (*Wellcome Trust*)

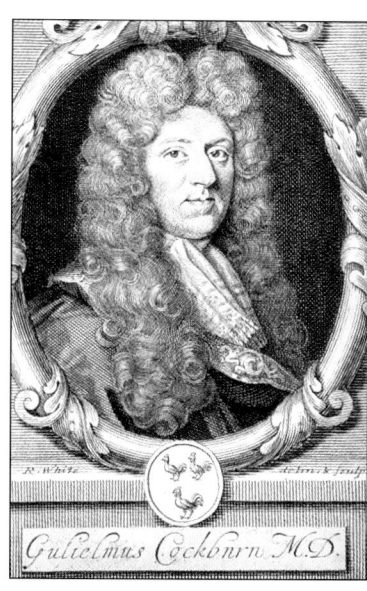

Dr William Cockburn (1669–1739). (*Wellcome Trust*)

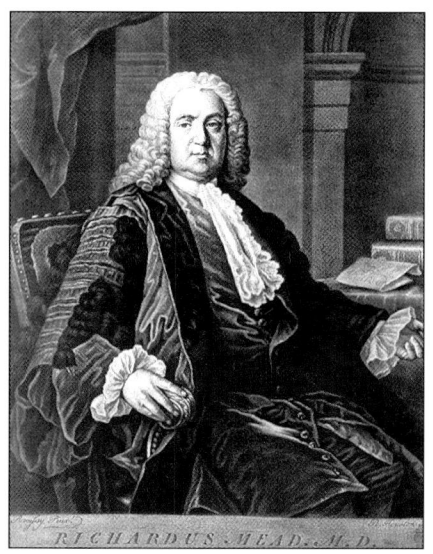

Dr Richard Mead (1673–1754). (*Wellcome Trust*)

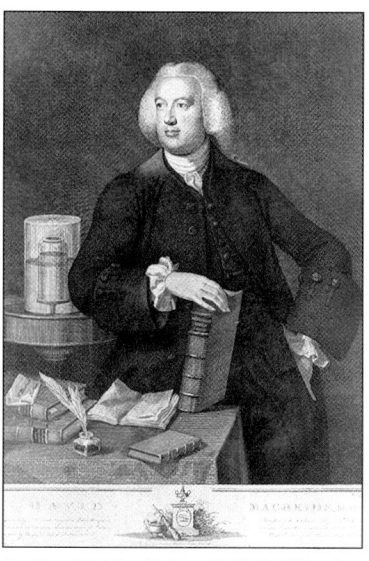

Dr David MacBride (1726–78), the favoured promoter of malt wort as a cure for scurvy. (*Wellcome Trust*)

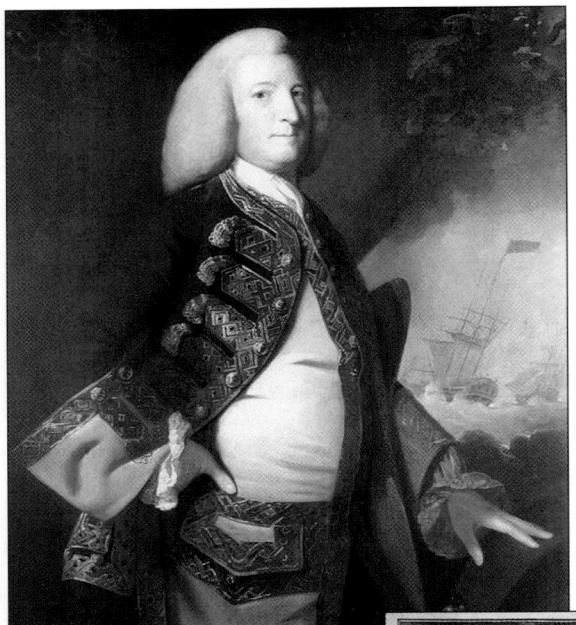

Lord George Anson (1697–1762), in a 1755 engraving after Reynolds. It was Anson's voyage of 1740–44 that prompted Lind's research into scurvy; he later dedicated his *Treatise* to Anson. (*Copyright: National Maritime Museum, London*)

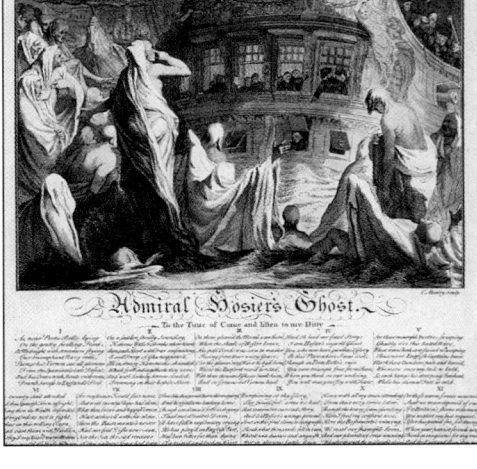

'Hosier's Ghost' depicts dire warnings of scurvy and fever in Hosier's Caribbean fleet in 1726. (*Copyright: National Maritime Museum, London*)

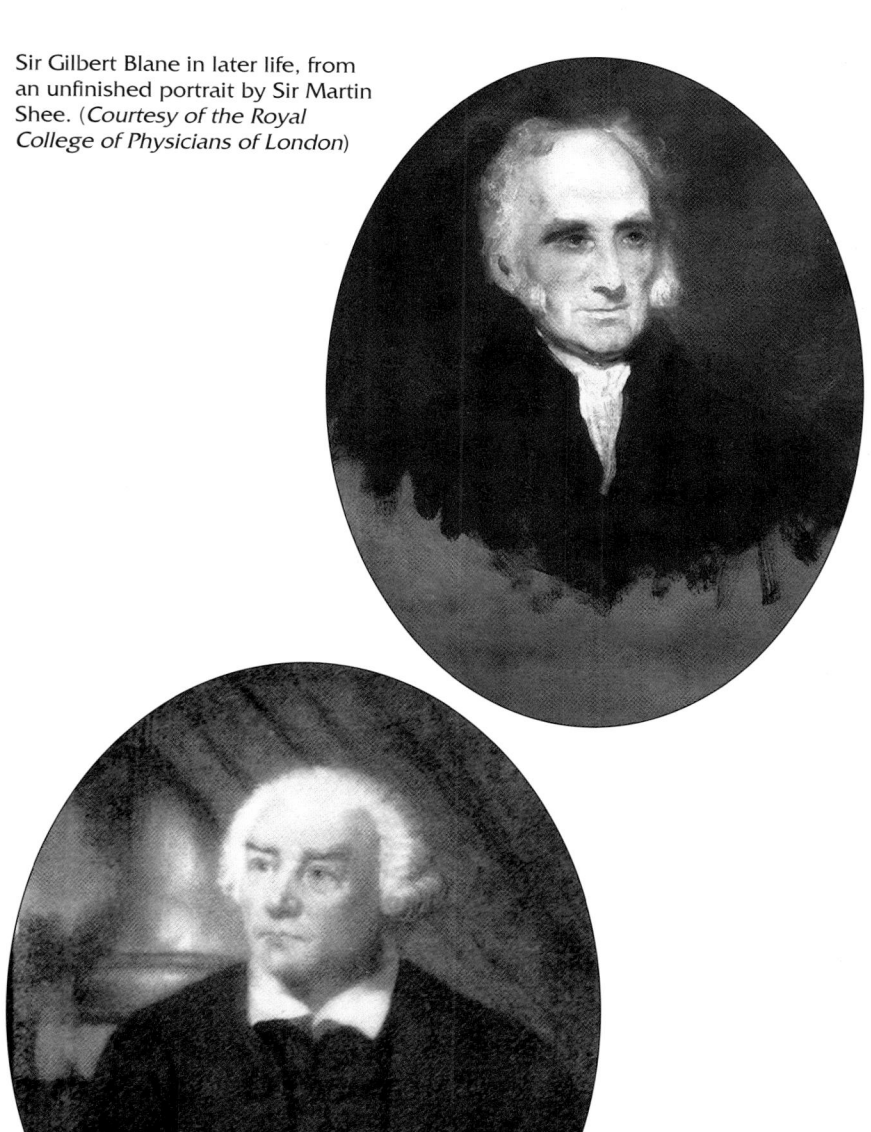

Sir Gilbert Blane in later life, from an unfinished portrait by Sir Martin Shee. (*Courtesy of the Royal College of Physicians of London*)

James Lind in later life, from a miniature portrait, c. 1790, by Alexander Gallaway. (*Courtesy of Bonhams & Brooks, London*)

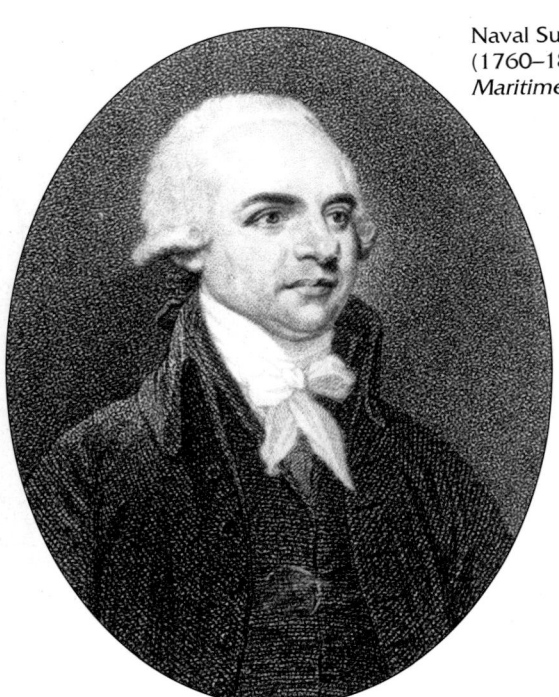

Naval Surgeon Dr Thomas Trotter (1760–1832). (*Copyright: National Maritime Museum, London*)

Lauchlan Rose (1829–85), founder of L. Rose & Company, manufacturers of Rose's Lime Juice Cordial. (*Courtesy of Cadbury Schweppes plc*)

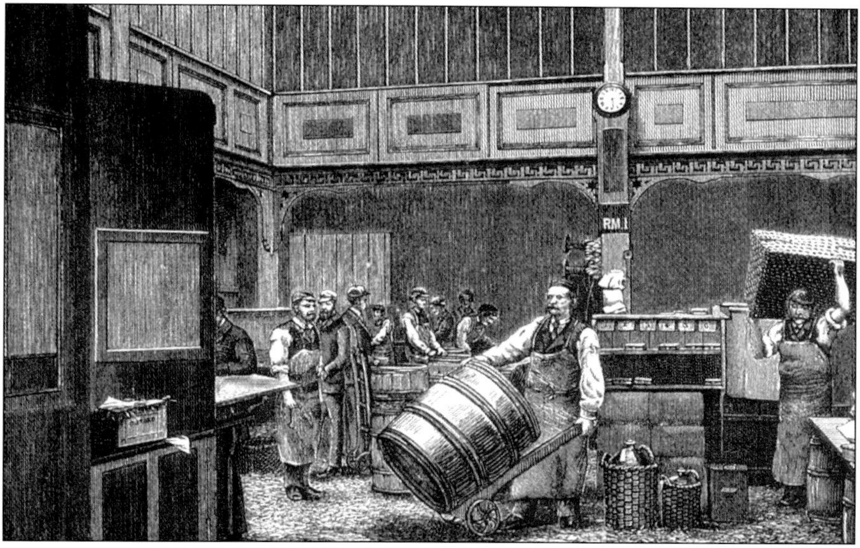

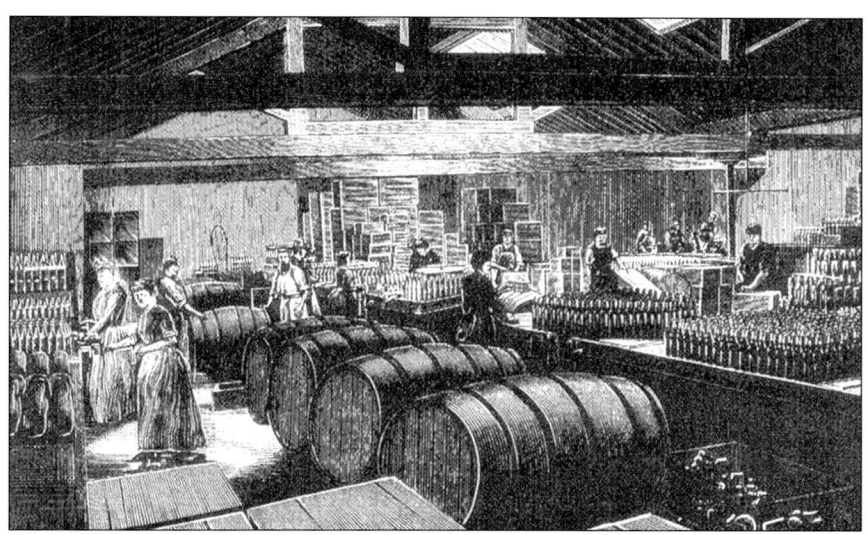

Lime juice packing at Evans & Company, Liverpool, c. 1898. (*Courtesy of the Trustees of the National Library of Scotland*)

Evans & Company's lime juice factory, Liverpool, c. 1898. (*Courtesy of the Trustees of the National Library of Scotland*)

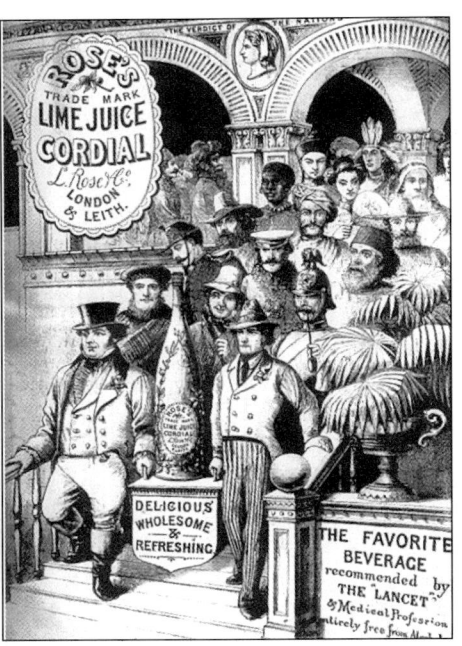

An advertisement for Rose's Lime Juice Cordial claims medical approval. (*Courtesy of Cadbury Schweppes plc*)

Issue of lime juice aboard ship in the Arctic, 1875, from a watercolour by Surgeon E.L. Moss. (*Scott Polar Research Institute, Cambridge*)

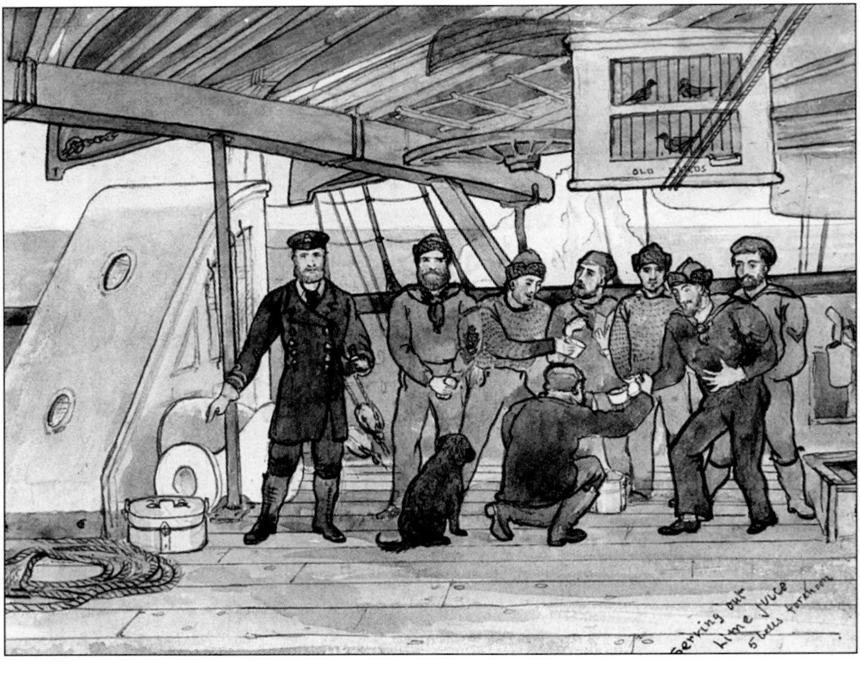

The bread is full of vermin, and other provisions destroyed by the heat of the hold. There are at present here (New York) in vessels provisions which have been on board 18 months without being looked at.[13]

Young sought a replacement of the endless oatmeal with the coffee and chocolate that were available to other fleets:

> I wish a substitute of provisions was made in lieu of the oatmeal; the people and public would reap an amazing advantage by it. I cannot conceive why in the West Indies the men cannot be allowed sugar, coffee and chocolate, in lieu of the oatmeal; they are a better breakfast for the men, and a much greater anti-scorbutic. I have given encouragement to this mode, but I find the purser too rapacious and robs the men, which has obliged me to stop it. If something is not done the men will be destroyed by the scurvy, which is more predominate in this squadron and in this country, West Indies, than ever was known.[14]

In the spring of 1781, when a large part of the fleet was patrolling against the French off Martinique, Blane was surprised by the severity of an attack of scurvy – 'such a degree as had never before been known in the West Indies.' Blane was puzzled as to why the virulence was so great in a hot climate. He concluded that most of the ships had not had a fresh meal for six months, nor had they been able to buy fresh vegetables for four months. One bold technique for dealing with scurvy on Rodney's flagship was nevertheless confidently put into effect by Surgeon Nathaniel Bedford:

> In the case of spongy gums I gargled frequently with diluted lime juice; in ulcers I used lime juice poultices; in constriction I gave one scruple of gum guiacum dissolved in one pint of warm spruce beer at bedtime.[15]

This combative technique was apparently highly successful, and Bedford reported that, 'not a single scorbutic neglected his duty.' It seems clear, however, that Bedford was only able to use lime juice in its curative rather than preventative role.

From Sir Samuel Hood on HMS *Barfleur* in the West Indies went a letter to John Montagu, Earl of Sandwich, and First Lord of the Admiralty in April 1781:

> The *Princessa* is so sickly, and her men dying so fast, I was obliged to order her to Gros Islet on the 21st to put the worst of the scorbutic men on shore.
>
> I thank God the *Barfleur* continues pretty healthy. I have got lemons and limes for my poor fellows from every place I could, which has prevented the scurvy from taking that root I am sorry to say it has in other ships.[16]

There was a new willingness that had not existed before to put matters directly before the Admiralty Board. Admiral Darby, having taken over command from Geary, complained in the summer of 1781 to the First Lord from his station aboard HMS *Britannia* on patrol in the Channel against the French:

> I do think it will not be proper to keep this squadron out long, as the scurvy attacks the people who had but little time in port this last; therefore, if not attended to, may lay several of the ships up for want of men.[17]

It seems that his warning was not heeded, for he sent another letter of complaint only three weeks later:

> I can't help observing to your lordship the Sour Crout is most expended, the beer at an end, and the scurvy making strong strides, many ships have been but short time in port, so that if these ships are kept out long they will be rendered useless for want of men.[18]

'POLICY AS WELL AS HUMANITY CONCUR'

Another letter to First Lord Montagu (the patron of David MacBride) was sent by Surgeon William Northcote on HMS *Prudent* off New York in August 1781. This was an extraordinarily frank letter from surgeon to First Lord, and Northcote began with a paragraph apologising for the liberty he felt he was taking. However, it appears here in full partly for its frankness and partly to show that there really did seem to be a move to insist that the hierarchy took the issue of scurvy with a new seriousness:

> As the Scurvy, my Lord, is the most prevalent and most destructive disease incident to seamen, and lemon and orange juice the grand specific in that most terrible malady, I humbly beg leave to recommend to your Lordship's consideration whether it would not be of infinite more service to the Navy, if the surgeons of His Majesty's ships were to be largely supplied with these most salutary vegetable acids instead of the present mineral acid (elixir of vitriol), which is of little or no use.
>
> Two thirds of our seamen die of the Scurvy and other diseases which take their rise from putrefaction, and for which the Peruvian bark, lemon and orange juice are the great and peculiar antiseptics; therefore, if our seamen could be preserved free from these diseases, they would seldom be endangered by any other.
>
> I beg leave to recall to your Lordship's memory that, by the returns made to the House of Commons in December 1760, out of 185,000 men raised for the sea service during the last war, above 130,000 died by diseases, and two thirds of those of the putrid kind.
>
> If the seizures of tobacco (instead of being burnt) were always sent to the dockyards to supply the ships destined for foreign service, it would be of infinite service to fumigate the ships frequently therewith, whenever there was a contagious disorder on board, and this without any additional expense to the Government.

> The vinegar supplied the Navy at present is good for little or nothing; it should always be the strongest that can be procured.
>
> Good, sound, rough cyder would also be of infinite use to scorbutics; and every ship should be supplied with some for their use only. Essence of malt and sour Khrout are also of great use. These and many other articles (which would be a means of saving the lives and preserving the health of our seamen, if put in execution), I recommended some years ago in an appendix to the 'Marine Practice of Physic and Surgery', to which I beg leave to refer your Lordship; and as the subject of this letter is a great National Concern, I have the vanity to hope that it will not be disregarded.[19]

Soon after Northcote's remarkable letter to the First Lord, Gilbert Blane accompanied the sick Rodney to England for a period of recuperation. Blane took the opportunity of being at home to compose and deliver his lengthy 'memorial' to the Admiralty Board in October 1781. He did not mince his words, but took the opportunity to lecture the board on the whole range of health and disease issues affecting not only the West Indies Fleet, but the entire Royal Navy:

> I beg leave to call to mind again, that 1,518 deaths from disease, besides 350 invalids, in 12,109 men, in the course of one year, is an alarming waste of British seamen, being a number that would man three of His Majesty's ships of the line; and what I advance is from a real conviction that a due attention to the above mentioned propositions would save more than two-thirds of the seamen that would otherwise die in that climate.[20]

His first demand was for better discipline and cleanliness among the men, and for ships to be maintained clean and dry. Second was the insistence on the proper supply of fruit and vegetables for the prevention of scurvy:

Scurvy is one of the principal diseases with which seamen are afflicted, and this may be infallibly prevented, or cured, by vegetables and fruit, particularly oranges, lemons and limes. These might be supplied by employing one or more small vessels to collect them at different islands, and such an expedient would prevent much sickness, and save many lives. I am well convinced that more men would be saved by such a purveyance of fruit and vegetables than could be raised by double the expense and trouble employed on the imprest service; so that policy, as well as humanity, concur in recommending it. Every fifty oranges or lemons might be considered as a hand to the fleet, inasmuch as the health, and perhaps the life, of a man would thereby be saved.[21]

Blane's clearly stated demand for the connection of policy and humanity could hardly have been missed by the board, nor could his equation of fifty oranges with the life of a seaman. He went on to demand the substitution of wine for rum; the provision of special dietary items for the sick; and government funding of certain medicines, especially the very expensive Peruvian Bark (naval surgeons of the period being personally responsible for the purchase and upkeep of medical supplies). He also wanted increased treatment of the sick aboard ship rather than in hospitals; the proper regulation of hospitals; the prevention of filth and overcrowding; and finally, the establishment of hospital ships. He was careful to remind their lordships that while scurvy in particular was not contagious and was fairly easily cured, one of its effects was to render sufferers liable, through weakened immunity, to death from other diseases.

At Blane's suggestion, Rodney had petitioned the Admiralty for supplies of 'Alkaline Salts', Peruvian Bark and the rob of lemons and oranges. However, in December 1781 a lengthy and wholly negative response to these requests went from the Commissioners of the Sick and Hurt Board to the Admiralty. It was pointed out to their lordships that the West Indies Station was well appointed with hospitals for the sick, and that surgeons at sea had all the medicines they could possibly need. The principal concern seems to have been to avoid spending any additional money on medical issues. The line was that if Rodney got what he wanted, everyone else would expect the same benefits:

> Dr James' Powder and Elixir of Vitriol are, at great expense, given by Government for the use of the sick on board; Bark is now proposed to be added and if granted will not be confined to the West Indies Station but immediately become universal, and we submit to their Lordships whether such a material innovation is to be admitted.[22]

The 'Alkaline Salts' referred to Dr Nathaniel Hulme's treatment for scurvy in which an acid/alkali composition produced a 'fixed air' effervescence in the stomach – the fizzy drink. The board noted that Hulme had never used this treatment at sea and said they would require practical proof of its value before using such a hypothetical remedy. This response really does seem to characterise the thinking that had prevailed for so long. If a remedy was an old one, it was nothing new; if it was new, it was unheard of and likely to be expensive:

> A very great variety of different substances, and preparations of substances, have been proposed; every man has his favourite anti-scorbutic which he presses upon the public with great earnestness, and extols with exaggerated praise. In the beginning the cure of this disease was not sought for from food but from medicine, and Elixir of Vitriol was to be the infallible cure. It was introduced into the navy and is now universally known to be of no manner of service in the cure of scurvy. We will venture to foretell the fate of the acid and the alkali will be the same because both are founded on wrong principles.[23]

The Commissioners stated that the citrus rob, 'supposing it to have all the virtues which it is thought to possess', was certainly inferior to the fresh juice, and that numerous captains had delivered negative reports. Mr Patten, surgeon on HMS *Resolution* reported that:

> The Rob of Lemons and Rob of Oranges were frequently given by way of prevention, but they by no means answered my expectation. Many were put on the Wort list after they had taken a spoonful of it every day for several weeks.[24]

Patten admitted that as well as wort, he was using portable soup, sauerkraut, sugar, sago and currants as antiscorbutics. The Commissioners advocated 'several preparations of food' which were being tried on a number of ships and which they declared to be excellent for prevention or cure as well as nourishing:

> We mean the Portable Soup, Malt or extract of Wort, and Sour Krout, and we think that no ship should go to sea without all of them.[25]

Then came the concluding condemnation of the rob of citrus; it was too expensive:

> Should their Lordships be inclined to favour the introduction of Rob of Lemons into the navy, we think it our duty to acquaint them that the process for making so large a quantity will require a very large and expensive apparatus, that it cannot be done but at one season of the year and will require a Clerk and a number of servants to attend solely to that business. The expense of ten chests of lemons made into Rob for the Resolution and Adventure amounted to £31-11-9d. The ten chests produced 83 pint bottles of the Rob, which is about 7/7d farthing the pint. If about 200 men had this quantity it may be judged what an immense expense it would be to supply a large fleet.[26]

In December 1781, with Rodney recovered, he and Blane returned to the West Indies to continue battle with the French.

This they did with some distinction, most notably in the Battle of the Saints in April 1782, when thirty-five ships of each fleet faced each other off Martinique. Excepting the effects of battle, Blane recorded reduced sickness and death at that time; the annual mortality rate was one in twenty, against one in seven when he joined the fleet. He put this down partly to good supplies of provisions, including sauerkraut, molasses and essence of malt. However, he made no mention of citrus fruit, and noted that 'the proportion of scurvy is somewhat increased.'[27] Rodney himself praised Blane's efforts:

> To his knowledge and attention it was owing that the English fleet was, notwithstanding their excessive fatigue and constant service, in a condition always to attack and defeat the public enemy. In my own ship, the *Formidable*, out of 900 men, not one was buried in six months.[28]

Blane later gave an instance of the rapid cure of scurvy using citrus fruits in a fleet of twenty-eight ships-of-the-line off New York in the autumn of 1782:

> In these the scurvy and scorbutic habit prevailed to a great degree; for though orders were given at Jamaica, where they lay for ten weeks previous to sailing for North America, for the purchase of fruit and other vegetables, very little could be procured on account of the extraordinary drought of the season. Fortunately a small prize vessel loaded with limes, lemons and oranges was carried into New York about the time the Fleet arrived, and the whole cargo was, by my advice, purchased for their use. In consequence of this and other refreshments served on board, few cases were sent to the hospital; and the men, as soon as they could walk, were sent on shore for a few hours every day for recreation, by which means their health, strength and spirits were restored in a few weeks.[29]

Blane feared that the saving of money was held more worthy than the saving of lives, and was forthright in promoting the fact that not only was citrus fruit completely successful, but it was cheap:

> The expense of replacing those who die, and of supporting hospitals, may with truth be stated at much more than a hundred times what the supply of fruit and other refreshments would cost.[30]

When the war ended, Blane returned to England with Admiral Francis Drake in *Princessa* in the spring of 1783 and almost immediately left the Royal Navy for a post as physician at St Thomas's Hospital in London. This was a hard-fought-for position, which Blane won by ninety-eight votes to eighty-four with the strong influence of Lord Rodney in his favour. Blane also began to build a substantial private practice among the upper classes. He had become a friend of the Duke of Clarence while in the Navy, and on his recommendation, Blane was appointed Physician Extraordinary to the Prince of Wales in 1785. He was to acquire further royal and international appointments in later years, all of which ensured a large and lucrative medical practice.

Blane did not simply retreat into the sinecure of just being a physician to the wealthy. Although no longer directly connected with the Navy, his expertise in naval medicine and public health was in demand by various branches of government, and in coming years he was to acquire prominence as the most distinguished and influential naval physician of all. He certainly gained the reputation of being a snob who revelled in his relationships with admirals, aristocrats and royalty. Several public archives have collections of correspondence between him and a wide variety of royal houses and statesmen, but the content is historically trivial. The index at the Public Record Office in London notes that such correspondence was of interest mainly 'for autograph value'. After the defeat of the

French at Martinique in 1782, he himself quite unnecessarily described, in a medical report of all places, his reaction with Rodney's titled flag captain:

> When Sir Charles Douglas and I . . . saw the French flag hauled down . . . stupefied as it were by an ecstasy of joy, [we] rushed into each others' arms and embraced.[31]

On the other hand, Blane treated his inferiors in a rather cold, reserved style that earned him the nickname 'Chilblain'.[32]

In 1785, he published the first of many important works on naval hygiene, *Observations on the Diseases of Seamen*. In this, he stated that the Admiralty had given proper consideration to his detailed memorial of four years earlier, and that most of his recommendations had been carried into effect. Sadly, the universal adoption of citrus fruit was not yet one of them. Blane himself had much to say in praise of the use of molasses against scurvy.

> The first trial of molasses was in the *Foudroyant*, and it answered so well that, in a cruise under Admiral Geary in 1780, this was the only ship free from scurvy, and out of 2,400 men that were landed at the hospital with this disease, there were none from this ship.[33]

However in his *Observations*, Blane followed Lind's conclusions closely, and in his section on victualling at sea he noted:

> . . . it was recommended to set apart a quantity of the best wines, and to be provided with brown sugar, dried fruits, barley, rice, sago and salep.[34] To these might be added eggs which, if greased and put in salt, may be preserved fresh for a great length of time. Carrots and other roots might also be preserved for the longest voyages by means of sugar; and green vegetables might in like manner be preserved by means of salt. But of all the articles, either of medicine or diet, for the cure of the scurvy, lemons and oranges are of much the greatest

efficacy. They are real specifics in that disease, if anything deserves that name. This was first ascertained and set in a clear light by Dr Lind. Upon what principle their superior efficacy depends, and in what manner they produce their effect, I am at a loss to determine.[35]

Blane was being too optimistic in thinking that the Admiralty had accepted his views on citrus fruit. They had been contacted by an East India Company surgeon who had tried to impress them with his hardly novel claim of preserving lemon and lime juice in brandy. The Sick and Hurt Board replied to this proposal in March 1786, referring to their earlier response to Blane's memorial:

> We have received your letter of 24th inst. enclosing one from Mr Stephen Matthews a surgeon in the East India Company service with an account of a remedy he has discovered for the Sea Scurvy, and signifying the directions of the Rt Hon. the Lords Commissioners of the Admiralty for us to take the same into our consideration and report to them our opinion thereon.
>
> We desire you will please acquaint their Lordships, the remedy proposed by Mr Matthews is not new, trials have been made of the efficacy of the acid of lemons in the prevention and cure of the scurvy on board several different ships which made voyages round the globe at different times, the surgeons of which all agree in saying the Rob of lemons and oranges were of no service, either in the prevention or cure of that disease, which we mentioned in our letter of the 18th December 1781. The methods already pursued with the preparation of substances such as the Portable Broth, Wort, Sour Krout are much more efficacious both in the cure and prevention of the scurvy.[36]

Not only was there a poor opinion of the rob, but there was a clear reluctance to give any further credence to the efficacy of fresh juice. Maybe the best route towards achieving success in the battle against scurvy would be to encourage informed discussion within the fleets, and hope that pressure for change could be generated upwards. One captain who had great concern for the health of his seamen, and who made informed remarks on scurvy among other subjects, was the infamous Captain William Bligh – a man who has had a worse press than he deserved. Bligh was a master navigator who was hand-picked by Cook, Nelson and Joseph Banks; he became governor of New South Wales, and was eventually promoted to admiral. On the ill-fated voyage of the *Bounty* in 1787, Bligh followed Lind's suggestion and hired a fiddler for the voyage in order to keep up the spirits of the crew. Bligh had strong views on scurvy, and carried copies of Lind's work in his cabin; although there is no evidence that he used oranges or lemons, he stated:

> . . . the scurvy is really a disgrace to a ship where it is at all common, provided they have it in their power to be supplied with Dryed Malt, Sour Krout and Portable Soup. With these articles properly issued, I am convinced no Scurvy will appear. Cheerfulness with exercise, and a sufficiency of rest are powerful preventatives to this dreadfull disease, a calamity which even at this present period destroys more men than is generally known.[37]

In 1790 the naval surgeon, Frederick Thomson published his *Essay on The Scurvy*. This was an interesting intervention because Thomson was neither a public figure nor especially senior within the Navy. While he recognised that he probably had little to say that was new, he was obviously determined to keep the subject of scurvy in public and professional view. In his opening remarks to the seven Lords Commissioners, he says pointedly:

> It happened to fall to my lot, during a long service in the Royal Navy, to see more distress and mortality arising from the Scurvy than from all other diseases and causes united.[38]

Thomson accurately blamed the delays in implementing the conclusions of Lind's *Treatise* on the problems of producing an effective rob of lemon juice. He thought that Lind had 'entirely exhausted the subject' and was obviously reluctant to put himself in the same league as Lind and Blane. Thomson was very keen on the use of hops, particularly in treacle beer or hop beer, and published a range of recipes for the use of hops in infusions, ointments and syrups. He also recommended malt liquors, porter, spruce beer, cider and wine. Fresh succulent vegetables, especially garlic, onions, celery and horseradish were all important; but the best antiscorbutics were fresh acid fruits, especially lemons, limes, oranges and their juices. He advocated an antiscorbutic drink made from cream of tartar, bruised juniper berries, ginger powder, powdered cloves, treacle and water. Thomson was scathing of those who claimed that salt caused scurvy. He cited the case of Shetland Islanders who in the winter of 1765–6 had been deprived by incessant storms of their normal supplies from Leith. There were few potatoes, and the islanders subsisted for six months largely on a diet of seaweed and a particularly salty fish called piltocks. He pointed out that during this emergency diet, which was both very deficient and simultaneously overloaded with salt, not a single case of scurvy had occurred.

Gilbert Blane followed Lind's enthusiasm for beer and other fermented drinks. The Navy allowed about a gallon of small beer per man per day, and Blane felt that, good as it was, it could only last in wholesome condition for a short time. He thought that 'one of the greatest improvements that could be made in the victualling of the Navy would be the introduction of porter.' While porter was often refused on grounds of cost, it could be kept in good condition in any climate for as long as required. He recalled that:

> I was furnished by Dr Clephane, physician to the Fleet at New York, with the following fact. In the beginning of the war two storeships called *Tortoise* and *Grampus* sailed for America under convoy of *Daedalus*, frigate. *Grampus* happened to be supplied

with sufficient quantities of porter to serve the whole passage, which proved very long. The other two ships were furnished with the common allowance of spirits.

The weather being unfavourable the passage drew out to fourteen weeks, and upon their arrival at New York the *Daedalus* sent to hospital a hundred and twelve men, the *Tortoise* sixty-two, the greater part of whom were in the last stage of scurvy. The *Grampus* sent only thirteen, none of whom had the scurvy.[39]

Blane continued to promote Lind's proposals within the Navy, and his influential contacts proved valuable. In 1793, he recommended to his friend Sir Alan Gardner (a member of the Admiralty Board just confirmed in command of the East Indies Station) that a large supply of lemon juice should be obtained. In December it was agreed by the Commissioners that:

> . . . putting a few chests of lemons, or a quantity of lemon or lime juice prepared for keeping on board the ships of the squadron as an antiscorbutic for the use of the ships' company in general would be a most salutary measure.[40]

The board wanted the citrus used in punch or negus (diluted, spiced sherry) in place of grog or wine, and the materials to be in the charge of the purser and administered under the supervision of the officer-of-the-watch:

> The daily allowance of each man for punch ought to be, together with his half-pint of spirit, three-quarters of an ounce of lemon or lime juice, two ounces of sugar (which also possesses antiscorbutic virtues) and one pint or one pint and a half of water at the discretion of the captain; and for negus when wine is served there ought to be added to the daily allowance of one pint of wine the above-mentioned quantity of lime or lemon juice and sugar, and one pint or one half pint of water. If due attention is paid to the preservation of the lemon

or lime juice by having it prepared and packed under our immediate direction, we judge that this improvement in maritime diet will powerfully check the appearance of scurvy and greatly contribute to the health and vigour of the crews.[41]

This was the first, cautious official sanction of citrus fruit against scurvy. Forty years had elapsed since James Lind had first made his detailed recommendations.

On 2 April 1794, the 74-gun HMS *Suffolk* sailed for India, under the command of Admiral Rainer, who had replaced Gardner at the last minute. Each man on board ship was given a daily dose of two-thirds of an ounce of fresh lemon juice taken with grog (a mixture of rum and water) and sugar. This continued throughout the voyage of twenty-three weeks and one day, during which time they were out of sight of land. When the ship arrived in Madras Road on 11 September, no man had died; there were fifteen men on the sick list, none in serious condition, and none with scurvy. Blane noted:

> [Scurvy] appeared in a few men in the course of the voyage, but soon disappeared on an increased dose of lemon juice being administered. Let this fact be contrasted with the state of the Channel Fleet in 1780 as described by Dr [John] Lind.[42]

The pressure in favour of citrus juice was beginning to tell in a number of places. Surgeon Leonard Gillespie, in charge of the hospital on Martinique, experienced the value of lemons and limes between 1794 and 1796:

> The benefits resulting from the supply of such articles to the navy during the course of the present war, and the number of lives which have thereby been preserved, are incalculable.[43]

One of the principal characters in the successful adoption of lemon juice – and another Lind disciple – was Dr Thomas Trotter, Physician to the Channel Fleet under Lord Howe. Trotter was born in Melrose in 1760, studied in Edinburgh, joined the Navy as a surgeon's mate, and was for a time one of Lind's juniors at Haslar. He had been appointed to the Channel Fleet in 1794, and immediately promoted Lind's antiscorbutic methods and his proposals for the supply of clean uniforms. He also sought his own improvements to pay, hygiene and food for ordinary seamen, and tried unsuccessfully to persuade the Admiralty to adopt vaccination procedures against disease. Trotter had published his own *Observations on Scurvy* in 1786, with a second edition in 1792. He expressed fierce support for James Lind's views, and condemned the Navy's favourite remedies for scurvy, Elixir of Vitriol, malt wort and even sauerkraut:

> . . . fresh, essential vegetables of all kinds will cure it, but those fruits abounding with an acid, such as the citric class, are more effectual than others.[44]

George, Earl Spencer, who had become Pitt's First Lord of the Admiralty in 1794, appointed Gilbert Blane one of the three Commissioners of the Board of the Sick and Hurt the following year. This appointment, at a salary of £300 per year, was to last for seven years, and it enabled Blane and Trotter to make rapid significant advances. Largely on the evidence of the voyage of the *Suffolk* to Madras, Blane persuaded the Admiralty, through the Sick and Hurt Board, to agree to the extended issue of lemon juice and fruit. This did not amount to a general order. The fruit was to be issued to commanders on demand, but Blane and Trotter would ensure that the demand was generated. In March 1795, Trotter persuaded Sir George Elphinstone to take supplies of lemons and juice on his squadron leaving to attack the Cape of Good Hope. The fruit was late in reaching the dockyard, and the squadron had to leave without it, with calamitous results.[45] During the year, other commanders throughout the Navy began to demand citrus fruit and juice. Trotter, keeping careful note of events, was aware of both an increase in the incidence of scurvy, and a shortage of lemons and limes as a result of the new encouragement of their use. In one incident where the supplies of fruit had not been delivered, Trotter himself went out into the local Portsmouth markets and bought fifteen cases of lemons:

> The reader may smile at the idea of a Physician of the Fleet attending the stalls at a vegetable market, or perambulating the country to calculate the produce; but it never appeared to me below the dignity of the profession.[46]

Trotter's enthusiasm for trawling the back street fruit stalls for the benefit of the nation's sailors did not obtain universal acclaim. One wealthy lady complained that she could no longer obtain oranges and lemons for her dinner parties:

> It's a shame that the nation's money should be expended this way. Captain P — tells me that these things are not good for sailors, but this physician can persuade Lord Howe to anything.[47]

However, the bandwagon was beginning to roll. In June 1795, Captain Cuthbert Collingwood of HMS *Excellent* (later Vice-Admiral Lord Collingwood) was only one of several commanders who wrote from Spithead demanding lemon juice:

> His Majesty's ship *Excellent* being ordered for foreign service, and her ship's company having been lately much afflicted with scurvy, from which they were relieved very much by the use of lemons. I have to request you will be pleased to direct that she will be supplied with lemon juice for the voyage and such other antiscorbutics as you may judge proper to cure or prevent the virulence of that disease; with which there are now a considerable number of men much afflicted.[48]

However, parsimony was still the natural state at the Navy Office. A few days after the request from Collingwood, in a letter from the Sick and Hurt Board to the Admiralty, concern was expressed at a similar demand to supply lemon juice to the North Sea Fleet under Admiral Duncan. The commissioners said that supplying juice to the home fleet on the same scale as was supplied to ships preparing for foreign voyages could not be managed. In any case:

> . . . our intention in recommending lemon juice as an antiscorbutic article of diet was that it should be given to the seamen after the small beer is expended, which we apprehend will seldom be the case in the North Sea.[49]

They did agree that a small quantity should be supplied to Duncan's fleet for use strictly as a medicine under the supervision of the surgeon. But the demands were becoming unstoppable. At the end of August a letter went from the Sick and Hurt Board to the Admiralty secretary indicating that the question of supply was actively under review:

> I beg leave to acquaint you, I have seen the persons who supply the Board with lemon juice, and that they have engaged to have five hundred gallons of that article ready this week; it shall be forwarded to Portsmouth with all possible expedition.[50]

In the summer of 1795, Lord Spencer, the First Lord, drafted official Admiralty instructions for an additional squadron being made ready to support the military campaign in the West Indies:

> As the force intended for the Leeward Islands may be looked upon as the main body of the whole British army, and its safe and speedy arrival as the grand remaining object of the present war, it seems necessary that it should be accompanied, during the whole of the passage thither, by a naval force so respectable as to preclude the possibility of any successful obstruction from any force the enemy may be able to send out.[51]

'POLICY AS WELL AS HUMANITY CONCUR'

Having been lobbied by Trotter, Spencer decided that the 'respectability' of the fleet was to include new instructions on the health of the crews, and he wrote down the new Admiralty view on the use of citrus fruit, which would also apply to the Channel Fleet then blockading Brest:

> From the report come today from Lord Bridport of the sickly state of his fleet, particularly in point of scurvy, a considerable supply of lemon juice and antiscorbutics of all sorts should be immediately sent out in some sloop or frigate to the squadron under Admiral Corwallis.
>
> Directions should also be sent to the Ports of Plymouth and to the eastward in conformity to the observations contained in Dr Trotter's letters. Supplies should continue to be constantly sent to Sir John Warren of fresh meat, vegetables and antiscorbutics, and a large quantity of seeds of quick growing vegetables should be also sent which, by being sown in the islands of Hédic and Houat, will soon give a fresh supply of the most antiscorbutic kinds of vegetables.[52]

It appeared that perhaps the battle against scurvy was about to be taken up by the Admiralty at last, even if only on the basis of instructions to individual fleets, rather than an official order applying throughout the Navy. However, this change of heart, encouraged by Gilbert Blane and brought about by Spencer, was tainted by an awful irony; it came almost exactly a year after the death of James Lind. The man who had good reason, forty years earlier, to expect the support and gratitude of the Admiralty had died at Gosport, not far from Haslar Hospital, on 13 July 1794 at the age of seventy-seven. He was buried at St Mary's Parish Church in Portchester. (His remains were later disinterred and reburied at an unconfirmed location in Ryde, Isle of Wight about 1819, when his son Dr John Lind retired from Haslar and built 'Westmont', now Ryde School. There is a tablet commemorating the 250th anniversary of James Lind's birth in St Luke's Church, Haslar Hospital, Portsmouth).

LIMEYS

Gilbert Blane later wrote unequivocally of the benefit to national prosperity brought about by this belated change of heart on the part of the Admiralty:

> Are we to thank for it a guardian angel, presiding and watching over the dearest and most valuable interests of our country? Or is it more rationally imputable to some of those profound and exquisite discoveries in science, mathematical, chemical, mechanical or pharmaceutical, with which the present age abounds above all others? No such thing. The scurvy has been prevented, subdued and totally rooted out, by the general use of lemon juice, supplied for the first time at the public expense in the year 1795, and which operated so speedily that in less than two years afterwards it became extinct, and has remained so.[53]

Despite the changing Admiralty attitude, new confusions threatened progress. Another naval surgeon, David Paterson, produced a flurry of mischief. His *A Treatise on the Scurvy* of 1795 (dedicated to Gilbert Blane) recommended a solution of vinegar and 'nitre', potassium nitrate, later commonly known as saltpetre. This evil brew he recommended in doses of up to a quart per night. His discovery he conceived to be 'of national importance', since he claimed it was a much more convenient means of curing scurvy than bothering with fresh fruits and vegetables which, as everyone knew, were difficult to obtain and impossible to preserve. He claimed, with the support of three other naval surgeons whose testimonials were appended, to have cured 180 cases of scurvy, 'without feeling any inconveniency for the want of lemons, limes or any kind of recent vegetable matter.'[54] He insisted that scurvy was caused by contaminated air, and calculated that in order to provide fresh air between decks in a 74-gun ship with a crew of 600, 556,800 gallons of air would have to be refreshed per night. Although Paterson's booklet was widely distributed among naval surgeons, little attention was given to it in the face of the new commitment to citrus fruit that was being shown by Spencer and others in the Admiralty. However, improvements were not to happen overnight.

Others moved into the more public side of the scurvy debate with dubious intent. In 1798, a London wine merchant by the name of David McBride (no relation to the earlier surgeon of the same name) vigorously promoted his Toc-Kay de Espagna wine as a preventative of scurvy (other wines were available for a variety of ailments):

> FOR THE SCURVY: two glasses four times a day, and bathing the ulcers with the wine, or keeping a linen rag to the ulcers wetted with it, will destroy the itchy or vicious humours, and soon bring on a smooth skin instead of the scaly, and it is the most effectual remedy yet discovered for that disorder either at sea or on shore.[55]

McBride waxed lyrical over his product, but hurriedly added the usual plea:

> When we say this, it is not with a view to promote the sale of this wine, but from compassion to thousands of our fellow-creatures, and a full persuasion of its utility; for we know that the proprietor of it does not wish any one to have a bottle of it, but such as may receive all the wished-for relief from its use.[56]

McBride was perhaps not wholly an opportunist, for he had taken the trouble to secure testimonials from Sir John Pringle, Professor Joseph Black and James Rodney, captain in the Navy and brother of Admiral Lord Rodney. He also obtained glowing correspondence between the surgeon of HMS *Sovereign* and Dr Johnston, one of the Commissioners of the Sick and Hurt, who declared, 'in the most unequivocal manner, that it is the best cordial and restorative that ever came within my knowledge.' McBride quoted Pringle as saying that, 'When the fever is protracted, with a low and slow voice, the sick have a particular craving for something cordial'. He confirmed his approval of the great Army surgeon's view by adding his commercial slogan, 'and nothing is so acceptable and cordial as wine.'

The use of lemons was still not the subject of a universal order, and some fleets were effectively out of regular contact with the Admiralty, and were therefore unable to react to or adopt the new methods. The commander-in-chief of the Mediterranean Fleet, Admiral Jervis, Earl St Vincent, protested his ability to stay at sea in San Firenzo Bay, Corsica, in March 1796 in a letter to First Lord Spencer:

> . . . nor can I keep the sea for any length of time, without the most imminent hazard of totally destroying the health of the people, among whom the scurvy breaks out after a cruise of six weeks in the most horrid shapes.[57]

In May that year, the Sick and Hurt Commissioners wrote to the Admiralty saying that they were now in a position to begin supplying the Victualling Board with lemon juice in bottles 'of uncommon strength' and packed in boxes. Eighty-eight boxes would supply 600 men for 6 months and require stowage space of 8 cubic feet. The board was 'under no apprehensions of its virtues though it should be kept for a very great length of time.'[58] They reported that 14,000 gallons of juice were in store, considered sufficient for 10,666 men for 6 months, and requested to be informed which ships were to be supplied so that proper communication could be made with their surgeons. However, war with Spain broke out, and supplies were immediately restricted. Clearly, there would be a major logistical problem in quantifying and obtaining supplies. However, in late 1796, Thomas Trotter noted that the condition of the Channel Fleet had improved significantly after the issue of the new instructions from Spencer:

> . . . the late occurrances [sic] in the Channel Fleet have sufficiently established the fact that scurvy can always be prevented by fresh vegetables and cured effectually by the

lemon or the preserved juice of the fruit. Whatever may be the theory of the sea scurvy, we contend that recent vegetable matter imparts a something to the body which fortifies it against the disease.[59]

It is interesting to note that, in his concluding uncertainty as to why lemon juice worked, Trotter was echoing Blane's remark of ten years earlier that he was at a loss to determine the principle that governed the efficacious action.

In September 1796, there was a tart correspondence from Blane and Dr Blair, his fellow commissioner, regarding supplies of sulphuric acid, portable soup, and essences of malt and spruce demanded by Dr Harness for Sir John Jervis, commander of the Mediterranean Fleet. They noted that 2,000 pounds of portable soup had been sent to Portsmouth for despatch, but rather acidly added:

> We beg to observe that essences of malt and spruce are not supplied by this office, but by the Victualling Board, and to refer to our letter of 11th of March last in which we gave it as our opinion that the supplying of essence of malt to His Majesty's ships should be discontinued.[60]

In Admiralty files there is an interesting indication of Blane's relationships with his colleagues on the Sick and Hurt Board which belies the version which Blane himself later gave. In his book on the improvements in naval health published in 1830, he made glowing reference to the contribution of the chairman, Dr Blair, in the introduction of lemon juice.[61] However, on 19 October 1796, Blane sent a vitriolic five-page letter to the Admiralty complaining bitterly about Blair's general attitude, procrastination, neglect of public duty and 'undue assumption of power.'[62] He also alleged that Blair was personally insulting to him. Four months later, Blair counter-claimed to the Admiralty that he did not know what Blane's complaint was about, and that whenever he tried to discuss the issue, Blane refused to answer. The battle obviously went on for a very long time, and while Blane's later opinion of Blair's contribution may be fair, it is clear that their working relationship was disastrous.

Demands for citrus juice were now coming from home and foreign fleets. In September 1796, Sir Richard Bickerton wrote from HMS *Ramilles* anchored in Yarmouth Roads:

> The scurvy having made its appearance in His Majesty's ship under my command in her last cruise, I am to request you will be pleased to order a liberal supply of lime juice to be immediately forwarded to her by the use of which having experienced its good effects I hope to check its progress; and if a moderate allowance could be made to the surgeon for the purchase of vegetables, I have his authority to say there is every reasonable hope that those now afflicted would be cured without putting Government to the expense of sending one to sick quarters.[63]

It is interesting that Bickerton referred to 'lime juice' whereas the Sick and Hurt Commissioners, in enclosing his letter to the Admiralty, referred to 'lemon juice'. This was a confusion that was to become significant, and will be addressed in the next chapter.

In December, off the coast of Ecuador, Sir Hyde Parker wrote to Lord Spencer:

> I shall cruise to windward as long as the state of the ships' companies will admit, but it is with infinite concern I feel myself under the necessity of stating to your Lordship that from the enfeebled state of the ships' crews in consequence of the fevers which we have all been subjected to, there is at present a great tendency to scurvy. The confined state of St Nicholas Mole does not admit of the seamen getting fresh beef nor limes or oranges, which almost every other part of the West Indies furnishes in abundance.[64]

Parker began to sound desperate seven months later, appearing to question the moves towards the use of fruit. He also expressed a view that Lind, Blane and Trotter would all have endorsed, that a more holistic change was necessary:

> The scurvy is again broke out with great violence, not only among the squadron but the troops in the garrison begin to be seriously affected with that disease, a proof of our distress for fresh provisions. The means recommended by the Sick and Hurt Board are bound to have no effect whatever, and I much dread the consequences unless we can procure fresh provisions sufficient to change the whole of the men's habits, as we have not been wanting of spruce, limes and other vegetables.[65]

Perhaps the most unusual document of many on scurvy appeared in 1797. *Remarks on the Scurvy* was written by the surgeon Robert Crosfield while he was incarcerated in the Tower of London on a charge of murder. It seems he had been arrested when the alleged victim was not in fact dead. Crosfield had run off to France, been captured, and held in the Castle of Brest. Later, he was held in a series of prison ships, and his descriptions of the conditions – including the incidence of scurvy – are harrowing:

> About the middle of April the scurvy made its appearance, and soon spread to an alarming degree, without any possibility of stopping its progress. The ships were, indeed, smoked with gunpowder and vinegar, cleanliness was endeavoured to be enforced, and vinegar was served out to such as chose to apply for it; but all in vain.[66]

Crosfield was in favour of the methods 'of the illustrious Captain Cook, whose plans are pretty now exactly followed in the British navy', but developed his own procedure for treating scurvy by the use of opium. He was clearly more certain than many other surgeons that scurvy was essentially a feature of diet, but was not convinced of the efficacy of vegetables, which he felt only enabled the digestion of salt:

> Were it otherwise, we should find that a little vinegar or lemon juice would cure the disease at sea; but the miracles said to be wrought by vegetables have in general been performed on shore, where fresh meat is likewise to be had, with the additional luxury of a pure and dry air.[67]

Despite Crosfield's enthusiasm, the methods of Captain Cook were slowly being overtaken as more and more fleet commanders adopted Spencer's instructions, and opium never made it into the surgeon's chest – at least as a remedy for scurvy. The full effects of the change in policy were to take two or three years to become apparent to the sceptics, but it is said that when First Lord Spencer visited Haslar Hospital in 1797 asking to see the scurvy cases, not one could be found.[68]

When Gilbert Blane published the second edition of his *Observations on the Diseases of Seamen* in 1799, he could add little to what Lind had said other than to reconsider the methods of preservation of lemon juice, which he insisted worked like 'what is vulgarly called a charm'. In early July, the Sick and Hurt Board received a letter from Rear Admiral Berkeley aboard HMS *Mars* in the Channel complaining that his crew were suffering badly from scurvy due to lack of sauerkraut and lemon juice. In their submission to the Admiralty, the board reiterated that despite their recommendation that all ships at sea should have lemon juice and sugar when small beer was finished, financial restraints had limited this to ships being prepared for foreign service and to the treatment of those already sick. They now insisted on changes:

> ... the stock of lemon juice now on hand is such as to afford a supply to the ships serving on the Coast of Great Britain and Ireland, over and above what is furnished for the use of the sick, and we are humbly of opinion that it would be for the

advantage of His Majesty's Service if their Lordships would please to give directions to the Commissioners of the Victualling to supply all ships on the said service with half the proportion supplied for foreign service and that the surgeons be directed to comply with the above cited article of their Instructions by selecting such men as may require lemon juice or sugar from the purser's stores in the proportion of one ounce of the former and two ounces of the latter to each man daily, after the expenditure of the small beer. We are farther of opinion that such a supply, together with the small supply of sour krout, which we beg also to recommend, will save great part of the expense now incurred in the several parts of England for vegetables furnished to scorbutic men.[69]

This was the final step in the long trail that led from the publication of James Lind's *Treatise* to the general supply of citrus juice to the entire Royal Navy. Blane and Trotter were being given the opportunity to ensure that production of lemons and lemon juice was increased and was not to be dependent on special pleading, but available to the entire naval fleet. Blane was in no doubt about the spectacular change in efficiency and economic benefit brought about by the new regulations:

It does not require any deep thought to perceive that at a time when a fleet, as we have seen, could not keep sea for more than ten weeks without being rendered unserviceable by scurvy, and that national protection required that when the channel fleet has been constrained to return into port in so short a time, another naval force, as nearly equal as possible, ought to be ready to replace it, for repelling invasion, or baffling the expeditions of the enemy. I was in the habit of saying that at present there was as much service in two ships as formerly in three; but one of the most distinguished sea officers that ever lived, declared to me, that it was his conviction that two ships now are equal to four of former times.[70]

The case can be made that, in strictly military terms, had it not been for Lind's rational dedication and Blane's popularity with the powers that be, the French Fleet may well have brought Britain to its knees. Blane went on to suggest that without the conquest of scurvy some of the other momentous changes that had been brought about in maritime affairs would have been thwarted:

> ... it is manifest, that without the supply of lemon juice, and the other means of maintaining health for a sufficient length of time, the advantages of copper sheathing, the facilities in finding longitude by chronometers, telescopes and astronomical tables, which do so much honour the human intellect, particularly to the age and country in which we live, would be in a great measure frustrated.[71]

Blane wrote in 1799 that, 'The great utility of the vegetable juices cannot be sufficiently impressed on the minds of those who direct the Navy.'[72] Impressing the minds of the Admiralty Board had been no easy prospect. It had been almost half a century since Lind had proposed the use of citrus juice; it was to be another half century before the Merchant Navy would be included in the new liberality. Other countries would be even more reluctant to act; the US Navy did not adopt citrus juice until a century after Britain. On the way to the successful eradication of scurvy, there were to be further disastrous mistakes and expensive cutting of corners that would cost yet more lives. The Admiralty Lords, relying too heavily on the advice of medical advisors who were far from disinterested, showed considerable weakness in failing to control the problem of scurvy. The great English philosopher and evolutionary theorist Herbert Spencer used Lind's treatment by the Admiralty as an example of the most outrageous, pig-headed bureaucratic indolence:

> ... two centuries after the remedy was known, and forty years after a chief medical officer of the Government had given

conclusive evidence of its worth, the Admiralty, forced thereto by an exacerbation of the evil, first moved in the matter. And what had been the effect of this amazing perversity of officialism? The mortality from scurvy during this long period had exceeded the mortality by battles, wrecks, and all casualties of sea life put together![73]

10

'Every Ship Shall Have on Board a Sufficient Quantity'

AT the beginning of the nineteenth century, with lemons (and to a lesser extent oranges) being issued regularly, there were to be two major problems. Firstly, there was the difficulty of supplying adequate quantities of fresh fruit, both at home and abroad; and secondly, there was still the obstacle of the preservation of juice. Neither the fruit itself nor 'fresh' juice could be successfully preserved for long voyages, and there was still a problem with what Lind had called the rob or concentrated juice. The Admiralty remained suspicious of its claimed efficacy, and in this case the adverse advice that it had been given on the subject was fair and objective.

Blane was in little doubt that rob was less useful than fresh juice, noting, 'if fire is used in preparing it, I know for certain that its virtues will be thereby very much impaired.'[1] It is now known that preparing rob by Lind's method, using heat, results in the loss of about 10 per cent of the vitamin C. Further storage of the rob for a month at room temperature meant that less than 15 per cent of the original vitamin content remained.[2] Both Blane and Trotter confirmed the value and rightness of Lind's recommendations, but neither had any more idea than Lind what constituted the antiscorbutic feature. It is also now known that even fresh lemons were not the most potent antiscorbutic that was available, with blackcurrant, for example, having about five times the vitamin C content of lemons. The notion of the

'EVERY SHIP SHALL HAVE ON BOARD A SUFFICIENT QUANTITY'

'acidic citrus fruit' was all that Lind, Blane and Trotter could rely upon for an explanation.

What is clear is that once the Admiralty began to advocate the issue of lemons and their juice, the incidence of scurvy dropped dramatically. Between 1779 and 1813, the number of scurvy cases fell by 75 per cent,[3] although cases still arose where supplies became exhausted or where ships were unable to obtain fresh reserves. By 1804, the annual consumption of lemon juice was 50,000 gallons, and between 1795 and 1814 almost 1 3/4 million gallons were issued.[4] Trotter wrote in 1803 that 'a case of scurvy requiring to be sent to hospital has not come under my observation since 1795'.[5] The number of cases of scurvy at Haslar can be seen from the table below, when by 1809 not a single case was recorded.

COMPARATIVE INCIDENCE OF SEA DISEASES AT HASLAR HOSPITAL[6]

Disease	1758–60	1780	1809
Total (physical and surgical)	5,743	9,818	573
Fevers	2,241	5,572	219
Scurvy	1,146	1,457	nil
Smallpox	53	42	nil
Consumption	360	218	137
Angina	10	3	1
Rheumatism	350	327	47
Fluxes	245	240	52
Asthma	40	61	9
Mania	19	16	24

The incidence of other sea diseases, notably typhus, was also falling at the time. The period of naval medicine that was covered by James Lind, Thomas Trotter, Gilbert Blane and Robert Robertson saw huge improvements in the treatment of disease in general. Much of that progress was the result of significant changes these men brought to the conditions in which seamen worked and lived.

In the first few years after the Admiralty issued advice on the use of lemons, there were three important naval actions which exemplify the benefits brought about by the resolution of 1759 on revictualling at sea, and even more by the new moves specifically to prevent scurvy. Without these decisions, none of the actions is likely to have succeeded. In 1795, the colourful Admiral Cornwallis (a teetotaller known to his sailors as Billy-go-Tight) was the first to be supplied with lemons in his blockading action at Brest. Three years later John Jervis, Earl St Vincent was similarly protected by citrus fruit in blockading Cadiz. The success of this blockade was used by Gilbert Blane as 'evidence of the high pitch of perfection to which it is practicable to bring the health of seamen in prolonged voyages.' He went on to state that the fleet:

> ... consisted of 24 ships of the line, besides smaller vessels, under the command of Lord St Vincent, and kept the sea from 27th May to 28 of September following, without one of them being in port – without the men having a single meal of fresh beef – and without sending more than 16 to an hospital. Let this state of things be contrasted with that of the Channel Fleet in the first years of the American War. It appears by a letter to me from Dr John Lind, of Haslar Hospital, that in one of these years there had been sent on shore from the channel fleet in the course of four months 6,064 men, almost all affected with fever or scurvy; and that on another occasion, after a ten weeks cruise, 2,500 men were brought into port ill of scurvy.[7]

In 1804, Nelson famously blockaded Toulon for eighteen months. Nelson had a lifelong aversion to salt, and was keen to acquire the best available antiscorbutics. (At the time of his death, his physician Dr Beatty noted that 'early in his life, when he first went to sea, he left off the use of salt, which he believed to be the sole cause of scurvy, and he never took it afterward with his food.'[8])

Nelson's surgeon at Toulon, Dr John Snipe, was given permission to complete a contract in Sicily for 30,000 lemons. Six months later he bid for 30,000 gallons of lemon juice at

1s per gallon. Negotiations failed, and he settled for 20,000 gallons at 1s 6d a gallon for the fleet, plus another 50,000 gallons to be delivered to England. Nelson had been given the instructions for having the juice produced on board ship, and he reflected at the time on the triumphant state of health of his crews, compared to what would have been expected only ten years earlier:

> When the thinking mind reflects on the ravages committed in our fleets by disease in times past and contrasts it with the present, we must be strongly impressed with sentiments of admiration and astonishment, and almost induced to say that mournful waste of the human species was more chargeable to mismanagement than anything unavoidable in nature or sea life.[9]

The Physician to the Fleet, Leonard Gillespie, was also impressed by the state of affairs aboard HMS *Victory*, as he wrote to his sister:

> As proof of the state of health enjoyed by the seamen, I may instance the company of this ship which, consisting of 840 men, contains only one man confined to his bed by sickness, and the other ships are in a similar situation of health, although most of them have been stationed off Toulon for upwards of twenty months, during which time very few of the men or officers (in which number is Lord Nelson) have had a foot on shore.[10]

In 1800, Thomas Trotter discovered that a druggist named Coxwell in London was experimenting with the production of lemon crystals. This was a potential answer to the overriding problem of trying to preserve the rob, and Trotter conducted his own trials at sea on board HMS *Superb*, concentrating the juice to an eighth of its original volume by freezing and removing the ice. He concluded that, 'it retains all the virtues of the fruit in its recent state',[11] i.e. fresh, and was encouraged that some fellow surgeons were reaching similar conclusions. In July, the Sick and Hurt Board arranged for supplies of the crystals to be sent for trials to Sir Roger Curtis on HMS *Lancaster* and to Lord Hugh Seymour in the West Indies. The board felt the crystals to be a doubtful remedy, and sought the results of Trotter's own trials. The commissioners reported that their own calculations found that the cost of using the crystals would be about the same as that for lemon juice.[12] However, Trotter was regarded as something of a maverick who was too ready to tell the board what to do rather than await instructions. He was eventually informed that the method of using crystals was too expensive. He retorted privately in his famous work *Medicina Nautica* with a sentiment that Lind might also have recognised:

> I can already see that the naval service is not likely to be soon benefitted by this ingenious discovery. There is a worm that cankers the bud of all improvements here.[13]

Trotter also demanded much better medical care for the entire seagoing community, in a plea anticipating regulations that would take another half-century to be introduced:

> A commercial nation like this ought to have a Board of Health to protect seamen on distant voyages, so constituted under legal authority that the power of gold could not abridge its benevolent spirit.[14]

In August 1800, Earl St Vincent, commanding the Channel Fleet, encouraged his surgeon, Andrew Baird, to report to the Admiralty on the use of lemon juice. Baird, writing from HMS *Royal George* off Ushant, wrote:

> ... the use of the citrus acid and sugar has been attended with the happiest effects, when its first use became general among the people of the *Ville de Paris*. I had upwards of twenty men

under cure of scurvy and fresh ones daily appearing, but before that ship quitted the fleet I had not a single case.[15]

Baird recommended the reduction of the amount of sugar to be added to what he called the 'sherbet', and the Sick and Hurt Board agreed.

The huge improvements that were nevertheless beginning to take effect did not attract much in the way of gratitude by the Admiralty. Lind had regretfully concluded that 'The Province has been mine to deliver Precepts; the Power is in others to execute'. Now, a disillusioned Trotter, who had done so much to bring citrus fruit into use, retired from active service at the age of forty-two in 1802 after twenty-three years, latterly as Physician to the Fleet under Lord Howe. Trotter had been with Cornwallis in 1795 when he suffered an injury from which he never fully recovered. Besides other works, he had written the massive three-volume *Medicina Nautica*, and was at the forefront of devising major improvements to the naval medical service that would commence in 1805. Coincidentally, Gilbert Blane left the Sick and Hurt Board the same year and returned to his lucrative private practice. In 1807, Trotter wrote to Henry Dundas, Viscount Melville and First Lord of the Admiralty, pointing out that surgeons now benefited from better pay and conditions, and that his labours had saved the country millions. He sought an increase of his pension to one pound per day, and a consultant position:

> I am certain that there are some departments, such as an Inspector of Hospitals, of Prisons, etc, where my knowledge of the duty is far beyond the experience of any other person, and where I could have it in my power to direct such changes as would make medical science more convenient to public advantage than it has hitherto been.[16]

The doctor who had scoured the market stalls for fresh lemons for the fleet was rebuffed – neither job nor increased pension was offered. Trotter – the part-time poet who decided that scurvy was an unconscionable evil after experience as a surgeon on a Liverpool slaveship – retired to private practice in Newcastle upon Tyne, where he died twenty-eight years later in 1832.

The trio of Lind, Blane and Trotter, as founders of the Royal Naval Medical Service, deserve a better and bigger public pedestal than they have so far secured. The significance of their efforts was well summed up in the US Naval Medical Bulletin in 1920:

> They struggled against stupidity, ignorance, prejudice and indifference in high places and low, the Admiralty and Forecastle; they had the hard task of seeking to break down immemorial custom; dared to challenge 'tradition'; hammered at the walls of a hierarchy as soul-chilling, as rigorous, as iron-bound, as any Brahmin caste; preached seemingly frivolous novelties to an insular conservatism that held hardships essential for hardihood.[17]

Nevertheless, considerable improvements were being made in the general victualling of ships, and there was a better understanding of the need for a balanced diet, which helped enormously to enrich the health of sailors, as a letter from Surgeon Peter Henry in Indonesia in December 1802 illustrates:

> The *Daedalus* has been the greater part of this year employed on the Moluccas station, the crew generally on salted diet during that time. The absence of scurvy while on that station can only be attributed to the great quantity of fruit and vegetables which they had access to at a very easy take. The men exchanged their overplus of rice daily for yams, pumpkins and sweet potatoes, with which they were able to make a hearty meal. During fifteen months the crew had only about six weeks fresh beef and only one scorbutic case appeared on the list, which clearly proves that the crew of a ship may remain free from scurvy on salt provisions ever so long when supplied with a due proportion of fruit and vegetables.[18]

'EVERY SHIP SHALL HAVE ON BOARD A SUFFICIENT QUANTITY'

In the summer of 1803, the Sick and Hurt Board reported to the Admiralty that there were 14,489 gallons of lemon juice in store, with a further 5,000 gallons in preparation. They also reported that they had been offered 50,000 gallons to be delivered between Christmas 1803 and May 1804 at a price of 8s per gallon, 'provided there should not be a war with Spain.'[19] They estimated that wartime consumption was about 40,000 gallons per annum, and noted that if war broke out, the price would rise to 9s a gallon.

* * *

Once the use of citrus fruit was finally established in routine operation, various self-serving individuals began to claim that they had been using it successfully for years. One senior naval surgeon, Dr John Harness of Greenwich Hospital, even had the impudence to hint that he was due the credit for the introduction of the remedy. He wrote in November 1805 to the First Lord, Charles Middleton, Lord Barham, pointing out that when it came to the great efforts to prevent sea diseases, 'the discovery of the effect of the use of lemon juice does not rank last in the list.' He disingenuously pleaded to be allowed to tell his lordship how this wonderful remedy came to be used so successfully, 'without exciting an impression on your Lordship's mind of my entertaining the most distant idea of assuming merit not due to myself.' In the summer of 1793 (when Blane and Trotter were working hard persuading fleet commanders to obtain and make daily use of supplies of lemons), Harness was a physician with Admiral Hood in the Mediterranean, where Toulon was under a blockade. He claimed that he had persuaded Hood to send a vessel into port for the specific purpose of obtaining lemons for the fleet. This had resulted in such a disease-free outcome that Hood ordered that in future no ship in his command should leave port without an adequate supply of lemons. (This was precisely the kind of reaction Blane was hoping for as he worked his influential way from commander to commander.) However,

Harness slyly suggested in conclusion to the First Lord, 'to this circumstance becoming generally known, may the use of lemon juice, the effectual means of subduing scurvy be traced.'[20]

This rather blatant attempt at self-promotion probably paid off for Harness. The Admiralty was then in the process of reorganising the Sick and Hurt Board. For years it had been plagued by inept administration and hopelessly incompetent financial management. Initial proposals had been for a split into two separate branches, a Medical Department and a Finance Department. However, the approved plan was to integrate the Sick and Hurt Board with Transport. Originally, the Sick and Hurt Board had responsibility for prisoners of war, but that had been transferred to Transport in 1796, and now full amalgamation was proposed. Harness had written to Middleton initially to complain about the proposals for merger, and about the various manoeuvres being mounted against him by his political enemies. Six weeks after his letter, when the amalgamations had taken place, Harness was appointed the sole medical commissioner to the new Board.[21] He is thereafter credited with introducing improvements in the conditions of service for naval surgeons, most of which had been planned by Trotter. (There was a later series of mergers in 1816 in which Transport was taken over by the Navy Board and medical responsibilities became subsumed within the Victualling Board. Dr Weir, then the sole medical commissioner, was prompted to complain to the First Lord that medical issues, on which he was uniquely qualified to comment, were being decided by the six unqualified victualling commissioners.[22])

It is clear that it took several years for the complete assimilation of the lemon juice regulation throughout the service. There were certainly logistical difficulties that resulted in administrative and operational changes. In February 1807, the Sick and Hurt Commissioners persuaded the Admiralty that, 'as lemon juice has now become a general of supply to His Majesty's ships' the responsibility for supplying it should pass from the Sick and Hurt Board to the Victualling Board.[23] Later, the

'EVERY SHIP SHALL HAVE ON BOARD A SUFFICIENT QUANTITY'

Victualling Board would also take on the duty of production as well as supply. Inconsistency in framing official orders was identified by the Board to the Admiralty in July 1807, when they enclosed a letter written by the surgeon aboard HMS *Belligerent* at Prince of Wales Island in which he reported the excellent results from using lemon juice and sugar:

> As their lordships will observe that the surgeon states that lime juice is allowed on that station only to the surgeons for the use of the sick, none being placed in the charge of the pursers to be issued with sugar to the ship's company at large, as is the practice in the Channel Fleet, we beg to recommend to their lordships that directions may be given to the several commanders-in-chief on this as well as on all other Foreign Stations to cause His Majesty's ships to be uniformly supplied with lime or lemon juice and sugar.[24]

There were also problems with bad lemon juice. In May 1808, the Admiralty ordered Dr Harness to conduct an enquiry into a scandal concerning bad supplies sent to the Channel Fleet from the Royal Hospital at Plymouth. It appears that the juice (in this case supplied into store at 2s 8d per gallon by a commercial producer) had been identified as inferior but reported as of good quality by the relevant official. This was another potential fraud that had come to light in the form of an anonymous letter to the Lords of the Admiralty, closely followed by a complaint from Captain Bedford of HMS *Ville de Paris*.[25]

There were also still occasional self-publicists who turned up out of the blue claiming to have found the immaculate cure for scurvy. In June 1808, Dr Richard Brooke, lately returned from thirty years on the Continent, wrote from Exeter to the prime minister, the briefly-in-office William Cavendish Bentinck, Duke of Portland. (Portland seems most remembered for having provoked a massacre while Governor of Madras by prohibiting beards and turbans among the Indian troops.) In his preamble, Brooke displayed formidable eccentricity by recommending that convicted prisoners should be punished by a form of 'home slavery', and by warning against Frenchmen in disguise. On scurvy, he claimed:

> I have brought from Italy the means of eradicating Scurvy from British Habits, provided that such Patients use gentle exercise in the open air. The medicinal means are small, but positively sure.[26]

Brooke did not describe the action of his magic pills, which came with no explanation or list of ingredients, and without testimonial or authoritative statement as to their function. Another remedy of national importance found its insignificant place in the compendium.

As the value of using lemon juice became widely accepted within the Royal Navy, the merchant fleet began to demand the same liberal issue of citrus juice. One branch of merchant shipping that made early use of fruit against scurvy was the trade in transporting convicts from Deptford to Australia. Vessels in that particular trade were provided with a surgeon and detailed instructions on the care of prisoners and their health, hygiene and living conditions. Specific instructions were given in relation to scurvy, and lemon juice, sugar, sago, oatmeal, peas, bread, wine and tea were ordered to be available to those showing any symptoms.[27] Often, many of the diseases suffered on these vessels were brought aboard from English jails. Dysentery, typhoid, typhus and smallpox were common enough, but if anything disrupted provisions, prolonged the voyage, or if lemon juice rules were ignored, scurvy would take hold with a vengeance. Despite the apparent liberality, there were serious outbreaks of scurvy in convict ships as in all other branches of the Merchant Navy until well into the second half of the nineteenth century. One vessel sailing from Dublin to Freemantle in 1853 had two thirds of her complement of convicts on the sick list with many of the more hideous diseases. Although the surgeon was prevented by foul weather from obtaining supplies at Cape Town, he later had a reprimand inserted in his journal:

> As the sickness and mortality which occurred in this ship appears to have been greatly increased by the general prevalence of scorbutic complaints, it is submitted that the surgeon be desired to state why he did not cause lemon juice to be issued more frequently than appears by his journal – *viz*, once every second or third day. And further, as the temperance men would not take lemon juice in wine, why he did not immediately cause it to be supplied to them as directed by the Instructions.[28]

The Merchant Navy was officially included in the regulation issue of lemon juice for the treatment of scurvy with the introduction of the Mercantile Marine Act of 1851. However, this did not immediately lead to improvements, for several reasons. The naval surgeon who delineated the medical aspects of the act left the same year to become a leading obstetrician, and displayed the same degree of confusion about lemons and limes as everyone else. The relevant part of the act stated:

> Every ship, except those bound to European ports, or to ports in the Mediterranean Sea, shall have on board a sufficient quantity of lime or lemon juice, sugar and vinegar.[29]

The juice was to be given on penalty of a fine of £20. The updated Merchant Shipping Act of 1854 doubled the penalty if the juice was inferior. Neither of these acts distinguished between lemon juice and lime juice, and the idea of vinegar as a substitute for either was absurd. Not until later legislation of 1894 was the reference to vinegar dropped (but so was the reference to lemon juice).

Shipowners continued where possible to flout the regulations. In 1863 Dr Barnes, Physician to the hospital ship *Dreadnought* at Greenwich, noted that half his patients were suffering from scurvy, one in twenty seriously. He accused international shipowners of:

> ... exhibiting the greatest amount of disregard of the safety and health of their crews. ... When it is remembered that the security of this country has on several occasions been imperilled by the disablement of the Royal Navy through scurvy, it may be presumed that the same cause will imperil the safety of our merchant ships. And there can be no doubt that many ships have actually foundered at sea because the crews were so prostrated from scurvy as to be unable to handle them when overtaken by severe weather.[30]

Many shipowners and captains tried either to circumvent the regulations, or to adulterate the juice in order to reduce expense. In 1865 after 'inquiries recently instituted by the Board of Trade in several cases of outbreak of Scurvy in Merchant Ships, in some even where it is manifest that the Owners have had every desire to provide for the health of the crew', new guidelines were produced. They required that supplies of lime or lemon juice had to be inspected and passed by a competent medical officer before sailing. Ten per cent brandy or rum was to be added to the juice, which was to be packed in one-gallon jars, covered with a layer of oil, and sealed. The dose was not to be delayed more than a fortnight from leaving port, and each man was to have a minimum of two ounces twice a week, to be increased when necessary.[31] Even after the regulations were formally strengthened by the act of 1867, defaulters were still active. The following year at Thames Police Court, Elisha Hitchens of the *Western Star* was fined £20 and costs after two men contracted scurvy, and one died, after a voyage from the West Indies.[32] In December 1870, James Farr, master of the *Princess Beatrice*, and its owners, were fined by a naval court after a dozen cases of scurvy and four deaths following a voyage from Aden.[33] There was an interesting administrative anomaly in 1871 when it was revealed that following the opening of the Suez

'EVERY SHIP SHALL HAVE ON BOARD A SUFFICIENT QUANTITY'

Canal two years earlier, 'a new excuse for the absence of lime-juice on board ship has been created, inasmuch as all vessels trading to the Mediterranean can legally claim exemption.'[34] It seems that vessels bound for China and India were claiming that they were entitled to exemption from carrying antiscorbutics by using the canal, since the rules exempted vessels sailing to the Mediterranean. In the same week that the Suez Canal anomaly was revealed, it was pointed out in the medical journal *The Lancet* that since the introduction of the new anti-scurvy provisions of the 1867 act, the incidence of the disease had fallen by 60 per cent. A month later, the Board of Trade issued a formal notice to owners and masters instructing that use of the Suez Canal did *not* confer exemption from the scurvy regulations, and that defaulters would be subject to the severest penalties.

The road towards the eradication of scurvy in the Royal Navy proved somewhat rocky. The momentum behind the introduction of lemons which had been induced in the 1790s began to dissipate, probably because both Blane and Trotter were no longer in the Navy, and Trotter in particular was not exercising the challenging approaches that had so discomfited the Admiralty. There were still disputes over some of the older remedies. In December 1812 Dr Robert Robertson, Physician at Greenwich Hospital, recommended that what he called Peruvian Bark Gingerbread should be given trials in the treatment of some fevers and scurvy among sick sailors from a squadron recently returned from Archangel. However, Dr Weir, the Medical Commissioner, and Dr Harness were wholly against the idea, and the trials were not allowed to proceed:

> ... the sickness prevailing in the Russian Squadron from Archangel is clearly of a catarrhal description attended with more or less of scorbutic acrimony in the circulating fluids and for the cure of which prompt and copious evacuations in the incipient stage of the disease assisted by vegetable acids, broth, etc have already been followed by the happiest effects.[35]

Dr Weir stated that, 'the administration of bark in any manner or form possesses no kind of specific virtue whatever in the prevention of fever', and that 'in all such cases it would be attended with the most pernicious effects.' A few years later came a request from Sir James Yeo of HMS *Inconstant* for supplies of port for mixing with Peruvian Bark as a measure against dysentery off the coast of Africa. However Their Lordships rather sniffily wanted to know 'whether it has been usual to send port wine to the Coast of Africa for similar purposes.'[36]

The biggest problems arose when the Admiralty, perhaps under political or commercial pressure, had to deal with the twin confusions of what constituted a lemon, and what was the word for a lemon. They perceived a means of saving money which resulted in another hundred years of suspicion and uncertainty in treating scurvy, a century during which the incidence of the disease increased again after its initial fall. The citrus fruit purchased and used by the Navy, and later the Army, was *Citrus medica, var. limonum*, known to us as the lemon, and supplies came from the Mediterranean, mainly Spain, where it had been introduced in about AD 1000. In 1493 Christopher Columbus brought citrus fruit from the Canary Islands to the island of Hispaniola, today part of Haiti, part of the Dominican Republic. It is likely that *Citrus medica, var. limetta* was also used by the Navy to a much lesser extent; this is known as the sweet lime, due to its almost total lack of acidity. War with Spain in 1796 ended the Spanish supply, and there was a momentary panic when the Admiralty wondered what to do. The Sick and Hurt Board wrote to the Admiralty Board saying:

> though we do not consider strong beer a substitute for lime juice and sugar for scurvy, yet as it is conducive, we recommend that the experiment be made of substituting it on some ships.[37]

It is interesting to observe that, even at this early date in the Admiralty's adoption of citrus fruit, the error was already established of referring to 'lime juice' although the overwhelming supplies were of lemon juice. New sources of lemons were soon established in Portugal, although these were unreliable and expensive, and negotiations were concluded in 1803 with preferred suppliers in Malta and Sicily. This change occurred as the Navy was wholeheartedly moving to the general issue of lemon juice to all ships, rather than only to the sick and to crews departing on long voyages.

From the beginning of the nineteenth century there was complete confusion in terminology between lemons and sweet limes, which both came from the Mediterranean. The term 'lime juice' was commonly applied to what was almost wholly lemon juice. It has been suggested that administrative confusion arose when Admiralty clerks confused the botanical expression *citrus limonum* as referring to limes. Other explanations have included the fact that the word for 'lemon' in Italian is *limone*, which happens to be the German word for 'lime'.[38] To those confusions was added the allegation that unscrupulous foreign producers (especially in Malta and the Indian subcontinent) were adulterating the raw fruit juice, leading to a deterioration or destruction of the (still mysterious) antiscorbutic agent. Since acidity was still the only feature that was identified as the potent characteristic, anyone wishing to adulterate the juice covertly could relatively easily do so by the addition of a spurious acid. Although James Lind had made oranges his prime recommendation, there is no evidence that they were ever seriously considered for use, in addition to or in place of, either lemons or limes. They were certainly used in some quantity, but never achieved prevalence in treating scurvy, which is a pity given that they contain more vitamin C than either lemons or limes.

The crucial twist in the convoluted tale of citrus juice was that there was a deliberate move away from lemons in favour of limes. This was probably at least partly due to the existing confusion between the two fruits, but it also had something to do with the promotion of British commerce rather than that of foreign producers. At any rate, the change was made from Mediterranean lemons to the West Indian lime, *Citrus medica, var. acida*. In 1846 the English Quaker family of Edmund Sturge of Birmingham bought the West Indian island of Montserrat and established huge lime plantations. The result of this was that by the midle of the century production of lime juice was entirely in the hands of British growers and producers in a part of the world that was firmly under British economic and political control. The Navy had completely substituted lime juice for lemon juice by 1875.[39] Unfortunately, West Indian limes were virtually useless against scurvy. Although they were acidic, as the botanical name implies (in fact they contain both more acid and sugar than lemons) and were therefore assumed to be potently antiscorbutic, their vitamin C content was about one quarter that of the lemon. This was enough to make the established recommended 'daily dose' ineffective. In some ships, lime juice worked, in others it unaccountably did not. There is one account from 1854 of a French naval surgeon whose ship was heavily affected by a scurvy attack. He was contacted by Surgeon Murray of HMS *Meander*, who regaled him with the virtues of lime juice. Murray offered eleven gallons of juice, which quickly put an end to the scurvy aboard the French ship *Cléopâtre*. The French Admiralty was so impressed that it immediately made it a general issue to the entire French Fleet.[40]

Nevertheless, by the middle of the nineteenth century, there was a perceived drop in the efficacy of citrus juice. To this effect was added problems brought about by the extended transportation times of limes from the West Indies, and decanting and settling times at processing plants in Britain. Processing techniques, involving the use of copper piping, almost certainly also resulted, through chemical reaction, in yet further reductions in vitamin C efficacy, echoing the problems that had been claimed as 'copper poisoning' by Dr John Travis in 1757. To cap it all, and against the expectations of the Admiralty, limes were more expensive than lemons.

There were reasons to assume during the nineteenth century that the incidence of scurvy would improve due to non-medical factors. Conditions at sea were improving significantly, both in terms of health and victualling, so that the use of antiscorbutics where scurvy was less intractable was consequently rather less urgent. Sailing was also becoming more efficient; the longitude problem was solved, copper sheathing of hulls had been adopted, and as steam power took over, the length of voyages reduced sharply. Scurvy began to be regarded as much more a problem for polar exploration, military campaigns and the whaling industry. However the reality was that confidence in the ability to treat scurvy fell so low that the whole issue of what caused the disease in the first place was reopened to dispute. Accounts began to appear of cases of scurvy aboard ships which had been liberally supplied with lime juice which, when tested, was found to be in good condition. It did not take too many such incidents before there was an upsurge of disaffection with the citrus remedy. The advent of food preservation by canning provided a new impetus for the dispute. There was ample scope for the discovery of flaws in those new processes, and the canard resurfaced of tainted meat as the cause of scurvy. Everything seemed to be going backwards.

There was no-one of stature left to carry the torch through the next stage of the battle against scurvy. Gilbert Blane had died in 1834, before the ill-effects were seen of the move towards limes instead of lemons. While he had been one of the commissioners of the Sick and Hurt, he had been consulted by the government on several major inquiries relating to public health. He was a consultant to the Turkey Company, which controlled the entire trade in that part of the world, and drew up much of the legislation which became the Quarantine Act of 1799. As the *Dictionary of National Biography* says, 'Hardly any department of state failed to resort to Blane's advice on one occasion or another.' Blane was knighted following his achievements in dealing with the aftermath of the disastrous Walcheren Expedition in 1809, when a huge military force on the Dutch island was devastated by malaria, typhus and dysentery. Blane later became Physician to George IV, to the Emperor of Russia, the King of Prussia and the US President. He had written widely on medical matters, particularly naval medicine and public health, and was responsible for great improvements in the administrative structure of numerous medical institutions, not least that of the Royal Navy.

The fact that after so many decades there was still complete ignorance of what constituted the antiscorbutic factor may have unconsciously dulled the prospect of further intellectual enquiry. The rigorous practical experiment favoured by James Lind, applied in the new field of organic chemistry, was what would eventually answer the riddle. That was the hope offered by Dr William Budd, the Bristol physician who contributed much to the progress of disinfection (and brother of the famous epidemiologist George Budd). As early as 1840, when writing of the efficacy of citrus fruit, he confessed his ignorance of the specific factor that conveyed the antiscorbutic effect, but suggested with remarkable prescience that:

> ... we shall probably not be deemed too sanguine if we anticipate that the study of organic chemistry will at no distant period throw some light on the subject.[41]

If 'scurvy fatigue' did indeed set in during the mid-nineteenth century, there was one major opportunity of progress when the government set up what became known as the British Scurvy Commission in 1877, the full impact of which is considered in chapter fourteen. One of the principal contributors to that enquiry underlined the one depressing certainty about scurvy, 'what may be the nature of the deficient element is at present altogether unknown.'[42]

It is probably the case that for sixty years, until about 1920, commercial lime juice was relatively useless against scurvy.[43] The disease reappeared in a variety of situations, and was being treated with erratic results. The trouble was, the antiscorbutic deficiency that was true of West Indian limes, which achieved superiority during this period, was also wrongly attributed to

Mediterranean lemons for the simple reason that the names were still being applied to the fruit with casual interchangeability. It does not seem to have occurred to anyone until much later that the increase in the incidence of scurvy may have been due to the change in fruit. There was a consistent lack of recognition of the fact that lemons and limes were different fruit, and that they may have had different characteristics. The political and economic factors in citrus production were of overriding importance.

It was not until the First World War, that the practical and political circumstances arose for new research on dietary deficiency. Infantile scurvy became a major problem throughout Europe, and scurvy was rampant in Russian, French and Serbian armies in particular. In London, the Lister Institute embarked on a series of experiments into dietary deficiency with a view to advising military planners on the nutritional aspects of field rations. Experiments were initially carried out using monkeys and guinea pigs to quantify the antiscorbutic properties of milk and dried milk. However, as will be detailed later, when assays were carried out using citrus juice, a century of confusion and inconsistent results would be rapidly explained.

Before that breakthrough occurred, the Merchant Shipping Act of 1867 resulted in a significant new chapter in the scurvy story. In itself, the new act simply tightened existing regulations, which as before were adhered to with varying degrees of enthusiasm. However, it was the indirect response provoked in a shipbuilder and grain merchant in Edinburgh's sea port of Leith that would make a difference. That same year of 1867 saw him secure a patent for a new method of preserving citrus juice without the use of alcohol or other adulterants. That improvement alone was also to lead to great improvements in the supply of the fruit. James Lind's 'rob' was about to take a leap into a future that would found a new world industry.

'Lime Juice and Wine Merchants'

LEITH was a prosperous town by the mid-nineteenth century that relied on shipbuilding and repairing, brewing and flour milling. Many small businesses were associated with the shipping trade – rope and sailmakers, brassfounders and chandlers. The Rose family was one of many that had been involved in small-scale shipbuilding for many years. Later, the family developed a sideline in the equipping and provisioning of ships, and in 1859 the shipbuilding was relinquished and the firm of Rose & Company concentrated on its activities as grain and flour merchants in Bank Street, Leith. The company built up considerable experience, not only of the practice of ship victualling, but also of the increasing complexity of rules and regulations that were applied by the Royal Navy and, with the passing of the Merchant Shipping Act of 1867, by the Merchant Fleet.

For centuries Leith had been the only port in Scotland, and grew from a prehistoric fishing settlement where the Water of Leith meets the River Forth. After its official status was conferred in 1329, commerce developed with France and the Low Countries, and later the Baltic and the Americas. Principal exports were whisky, coal, iron, hides, paper and linen traded against the import of sugar, grain, wine, spices and timber. Leith was almost destroyed by the English in the sixteenth century, but survived and became the seat of government, when French troops were garrisoned in the town to protect Mary Queen of Scots. The port then acquired a walled fortification to protect its naval dockyards. A century later it was nearly wiped out by the plague; and then it witnessed the launch of the disastrous Darien Expedition to Panama – that most infamous of ventures that foundered in disease, personal feuding and political chicanery.

Scotland's first dry docks were constructed in Leith in 1720, and the town gained even greater concentrations of merchant and naval facilities while at the same time managing to present rather a fashionable face to some of Edinburgh's wealthier businessmen who established homes in the vicinity. Many of these families were in the ship victualling and foreign trade business. W.E. Gladstone's family were flour and barley merchants; the Melroses were tea importers; and the Rose family, having changed their field of business from shipbuilding, were firmly established as grain merchants and ships' suppliers. Over a number of years, there were changes of name (Rose & Morrison, Rose & Milne) as partners came and went, and by 1871 the company, now in Mitchell Street, reverted to the name L. Rose & Company, 'lime juice and wine merchants.'[1] It was in this unlikely setting that the world's first soft drinks industry was conceived.

Lauchlan Rose, the head of the firm, who was born in 1829, was familiar with the regulations and legal conditions under which lime juice had to be supplied to all vessels sailing from British ports. For preservation, it was fortified by the addition of 15 per cent demerara rum, and supplied in 4-gallon jars covered in wickerwork, sealed and capsulated. Regulations were tightly controlled, and most ports had an official inspector of lime juice who was responsible particularly for naval supplies. Rose was aware of the problems associated with attempts to preserve the juice, and considered that preservation by the addition of alcohol was hardly an ideal adulteration. It appeared to him that, quite apart from any medical considerations in regard to the treatment of scurvy, existing methods did not enable the consumption of truly fresh fruit juice. In about 1865, Rose decided to concentrate his efforts on the production and supply of lime juice for the shipping trade. He had an eye on the possibility of producing a sweet fruit juice suitable not only for use at sea, but also for public consumption. At the time, there was no such thing as a non-alcoholic fruit drink, or anything resembling a soft drinks industry. Rose was taking a bold, imaginative step in making lime juice available and acceptable as a refreshing drink for the public rather than just an adulterated medicine for seamen. However, sweetening the juice and putting it in bottles suitable for the domestic market was one thing, but there was still the problem of preventing it from fermenting. Alcohol did that to a limited degree, but was no more acceptable to the public than the use of olive oil.

The invention of practicable methods for the preservation of foodstuff is usually credited to Nicolas Appert. Son of an innkeeper, he was a chef, confectioner and distiller from Massy, near Paris, who won a F12,000 government award in 1800 for his invention, which was initially intended to be principally of military interest. His system of 'sealing the seasons' by using hermetically sealed glass containers was highly successful in preserving a wide range of fruit, vegetables, soups and dairy products.[2] He established a huge cannery which remained in business until 1933. Appert in effect invented the sterilising autoclave, and later devised the first stock cube (if we discount portable soup), but died in poverty in 1841. In 1810, the Englishman Peter Durand patented a method of preserving food in tin cans, and enjoyed great financial success supplying the Royal Navy.[3]

In 1867, the year when the Merchant Shipping Act finally made it compulsory for all British shipping to carry fresh lime juice, Lauchlan Rose registered a patent for 'an improved method of preserving vegetable juices'. He had observed wine casks being fumigated by the burning of sulphur candles, and discovered by experiment that sulphur salts acted as a preserving agent for fruit juice. His principal patent application stated:

> I now propose in the preparation of lime juice, lemon juice, and other like vegetable medicaments to employ sulphurous acid or sulphurous gas. The acid in a liquid state is mixed with the juice in an air-tight vessel or cask, and allowed to

stand for a few days until the acid has acted upon the vegetable matter in the juice. Afterwards the vessel or cask is exposed, and any fumes not absorbed by the juice allowed to escape until the juice has attained its natural flavour. When the gas is used I cause it to circulate over and through the lime or other juice while exposed in air-tight casks or other air-tight vessels until the result required is accomplished.[4]

By 1879 Rose had registered a further nine patents for various improvements in bottles and stoppers, and his new venture seems to have been immediately successful. He managed quickly to fulfil his idea for a sweet, popular product aimed at the domestic market. He used attractive bottles heavily embossed with a representation of lime leaves and fruit, accompanied by well designed labels – trademark devices which he quickly registered. Rose's Lime Juice Cordial was one of the great success stories of the nineteenth century that has continued into the twenty-first. Not only was the Admiralty and the Merchant Shipping Act satisfied; there was great public interest in buying a sweet, tasty bottled fruit juice which had more than a hint of medical approbation (one advertisement quoted the approval of the lack of alcohol by *The Lancet*). While maintaining production at Queen's Dock in Leith, Rose moved his headquarters and main production centre to new premises at Curtain Road and Worship Street, Finsbury, north London, in 1875.

Rose was not the first to produce lime juice commercially. The Sturge family had established lime-growing estates in the West Indies twenty years earlier, and there were to be half a dozen smaller British companies involved in the trade, both at home and abroad. Edmund Sturge was a manufacturing chemist in Birmingham, where he had been producing citric acid since 1826. In 1852 he contracted with Francis Burke from Montserrat to grow limes on the Woodlands Estate. Montserrat, with a rich volcanic soil, was ideally suited to the growing of limes, and the venture was probably prompted by times of fervent temperance and by the possibility of producing a popular non-alcoholic drink. With his brother Joseph, Sturge purchased other estates and converted sugar plantations to lime growing. In April 1869 the family raised £36,000 in capital and registered Sturge's Montserrat Company Ltd (changed in 1875 to The Montserrat Company Ltd) to control their extensive business. The objects of the company were:

> ... the purchase of the Olveston and Woodlands estates and of certain warehouses in the town of Plymouth in the Island of Montserrat in the West Indies; the planting and growth of lime trees on such estates and lands; the production of lime juice and other products therefrom; the stocking of the same with cattle, horses and animals; the growth of sugar and other colonial products therefrom.[5]

In 1869 Sturge entered into a contract with Evans & Sons of Liverpool, a long-established firm of manufacturing chemists that had its origins in London in about 1800. Evans was to be the sole consignee and bottler of the entire output of Sturge's lime-growing estates – a volume of about $1/4$ million gallons annually.[6] The raw squeezed juice was shipped in casks to Liverpool, where it was allowed to settle and clarify before being bottled. Most of this production was destined for use at sea, but the company's advertising suggests that some at least was available for the domestic market since 'as a non-alcoholic drink during warm weather, Lime Juice is steadily growing in favour.' There is no indication that this juice was preserved against fermentation in any way, so their claims that it lasted in good condition for almost any length of time may not be credible. Evans also produced a popular lime sauce, 'claimed to be cheaper and more dietetic than any other condiment for the table.' Another advertising line used by Evans for its sauce drew on the remark by John Woodall in 1617:

> I dare not write how good a Sauce it is at meat, least the Chiefe in the Ships waste it in the great Cabins.[7]

'LIME JUICE AND WINE MERCHANTS'

Not all the colonial enterprises aimed at producing lime juice had the immediate success of the Sturge family. In 1887 The Montserrat and Antilles Produce Company was bought from some entrepreneurs by a solicitor, an MP and a merchant. Their proposed product range was wide: lime juice, lime juice cordial, guava jelly, chutneys, tamarinds, tamarind zest or sauces, and other sauces and condiments of the same nature.[8] The new arrival did not last long, however, and was out of business within five years. It had gone classically 'bust', with insufficient assets to cover debts.

Lauchlan Rose imported raw juice direct from the West Indies and also purchased from brokers in London. However in 1893 he guaranteed his source of supply by buying the Bath Estate near Roseau, the principal town in Dominica, the largest of the Windward Islands. The estate produced 20,000 barrels of fruit a year, and other estates at Soufriere and St Aroment were added to expand the growing acreage. In 1924, growing estates were also bought in the Gold Coast (now Ghana); the company sponsored the planting of these estates by local native farmers, and built a processing factory to guarantee benefit to the local economy.[9] The West Indies limes fruited twice a year, so juice production for Rose & Company was virtually non-stop throughout the year.

At about the same period in the 1920s, the fortunes of the Montserrat Company were on the wane. Apart from the fact that the islands had been subjected to a devastating series of hurricanes over a number of years, the company had the added duty of operating in very close association with the colonial administration. Its responsibilities were therefore much more diverse than those of Rose & Company. Partly in response to the ravages of weather and the competition in lime juice production, the Montserrat Company moved increasingly towards cotton production, augmented later by the production of rum and tomato paste. As a result, the cultivation of limes was gradually relegated to a minor activity. The attempt to diversify was not successful; eventually the new products were abandoned, and the Montserrat Company was sold in 1961 to a Canadian real estate corporation.

Rose & Company also experienced difficulties. Their estates suffered from the 1920s Depression, from hurricanes and botanical disease. In addition, by 1930 the Admiralty was trying to use synthetic ascorbic acid, to the potential deprivation of the fruit and juice-making industries. However, instead of following the Montserrat route of diversification, Rose & Company expanded the range of its prime product. The great boost was given by the production of lime marmalade, which was enormously popular; this was aided by the promotion of gin and lime as a popular social drink, and the 'discovery' that lime juice could act as a hangover cure. This latter supposed property became the focus of a successful and long-running advertising campaign which ran well into the post-Second World War period. [10]

After the scurvy mystery was eventually solved in the 1920s, the need for lime juice by the Royal Navy and the Merchant Navy ended. Rose & Company went from strength to strength in the domestic market, and apart from its world-famous Rose's Lime Juice Cordial, it produced Rum Shrub, Ginger Brandy, Orange Quinine Wine, and its famous Lime Marmalade. Fearful of wartime bombing, production was moved 20 miles from London to St Albans, in Hertfordshire, in 1939 – and the following year the old factory was flattened in an air raid. During the war, lime juice in the UK was produced by the pooled resources of various companies to an austerity recipe required by the government and sold under a generic label. In the post-war years Rose's recovered its pre-eminence and continued to flourish; in 1957 it was bought and marketed by the Schweppes Company (now CadburySchweppes plc).

One of Rose's publicity booklets from 1959 paints an anachronistic and distinctly paternalistic picture of life on the plantations at that time:

> Limes are picked in the early hours of the morning, before the heat of the day. There is a carefree picnic atmosphere about

lime gathering on the plantations. As they move about beneath the trees the coloured workers laugh and joke among themselves and sing music-hall songs or hymns with equal fervour. Then, basket on head, they make their way to the nearest plantation road where their loads are transferred to lorries for transport to the mill.[11]

The fruit was washed in running water before being crushed between granite rollers. The entire product of the milling process, juice, pulp and essential oils, was packed in wax-lined casks, without the addition of any preservative, for transport to Britain. Although the import of this raw juice satisfied the huge production of lime juice in the UK, the bulk of the output of the West Indian estates was devoted to the production of citric acid, and this was a highly lucrative market for the company. Later, citrate of lime was produced in Dominica, although an attempt to produce citric acid entirely in the islands was not successful due to climatic conditions. Citric acid (still not yet the mysterious substance that prevented scurvy) had first been isolated from lemons in 1784 by the Swedish chemist Carl Wilhelm Scheele, and was used in confectionery, soft drinks manufacture, metal-cleaning compounds and as a food stabiliser. It had no role in attempts to treat scurvy.

In very recent years, the rights and licences of Rose & Company in various countries were shared between CadburySchweppes plc and the eternally present Coca Cola Enterprises. Today's label now declares that 'Rose's cordial is now available in Original Lime, Zesty Orange and Cloudy Lemon'. So not only can Rose's Lime Juice claim that its genesis was a unique feature in the story of scurvy, but it is a remarkable survivor in the increasingly difficult international commercial market. It is a pleasing whimsy that the endeavour of a ship-chandler from Leith produced the first preserved juice that satisfied not only the vital needs of those at risk of scurvy, but led to its becoming the world's first and still-surviving branded fruit drink. Today the bottle (plastic alas – gone is the heavily embossed glass) carries the same label design recording the date of Lauchlan Rose's first patent. The original lime-branch trademark device celebrating the battle against scurvy in the Merchant Navy is a unique part of history surviving in the commercial world.

The popular success of Rose's Lime Juice Cordial had a singular effect on the public consciousness. Together with the impact of the use of fresh limes and lime juice at sea, there arose a particularly colourful effect on language. The word 'limeys' is still recognised today as a term (sometimes of abuse) for the British. It was during the second half of the nineteenth century that English, and latterly British, sailors began to be referred to by their American counterparts as 'lime-juicers', although the origin of the term may be Australian. *Partridge's Dictionary of Historical Slang* gives the first date of this nickname as 1859, and the following year for its reference to an English sailing ship, as in 'They would not go on a "lime-juicer", they said, for anything' (*Pall Mall Gazette*, 1884). The *Oxford English Dictionary* also gives the date 1859, but this time the locus is Australia and the reference is to someone (a 'new friend') just off the boat from Britain. The 1867 Act finally confirmd the overdue commitment to the use of lime juice in the Merchant Navy, as was illustrated in such popular songs as 'The Lime Juice Ship':

Now when ye join a merchant ship ye'll hear yer Articles read.
They'll tell ye of yer beef an' pork, yer butter an' yer bread,
Yer sugar, tea an' coffee, boys, yer peas an' beans exact,
Yer limejuice an' vinegar, boys, according to the Act.

Later, as the nickname came to be used in the USA in a less affectionate manner, it was shortened to 'limeys', and still related to British sailors and by extension became a pejorative term for anyone from Britain; occasionally Britain was referred to as 'limey-land'.

It was not long before the term came to be used as a term of insult. The Oxford *Twentieth Century Words* quotes R.D. Paine in

'LIME JUICE AND WINE MERCHANTS'

1918 thus, 'Squads of the American Navy patrol began to stroll about . . . displaying no sympathy . . . loudly announced that he could whip any three "Limies" that ever trod a British deck.'[12] Rawson's *Dictionary of Invective* gives an example from *Strange Passage* by Theodore Irwin in 1935 which ensures that we get the full flavour of the insult by ensuring that it is delivered, if by no other means, by association: 'Then out with you, go back where you came from, you dago, you hunky, you scoovy (Swede), you heine, you mick, you sheenie, you limey!'[13] Rawson also offers, from Leonard Moseley's *Marshall: Hero for our Times*, the following example:

> General Joseph W. Stillwell . . . was a rabid hater of the British and became angry with the way they deliberately diminished the importance of the Chinese effort. 'It was wonderful the way we slapped the Limeys down,' he said afterward.[14]

The folk wisdom that 'names will never hurt me' is questionable when the epithet takes on a pejorative character. It is surely preferable to take pleasure in the curious little coda to James Lind's work that had a slang word originating, if not on the mess-deck, at least on the dockside. That it found its basis in a somewhat obscure quasi-medical treatment, and survived and transformed itself into a term of wry affection for an entire nation is a pleasing quirk of linguistics.

12

'The British Army Were Allowed to Rot of Scurvy'

ALTHOUGH scurvy was classically a sea disease, and both Lind and Blane were solely concerned with its maritime form, it was also a widespread disease on land. Scurvy was a disease of explorers, armies, besieged populations, and a constant companion of those who lived on the periphery of life – those in cold, wet countries with poor cultivation and diet. In later manifestations, it has been a disease of infants, the elderly and of refugees.

One of the greatest movements of people generated by a single incident was what is known as the Gold Rush, which began in California in 1848 and lasted, on and off, for the next half-century. In the first two years alone over 100,000 men and women – rogues, cobblers, lawyers, tailors, cooks, doctors and sea captains – trekked from the four corners of the world, by sea and overland, to a grim existence in some of the most inhospitable areas of North America. The most impatient travelled by ship to San Francisco, commonly from New York via Cape Horn with stops for revictualling at Rio de Janeiro and Valparaiso – an 18,000-mile voyage. They often succumbed to scurvy while at sea, for all the reasons with which this account has been familiar. Some others shortened their journey but risked tropical disease by crossing from Atlantic to Pacific by the Panama route. Using the 'northern route' from Missouri, they traversed maybe 2,500 miles across a landscape with no roads,

'THE BRITISH ARMY WERE ALLOWED TO ROT OF SCURVY'

before crossing the South Pass of the Rocky Mountains at a height of 7,000 feet. These people were martyrs to all manner of disease, and scurvy was not the least of them.

Typically, the trekkers carried flour and salt beef or pork as their main dietary items augmented, by those few who had done any kind of informed preparation, with pickles and vinegar as basic antiscorbutics. Grasses, wild onions and fruit picked by the trail were also used deliberately against the possibility of scurvy. At Fort Laramie – last stop before the Rockies – there had been recurrent ravages of scurvy in 1858, and one surgeon used a concoction of the juice of cactus plants flavoured with whisky and lemon juice to combat the disease.[1] By and large, food was difficult to obtain and even harder to preserve. Essentially, the itinerant gold miner's diet was similar to that of the sailor, but since they had to carry everything, much less varied.[2] Often, much of what was carried on the trail was discarded at Fort Laramie before starting the climb into the Rockies. Those who had already suffered left themselves further exposed by thereafter carrying dangerously insufficient supplies. There were many diaries kept by pioneers that contain descriptions of the most piteous cases of scurvy; people abandoned dying in the snow at the side of mountain tracks, and adults and children so crippled as to be unable to walk. Surprisingly, a number of travel guides were available. Charles Darwin's cousin, Francis Galton, the noted explorer, anthropologist and expert on statistics, eugenics, heredity and fingerprints, had something to say about scurvy in *The Art of Travel, or shifts and contrivances available in wild countries*:

> Scurvy has attacked travellers even in Australia, and I myself have felt symptoms of it in Africa, when living wholly on meat. Any vegetable diet cures it; lime juice, treacle, raw potatoes, and acid fruits are especially efficacious.[3]

Galton also recommended sprouted seeds and raw meat, as was commonly used by the Inuit.

In the mining camps, there was sometimes the possibility of potatoes, beans, rice, onions and game to a greater or lesser extent, with occasional dried fruit. Many of the gold seekers died from starvation, scurvy, cholera or associated disease, either because they were simply too destitute or because they were too isolated for anyone to know of their plight or be able to assist.[4] Against scurvy there were favourite nostrums and quack remedies, and there are reports of the enthusiasm by entire camps for burial up to the neck in earth, with only a couple of old men left to guard against bears and coyotes.[5]

Scurvy was popularly blamed on salted, fatty meat and lack of fresh vegetables, and its effects were relentless. One account from Sutter's Fort in 1850 talks of a death rate of eighteen to twenty men per day over a period of five months. The commonest cause was scurvy, followed by dysentery and typhus.[6] One doctor from New Orleans, who took the Cape Horn route to seek his fortune, was appalled by the extent of the disease. He claimed in 1850 that scurvy was a disease of the blood caused by a lack of sodium and potassium. He alternatively surmised that putrid food could cause the disease, thereby hinting at the 'ptomiane poisoning' theory that was to gain ground a few decades later.[7] Anthony Lorenz, the historian who studied in depth the incidence and effects of scurvy in the Californian Gold Rush, made a conservative estimate that 10,000 men died from scurvy, with half of them succumbing in the first two winters alone.[8]

* * *

The Crimean War of 1854–6 (described by the English barrister and historian Philip Guedalla in 1943 as 'one of the bad jokes of history'[9]) produced another situation in which scurvy had terrible consequences, in this case greatly exacerbated by administrative and logistical incompetence. Many British troops were in the advanced stages of scurvy even before landing at Crimea, on the northern shores of the Black Sea, and 1,600 men were admitted to military hospital with scurvy during the first winter. Military surgeons demanded better supplies of fresh food and lemon juice, but supplies failed due to transport difficulties.[10] On more than one occasion, supplies were thrown overboard because they were not dispatched to anyone in particular:

> Of 340,818lbs of vegetables stated to have been issued to the troops in November, 336,000lbs, shipped by the *Harbinger*, left the Bosphorus in a very bad state. That vessel reached Balaclava on the 9th, and lay there until the 24th of that month because the captain could get no-one to take away the cargo. In the meantime the vegetables rotted, and were either thrown overboard or scrambled for on deck.[11]

Florence Nightingale, the outspoken English nurse and hospital reformer, was enraged at the incompetence of the administrative system, comparing the obstruction that existed between the victualling officers and medical staff to that between surgeon and purser on board ship.[12] Unwholesome coffee was issued at one stage to troops in Balaclava while there was 173,000 lbs of fresh tea in store; and in one disastrous interdepartmental wrangle, twenty thousand pounds of lime juice arrived at Balaclava in early December but was not issued to the ravaged troops until February.[13] The Crimean War was the first major conflict to which journalists had uncensored access. When *The Times* began to publicise what was going on, there was a huge public and political outcry, and major improvements were brought into effect. Colonel Alexander Tulloch, the Government Commissioner appointed to enquire into the disastrous management of supply and distribution in the Crimea, was scathing in his 'Chelsea Board' report of 1857:

> It can hardly be doubted that it was the duty of the Commissary-General to keep the General Commanding informed of the supplies of every description in his possession which could be rendered available for the use of the army, and

to call his attention to the expediency, from time to time, of making such changes as they admitted. Had he done so, it might probably have brought out the fact that, while thousands were suffering from scurvy and scorbutic diarrhoea in their worst forms, 20,000 lbs weight of lime-juice were lying in his custody unused for nearly a couple of months – and that while Lord Raglan was authorising the stoppage of rice and biscuit, in the belief that there was not a sufficient quantity of either in store, Mr Fidler had, according to his own statements, abundance of both.[14]

The enquiry was equally furious with the attitude of the Commissary-General after he had been informed that scurvy was rampant and had been urged by the Quartermaster General to act promptly in obtaining fresh vegetables:

. . . he stated that it was not his duty; that according to the usage of the service vegetables were provided by regimental arrangement. Without explaining how the unhappy regiments on the plateau of Sebastopol could 'arrange' in their own behalf he made objections to purchasing potatoes which were for sale in the harbour; and in the vicinity of the market of one of the largest capitals in Europe, where vegetable diet forms a considerable proportion of the food of 650,000 inhabitants, for some months the British Army were allowed to rot of scurvy for the want of a commodity which there is little doubt he could have procured them.[15]

After supplies were properly managed, the incidence of scurvy dropped dramatically, although many British surgeons, and the official reports on the matter, repudiated the supposed efficacy of lime juice, in favour of theories of protein deficiency. It was reported that lime juice had in many cases failed to prevent or cure scurvy, whereas milk, eggs and soup rich in gelatine were more useful.[16] While the British medical situation eventually improved, that of the French Army and Navy worsened dramatically. Although better managed and supplied, the French Army was less well protected against the Crimean winter; they also blamed neighbouring marshland and bad ventilation. At one point the French Fleet in the Black Sea had 4,000 men aboard six battleships with a quarter of them down with scurvy and the possibility of vessels having to be withdrawn. At the end of the war, the French recorded a total of 23,000 scurvy cases in some of their hospitals. In March 1856 alone, there were 4,000 cases in the hospitals of Constantinople and 650 cases in field hospitals.[17]

* * *

The American Civil War of 1861–5 had dreadful consequences due to disease. Figures for the southern Confederate armies are uncertain, since the south was generally disorganised, blockaded and starving. It is recorded that in the Union armies of the north, where conditions were better, there were 47,000 cases of scurvy. Although only 7,000 deaths were directly attributed to that disease, another 45,000 deaths from dysentery and diarrhoea followed from severe scurvy.[18] There were outbreaks of scurvy throughout the entire area of military operations, and occasionally they extended in gravity to include 'night blindness'. There had been no traditional reliance on using citrus juice in the US Navy, and that lack of experience prevailed in the various armies during the war. Potatoes (raw and boiled), fresh vegetables, lemonade and occasionally molasses with any available acids constituted the main remedies. The prevailing notion of the disease in Army medicine seemed to be that it was a potassium deficiency, to be treated by the administration of suitable mineral salts. However on at least one occasion, in Massachusetts, the disease was halted by the provision of 1,500 boxes of fresh lemons.

The worst conditions were to be found in the many prisoner-of-war camps, where diseases of medieval harshness were to be found. There were dozens of camps on both sides of the conflict, holding prisoners, deserters, 'spies', bounty jumpers and even suspect civilians. They were disgusting, overcrowded, deeply unhealthy places where brutality wrought damage over and above disease and malnutrition. In one camp for Confederate prisoners in New York State, boiled rat was considered a delicacy, and the commandant regarded it as a 'waste' to give medicines to prisoners. Probably the most notorious was the Confederate camp for Union prisoners at Andersonville, Georgia, whose commandant was eventually tried for 'wanton cruelty'. He was tried before a military commission, sentenced to death, and hanged in Washington. Hundreds of men died in the camp every week, and one inmate counted 235 bodies dumped on one day alone in August 1864.[19] The mortality rate was 9 per cent per month, and three thousand men died directly of scurvy. Thirteen thousand Union prisoners died there from disease and malnutrition out of a total of 30,000 men who died in captivity in all Confederate camps. Dr John Bates, an assistant surgeon at Andersonville, spoke of his experience of scurvy:

> The effect of scurvy upon the systems of the men as it developed itself there was the next thing to rottenness. They would go on crutches sideways, or crawl upon their hands and knees or on their haunches and feet as well as they could. Some could not eat unless it was something that needed no mastication.

Bates was giving evidence in support of the prison governor, and seemed willing to put both the disease and the deaths arising from it down to the external circumstances resulting from the war:

> It seemed to me I did express my professional opinion that men died because they could not eat the rations they got.[20]

* * *

In the late 1840s, a horticultural blight broke out across Europe from Poland to France and Belgium and spread to Britain and Ireland. The primary casualties were potato crops, but the ensuing famines that engulfed some of Europe's rural areas were appalling, with death, disease, starvation and emigration in their wake. The role of the humble potato in the diet led to scurvy and other diseases erupting in cities. In Ireland, the effects were catastrophic, since most of the rural population relied heavily on potatoes in their diet. The colonial British Government refused to intervene sufficiently to prevent mass starvation, and in the next five years more than 1 million people died from typhus, cholera, scurvy and dysentery.

In Scotland and England, the effects were much less severe since the spread of dietary staples was much greater. Scurvy broke out first at Perth Prison in the winter of 1845, where 15 per cent of the population was affected; soon, it spread to Skye and the Highlands, Edinburgh, Glasgow and elsewhere. The government, perhaps conscious of the political effects of denying Ireland sufficient assistance, sent aid to the rural areas of Scotland where starvation was a greater hazard. One effect of the potato blight was to raise the price of vegetables and dairy products to levels that the poor could not afford, thereby exacerbating the initial effect of the famine. The Treasury advisor who was sent to report on the situation in the Highlands was sympathetic to the plight of the people and was very energetic in securing political and practical relief from starvation and the attendant diseases. Food depots were established and supply ships were sent to Tobermory.[21] Two of the long-term effects were rural depopulation and an increase in assisted passages to Canada and elsewhere.

In Glasgow, 122 scurvy cases had been admitted to hospital by the end of 1847 and 143 in Edinburgh. Those afflicted were mostly navvies working on railway construction who had been exposed to a poor diet.[22] Hardly anyone had dealt with the disease. The President of the Royal College of Surgeons of Edinburgh studied the outbreak. He concluded that the Perth prisoners had been used to a good diet but that, as a result of the famine, had been denied potatoes and milk, the latter item being replaced by syrup and water. His theory – not universally accepted by his peers – was that the lack of milk, together with a diet high in sugar and starch, had contributed to the incidence of scurvy.[23] There were new arguments over the observation that while many 'scorbutic diets' were low in potassium, the accepted antiscorbutic vegetables contained high levels of that mineral. New theories were on the rise again.

These examples show how scurvy maintained its horror in a range of circumstances throughout the nineteenth century. There were still others that continued the scourge until after the First World War. In 1870 the city of Paris suffered an eighteen-week siege during which there was intense food and fuel starvation and an explosion of scurvy. The outbreak appeared in contradictory circumstances and provoked an intense medical debate that continued for decades. Prisons and hospitals showed an incidence of scurvy varying from zero to 90 per cent with the most modern and well ventilated exhibiting the worst cases; idleness was blamed. At the city's military defences, on the other hand, overwork, lack of sleep and poor physical conditions were blamed. Yet again, relatively fit, well fed middle-class citizens succumbed. The cause-and-effect arguments had considerable evidential support, but were highly contradictory, and raged for years, with suggestions that scurvy was still extant in the city fourteen years later. The principal propositions in the long-running and unresolved argument were those of contagion and faulty nutrition.

* * *

In the Boer War, from 1899 to 1902, there was again a remarkable apparent contradiction in the incidence of scurvy in the concentration camps and military establishments. Most of the outbreaks actually occurred after the peace, when food restrictions had been lifted. One British Army surgeon conducted detailed research in which he analysed the situation within four population groups; the burgher concentration camps, European soldiers, African natives attached to the British

Army, and African natives attached to civilian departments. He concluded that the disease was caused not by dietary deficiencies but by lack of cleanliness.[24] At the same time, during the Russo-Japanese War of 1904–5, there was an appalling incidence of scurvy when, following the siege of Port Arthur (now the Chinese port of Lü-shun), half of the garrison of 17,000 men had the disease.[25]

On land, scurvy continued to be a problem in the First World War, with the Russian and Serbian Armies badly affected. The British Army suffered from scurvy and a number of other dietary deficiency diseases in the former Mesopotamia (Iraq).[26] Because of the massive disruption, scurvy was a considerable problem in the civilian population, especially among children. On the battlefield, there was some reliance on the use of juice squeezed from fresh vegetables – swede turnip showing some success – and germinated pulses. As we shall see, work was taking place in a number of laboratories into improving the nutrition of combatants, and it was this work that would provide the answers to the scurvy problem. For the moment, however, the practical means of coping were as precarious as ever.

Alfred Hess, a paediatrician from New York with a particular interest in infantile scurvy, published his review of the disease in 1920, and described very graphically the continuing fragility of the world's ability to deal with scurvy:

> It is important for us to realise that we are still dependent on the annual crops for our protection from scurvy; in other words, the world is leading a hand-to-mouth existence in regard to its quota of antiscorbutic food.[27]

13

'The True Antiscorbutic is Purity of Food'

IN the late nineteenth century, the treatment of scurvy at sea was still confused, with the disease continuing to erupt in circumstances where it was thought that appropriate measures had been taken. The substitution of limes for lemons resulted in there being more scurvy at the end of the century than there had been fifty years earlier. As confidence in the citrus remedy fell further, the use of alternatives increased. In the 1860s, the Admiralty's willingness to reconsider the value of beer as an antiscorbutic was taken up in practice by whaling ships and by the expeditions that began to seek out the North-West Passage, which it was hoped would provide a short route from North America to the Far East. This was the same legendary route that had entranced explorers since the time of Jacques Cartier. Since those times there had been a great reliance on various forms of 'beer'. In Cartier's case, it was one of the better performers – spruce beer; this was strictly speaking a misnomer, for the *sprossen-bier* was made with the green buds, or *sprossen*, of the fir tree. The critical factor in its efficacy was probably the necessity to pick and boil the buds very fresh. The name 'spruce beer' was often applied to beers made entirely without freshly picked *sprossen*, so it came to be that several scurvy remedies retained a specific in their names long after that element had ceased to be in use. One officer in the Arctic spoke of making spruce beer when his ship was many degrees of latitude beyond where fir or spruce could grow. What he had been drinking was sugar or malt beer flavoured with a commercial (and probably ineffective) 'essence of spruce'.[1]

'THE TRUE ANTISCORBUTIC IS PURITY OF FOOD'

The Russia Company, the Hudson's Bay Company and the North West Company in Canada all saw their economic prosperity compromised by scurvy as a result of exposure to near-Arctic conditions. Ships entering Hudson Bay itself had to travel well into northern sea-ice areas in order to reach their destinations on the southern shores. One account survives from the early seventeenth century, before the company was incorporated, of a Danish vessel in the bay attempting to penetrate ice that was 'forty fathoms deep'. Sixty-one seamen died, and only the captain and two others survived.[2] It is recorded from the company's earliest times in the seventeenth century that some lime juice was used as an antiscorbutic.[3] There was also an abundance of fresh game available, potatoes were fairly easily grown, and wild dandelions were the source of an effective antiscorbutic beer. Spruce beer was commonly used, although apparently the local speciality was to add gunpowder to boost the efficacy. There was also a local cure-all tea known as 'wishakapucka' that was employed against just about every ailment.[4]

Similarly exposed were the whalers who set out from small ports between Leith and Stromness in Orkney, bound for the icy wastes of Baffin Bay. Many of the men who sailed these ships had spent seasons working with the Hudson's Bay Company, which recruited widely in the Orkney Islands. They suffered badly from scurvy, and in the winter of 1836/7, five whalers were ice-locked for the entire winter in a disaster from which the British whaling industry never fully recovered. There had been a near-disaster in 1830, when nineteen British and one French whaling ship had been crushed. All eventually escaped, but lessons went unlearned and provisioning of these ships continued to be basic, with no allowance for such frivolities as antiscorbutics:

> The death-monster scurvy now began to harass the greater part of the men. When beef was used, the suffering was dreadful, and the salt and cold frequently caused the blood to flow. On the 18th, twenty-one men were ill of scurvy, some of them suffering most severely. To add to the misery of all on

board, the ice again gave way and threatened to squeeze every one of the vessels.[5]

That description came from the *Dee*, which suffered the deaths of forty-six men, whose bodies were sewn up in blankets and pushed through holes in the ice to a watery grave. There was considerable public outcry about the catastrophe that winter, and the government, the Admiralty and the shipowners all attacked each other over the whalers' appalling conditions. One anonymous naval surgeon vented his anger in the press:

> The owners . . . could not say that such a prevalence of disease and such a mortality was not to be expected, when they had the melancholy example before them of the fatal effects of scurvy during the preceding seasons, notoriously caused by want of nutritive food, and a total neglect of all means of cure.
>
> Did they make any change in the provisioning, so as to endeavour to preserve health in future? Did they use any precautions to prevent disease? Or did they send any better means to cure it when it did occur? No: These seem to have been matters of no moment with the gentlemen dealers in oil in the enlightened year 1837.[6]

On some polar voyages from the mid-nineteenth century, Allsopp's Pale Ale was carried in casks in considerable quantity; in addition, malt and yeast were used to brew small beer on board ship. Commercial pale ale made for export (and long life) may have already lost any antiscorbutic value before leaving port, and new 'high-tech' kiln-dried malt was certainly useless against scurvy in comparison to freshly germinated malt. Similar problems with commercial production were confirmed much later in 1918 when a study was made of scurvy in the South African Native Labour Corps stationed in France. It was recommended that, in preference to commercial beer, they should have ready access to 'kaffir beer' which the labourers produced themselves from germinated maize.[7] However, as far as the Royal Navy was concerned, there were potent traditions associated with beer, especially among men sailing in the Arctic, so it was happily adopted as the new antiscorbutic of choice, and was specifically sought even if lime juice was carried.[8]

Many surgeons took against alcohol in any form, some from a moral position and others from having seen it heavily abused at sea. Alexander Armstrong, later to become Medical Director-General of the Navy, was totally in favour of its use against scurvy:

> In every case I gave wine to as large an extent as my resources would admit, and I believe that it assisted very materially in the treatment; but I should certainly give a preference to ale or porter over wine had they been available, as I believe they are valuable auxiliaries in this disease.
>
> Beer was always relished much more than any other beverage, and in Polar Service it ought to be given as frequently as the resources of a ship will permit. Spruce beer is likewise useful, but I consider it secondary to either ale or porter. No ship going on service, where scurvy is to be apprehended, should be unprovided with the means for making these valuable beverages.[9]

When Sir John Franklin's ill-fated expedition left the Thames in May 1845 bound for the northern wastes in search of the North-West Passage, brewing equipment was carried with *Erebus* and *Terror*. The expedition was lavishly provisioned, there was sophisticated equipment for water desalination and steam heating, and both ships were strengthened against pack ice. All 128 men were fit and well-trained, and there were among them 2 experienced surgeons and 3 assistants. Confidence at the Admiralty was high to the extent of completely disregarding the value of having contingency plans in case of accident, disease or other calamity. Provisions were said to be capable of lasting for twice the planned length of the voyage, which at three years was thought to be overgenerous in any case. The expedition carried

9,300 lbs of lemon juice, as well as good supplies of onions, cranberries and preserved vegetables of various kinds.

The two ships were last seen that July north of Baffin Island, but after two years no word had been received of the expedition's fate. Any hope of mounting a desperate rescue was already far too late, but with substantial rewards offered for information, many search expeditions were despatched over the next twelve years, without any success. The subject became a *cause célèbre*, and provoked huge public interest. Many British expeditions apparently relied on lemon juice, at least to some extent, but those organised by Americans such as Henry Grinnell, had never adopted the citrus habit; they relied on beer and the old standby of potatoes and molasses, with disastrous results.[10] The US Navy surgeon, Dr Elias Kane, who had been surgeon aboard one American expedition in 1850 and commander of another in 1856, obsessively attempted to produce beer and other fermented drinks as a possible cure for scurvy. His attempts on one voyage were desperate, since there were only three men including himself who were fit enough to rise from their bunks. His efforts, however well-intentioned, were wholly out of proportion to the likely beneficial results, and the Americans were kept alive only by reasonable supplies of fresh meat.[11]

In 1850 three graves were found on Beechy Island, with wooden markers bearing the date 1846. This gave a powerful impetus to a last expedition to determine once and for all the fate of Franklin and his crew. The British Government, heavily committed to events in the Crimea, gently spurned the opportunity to promote and pay for such a venture. Lady Franklin decided to mount the expedition at her own expense, and the small steam yacht *Fox*, commanded by the Arctic veteran Captain Francis Leopold McClintock, left Stromness in the Orkney Islands in 1857. *Fox* was well supplied with the means to brew beer on board, and also 'as much of Messrs. Allsopp's stoutest ale as we could find room for.'[12] After two years of searching and establishing links with Inuit traders who had collected pathetic Franklin relics over the years, McClintock was finally successful in discovering something of the fate of Franklin and his crew. Skeletons and fragments of diaries were found on King William Island which enabled at least some of the history of the original expedition to be plotted. The ships had become ice-bound and were crushed, and Franklin and 23 others had died. The 105 survivors abandoned the ships and attempted to trek across the icy wastes, resorting in desperation to cannibalism, according to some accounts.[13] They all perished, and it was thought probable that scurvy and pneumonia were the joint causes. However modern methods of analysis produced startling new theories.

Forensic examination of remains in 1981 showed that while Inuit bones showed lead levels of 22–36 parts per million, a hair sample from a Franklin crew member gave levels in excess of 600 ppm.[14] Although tinned meat carried by the expedition had passed rigorous inspection at the Royal Clarence Yard at Deptford, it was suggested that poor lead-soldered joints had resulted in spoiling of the meat and, probably, lead poisoning. This would most likely not have been fatal in itself, but enough to have weakened the men sufficiently for scurvy and the rest to take catastrophic hold. It was a terrible irony that this new food preservation technology was what many hoped might answer the problem that had been so difficult to solve for citrus juice. The new reliance on small beer and canned meat seemed frustratingly misplaced.

Ideas again became chaotic, and occasionally exotic, and everyone seemed to be on the lookout for a new answer. James Lind's proposals for maintaining a cheerful outlook as a measure against scurvy also received new attention. Alexander Armstrong wrote in 1858:

> The promotion of hilarity and cheerfulness has always appeared to me to exercise a most salutary influence among seamen; and it has, I think, a strong preventive influence over the disease under consideration. I have always remarked what an exhilarating effect music exercises on the mind and feelings

of those within its influence, and . . . I am satisfied much good could not fail to accrue, if all ships were provided with Bands.[15]

As ever, there were some oddities. Correspondence to the *Geographical Journal* by the Norwegian arctic explorer Fridtjof Nansen in 1893 provoked a response from a Major Raverty, who recommended the use of henna *(lawsonia enermis)* against scurvy. He claimed that the well known Oriental shrub which had been used for centuries in Central Asia as a hair dye and skin decoration had been successfully used against scurvy at the siege of the town of Uk in Sijis-stán in 1227. The dye, in the form of hennotannic acid, had been accidentally ingested by a scorbutic patient, who then made a full recovery within four days.[16] The remedy (apparently also used in the treatment of jaundice, smallpox and leprosy) thereafter became a standard for the cure of scurvy in that part of the world. It was unheard of anywhere else.

The fate of the Franklin crew had fuelled wild talk of the 'real' causes of death. Suggestions that they had been poisoned by bad meat became so public and controversial that there was an official enquiry into the activities of the commercial suppliers of most of the tinned meat; they were absolved of any blame. However, the 'ptomaine poisoning' theory gained ground and was to be at the forefront of the scurvy issue for some years. The term was coined in 1870 by an Italian toxicologist, and referred to an acute gastro-intestinal illness brought about by food contaminated by natural poisons, chemical contaminants or bacteria. Chemical contamination could, in the case of tinned meat, include lead from soldered joints. Bacterial contamination could also occur due to inadequate sealing of the tins. Fridtjof Nansen was a staunch believer in this answer, and went further by claiming that ptomaine poisoning led directly to scurvy. The simple view was that eating fresh meat was good, but consuming preserved meat and lime juice was deadly. According to Nansen, if tinned meat was tainted, only the worst-affected tins should be used since the ptomaines that caused scurvy were destroyed by the fermentation established within the foul meat.

'THE TRUE ANTISCORBUTIC IS PURITY OF FOOD'

By 1900, scurvy was held to be caused by a deficiency of either potassium salts or organic salts; alternatively, reduced blood alkalinity caused by the lack of malates, citrates and lactates in the diet was the culprit.[17] The Department of Pathological Chemistry at the University of London had responded to the experiences of polar explorers by claiming in 1896 that 'scurvy is a disease due to want of proper ventilation and want of proper blood nourishment; in fact, scurvy begins with anaemia, and its great antidote is fresh blood.'[18]

Inevitably, the eternal 'state of the blood' fad regained popularity as a theme in the new rush to make sense of the scurvy issue. A new 'anti-fruitism' campaign was begun. Sir Almroth Wright (1861–1947), the bacteriologist and professor of experimental pathology at the University of London, was convinced that scurvy resulted from acid intoxication of the blood and was especially concerned to prevent the use of lime and other citrus juice in its treatment. He insisted that the only means of preventing scurvy was the regular use of fresh vegetables. In his role as Professor of Pathology at the Army Medical School at Netley, about ten miles from Haslar, Wright conducted a series of experiments on severe scurvy cases returned from the Siege of Ladysmith in February 1900. None were given vegetables, and most he treated with sodium acetate, sodium lactate or sodium bicarbonate, and he claimed substantial improvements and cure in most cases:

> . . . the proper prophylaxis and treatment of the condition would consist in the administration of salts of oxidisible organic acids, inasmuch as such treatment would lead by the most direct means to the retention or restoration of the normal alkalinity of the blood.[19]

Wright's views were held in some regard by some surgeons on polar expeditions. Dr Edward Atkinson, who travelled in the Antarctic with Scott, was known to carry out litmus tests on the blood of members of sledging parties before and after each journey. He drew blood and added dilute sulphuric acid until the point of neutrality was reached, and by comparing the results claimed to be able to identify those who were beginning a scorbutic period.[20]

A startling claim as to the cause of scurvy was made in 1911 by the medical officer of the Booth Shipping Line, who insisted that scurvy was caused by parasites living on cockroaches. He condemned the use of lime juice, and claimed, with some reason, that it had gained its supposed value simply because it was acidic.[21] Yet others, including Frederick Jackson, an experienced British Army officer and explorer, and Dr Reginald Koettlitz the senior surgeon of Scott's 1901 expedition to the Antarctic, blamed everything on the food. Both men held the view that there was no antiscorbutic value in any food or medicine, and that the only thing to be done was to ensure the absolutely total freedom from contamination of all preserved foodstuff.[22]

In 1900, Jackson collaborated with Vaughan Harley, Professor of Physiological Chemistry at the University of London in conducting experiments with monkeys on tainted meat, financed with the help of Lord Lister, President of the Royal Society. In their preamble, they stated that the efficacy of fresh vegetables and lime juice against scurvy required modification. To support this they gave several instances, some from personal experience, of expeditions or communities which had neither vegetables nor juice and, despite harsh and enduring conditions, had not suffered from scurvy. Intriguingly, they several times stated that such groups often had access to fresh bear, walrus, reindeer and other hunted meat. These meats contain a little vitamin C, and the offal somewhat more. In Inuit communities such meat formed a very large proportion of the diet, and they may have acquired sufficient vitamin C simply by reason of the volume of meat eaten. Jackson quoted one account from a visit to northeast Russia:

> Six Russian priests, whose religion forbade them to eat reindeer or other such meats but allowed them to eat salted

fish, were left in a hut by the wealthy mine-owner to pass the winter. A small Russian peasant boy was left to wait upon them. The priests lived almost exclusively on tea, bread and salted fish; the boy lived upon similar food, except that instead of the salted fish he ate reindeer meat. None of them had any vegetables. In the following May, when the Samoyads and peasant traders returned, they found that all six priests had died from scurvy, whereas the little boy who had lived upon fresh meat and not eaten salted fish was alive and well and had buried all his late masters in the snow.[23]

What the Edinburgh-trained Harley undertook in the laboratory was the second controlled clinical trial related to scurvy, 150 years after James Lind's experiments aboard HMS *Salisbury*:

> In the first the monkeys were given, daily together with boiled rice, 50 gms. of meat from a freshly-opened tin together with maize; in the second group the same food matters were given but the meat was obtained from tins which had been opened for a few days and had stood in the laboratory; in the third group the monkeys were given exactly the same diet as in group two, except that each received daily either an apple or a banana. In the first group no signs of scurvy appeared, but in the second and third symptoms showed themselves which were considered characteristic of scurvy.[24]

The conclusion, presented in very public fashion to the Royal Society by its president was that:

> ... the presence of fresh vegetables or lime-juice is not alone sufficient for the prevention or the cure of scurvy and that we must regard the condition of the food in general, and especially the state of preservation of the meat, as the <u>essential factor</u> in the etiology of the disease.[25]

The verdict was by no means widely accepted. It appealed to those who already supported the 'ptomaine poisoning' theory, but those who did not were duly excited into action in support of alternative explanations. There were suggestions from some that the monkey experiments had not been properly rigorous. Navy surgeon W. Home, who had said 'I cannot be quite certain that I have ever seen a case [of scurvy],' wrote to *The Lancet* from HMS *Minotaur* at Portland:

> ... they did not take care to administer ptomaines only, but as the 'sour-smelling meat' on which the second lot of monkeys were fed had not been sterilised, only as they say 'gently heated' the monkeys got not only ptomaines but also the living bacteria which produced the ptomaines.[26]

Home's complaint was that the experiments were so designed as to be unable to exclude the likelihood that the bacteria of putrefaction were transferred directly from the meat to the monkeys mouths. His own theory was that scurvy was:

> ... essentially an infection of the mouth with micro-organisms out of decayed food, antagonised by lime-juice and fresh vegetables which act as antiseptics.[27]

Home was very much one of the proponents of the idea that lime juice was useful principally as a mouthwash at bedtime, in much the same way that natives of hot climates lessened their symptoms by 'eating curries and chewing peppers and other "hot things" – that is, aromatic antiseptics.' His only uncertainty was why the humble potato, raw or cooked, was such a good antiscorbutic since it was no good as an antiseptic.

The potato, long revered with some justification as an antiscorbutic, was popular with polar explorers, and these were the men who were the pioneers in using it in newer preserved forms. Alexander Armstrong, surgeon on an Arctic expedition in 1850, was very much in favour of the potato against scurvy in both forms:

'THE TRUE ANTISCORBUTIC IS PURITY OF FOOD'

I have had no personal experience of its efficacy in this disease in the fresh state, but in the form of Edwards' Preserved Potatoe, as supplied to us, I can bear the most ample testimony to its excellence. It was most agreeable as an article of food, possessing all the taste and flavour of the fresh tuber, and I believe it exercised a most beneficial influence on the health of our crew, and I can also affirm that it was universally better liked than any other vegetable with which we were supplied.[28]

In 1902, the retired naval surgeon Dr Alexander Turnbull was impressed by the fact that Nansen's expedition of 1893–6 had been wholly free of scurvy:

... has not Nansen, acting under the direction of Professor Torup, of Christiania, established a 'proper antiscorbutic diet' by the scrupulous care with which the provisions of the *Fram* were selected and prepared, by sterilising even in some cases? I submit that he has.[29]

Turnbull insisted that:

From the time of Woodall (1636), Lind, Trotter, and Blane lemon or lime juice has been erroneously accepted as a certain curative of scurvy, and not as only a remedy for the disease, which cannot be questioned.[30]

He explained the improvement in seamen's health by better regulations and victualling; the Merchant Shipping Act of 1867; and the decline in sailing vessels and the increase in steam propulsion, both of which produced faster, shorter voyages. Nansen's men had shot large amounts of game, and had relied on that and purely 'medicinal' versions of lime juice. For two winters, they had been away from their ship with only four months' supplies and some lime tablets as medicine:

For about a year they were dependent on their rifles for food – bear, walrus and bird meat only. Not only did they not suffer from scurvy, but at the end of the time on arrival at . . . San Josef Land, they were in robust health, and had gained a stone in weight since leaving the *Fram*.[31]

Turnbull contrasted another expedition which had become ice-bound in the same latitudes:

. . . trusting to the daily ration of 'lime-juice' fresh and unconcentrated, administered under Dr Koettlitz's supervision to act as an antiscorbutic – according to the Merchant Shipping Act – [they] refused the bear meat, which they termed 'scran', and lived on the ship's salt and preserved meats. They all suffered from scurvy and two died of the disease.[32]

Turnbull was adamant in condemning both lemon juice and lime juice: 'I submit the true antiscorbutic is purity of food.' This aspiration was entirely desirable from the general nutritional and health points of view, but in relation to scurvy belonged with some of the medieval notions.

Further momentous polar expeditions took place, with varying success – medical and otherwise. Robert Falcon Scott led an expedition to the Antarctic in 1901–4 during which lime juice was carried but hardly used, since it was now regarded with disfavour, the 'ptomaine poisoning' theory being now in vogue. Their preserved vegetables and fruit were deficient and probably overcooked, and sledging parties were badly affected by scurvy. One of the worst sufferers was Ernest Shackleton, who had to return home in a relief ship. At the time scurvy broke out, major parts of the diet had been tinned, and in panic the use of tinned food was stopped. The surgeon wisely increased rations of fruit and lime juice, and greater reliance was placed on seal meat and other game, which Scott had originally refused to allow to be killed on the grounds of cruelty.

'THE TRUE ANTISCORBUTIC IS PURITY OF FOOD'

Shackleton led another Antarctic expedition from 1907–9 which was largely unaffected by scurvy. This may have been due to the crews being in better initial health and having improved nutrition. There was much greater consumption of seal and penguin meat, and sledge parties also benefited from pony meat, all of which provided some vitamin C.

Scott led the famously disastrous Antarctic expedition of 1910–13. Again, lime juice was deprecated, although the expedition had the advantage of better supplies of tinned foods, including for the first time tinned tomatoes, which are high in vitamin C. Scurvy was a considerable problem on sledging parties, but in terms of the total extent of the catastrophe, it was as nothing. The entire party died from lack of food, frostbite and exposure and severe scurvy was almost certainly an additional factor.

By the time of Shackleton's next and heroic Antarctic expedition of 1914–17, ideas about scurvy had shifted a little. The notions of 'ptomaine poisoning' had been abandoned in favour of the old certainty that the disease was some form of dietary deficiency. Improvements had been made in the manufacture of some of the potential antiscorbutics. Tinned foodstuffs had improved steadily. Dried milk, which was a good source of vitamins including a little vitamin C, was available, and lime juice, while distrusted when produced by the older techniques involving boiling, was being concentrated using new vacuum procedures. The juice was supplied in small sealed 'one-per-day' capsules which were easily carried and used, and avoided the earlier spoiling.

Shackleton and his 28-man party aboard *Endurance* aimed to make the first crossing of Antarctica. But their ship was crushed by pack ice in the Weddell Sea, losing most of the stores, including antiscorbutics. The party was stranded for months on an ice floe; they sailed in an open boat to Elephant Island, where most remained while a small group continued across the Southern Ocean to South Georgia. After traversing the island, Shackleton sailed back to Elephant Island to rescue his main party. It was a truly remarkable story of human survival in the most awful of conditions.

LIMEYS

By the beginning of the First World War, the lack of confidence in the remedy for scurvy was such that the situation equated to that of 150 years earlier. Personal theories were promoted; exotic ideas were attempted; old ideas were dusted off and reinvented, and the blunderbuss technique of trying every available 'remedy' was resorted to yet again. Crews put to sea or ventured on to the ice with no clear expectation of relief.

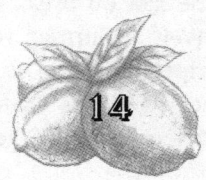

'A Sufficient Explanation of the Anomaly'

BY the early twentieth century, the citrus remedy was widely regarded as wholly unreliable. The uncertainty and disagreement were as great as they had been three centuries earlier, when John Woodall said that 'the causes of this disease are so infinite as they farre pass my capacity to search them all out'.

There were many who held prejudiced opinions on the issue, but others insisted on being more open to investigation. A surgeon working with the Royal Army Medical Corps in the Transvaal during the Boer War had produced an analysis of a bad outbreak of scurvy in a prisoner-of-war camp. He pointed out that he had no particular previous interest in scurvy, and had approached his experience with an open mind – a condition which he pleaded his peers would adopt in hearing his account. He concluded:

> . . . the condition known as scurvy in adults is not brought about by the absence of any particular kind of food from the dietary but is more probably a specific infection of bacterial origin.[1]

In the Royal Navy, where conditions in general and victualling in particular were improving dramatically, only three cases of scurvy were reported during the entire period of the First World War. The surgeon who made that report had noted that in the Navy, the use of lime juice had been regarded as useless for the previous two decades.[2]

What is regarded as the last outbreak of serious scurvy at sea was in 1917 aboard the *Wolf*, a German Navy vessel patrolling in the South Atlantic. Descriptions of the eruption of scurvy on that vessel, appearing in *The Cruise of the Raider Wolf*, are a match for anything that Jacques Cartier wrote 400 years earlier:

> Some went blind . . . And they stank: their sores stank. The unfortunate wretches were simply rotting alive . . . None of us had seen scurvy before, and the old sea tales of this disease had seemed ridiculously exaggerated. But the foul symptoms of a serious outbreak of scurvy could never be overdrawn. This curse is an unholy combination of all the worst features of dysentery, syphilis and dropsy.[3]

The year after the dreadful incidents aboard the *Wolf*, an investigation into 'the antiscorbutic principle in limes and lemons' was mounted at the Lister Institute of Preventive Medicine in London. As part of its work on military nutrition, the institute had conducted a series of investigations into the antiscorbutic properties of various foodstuffs over the previous two years. They stated their starting point in the new inquiry:

> Scurvy, in accordance with the view of ancient tradition, has been shown to be a deficiency disease, occasioned by absence in the diet of an unknown accessory food factor, or 'vitamine'. This factor is present in living vegetable and animal tissues, in largest amounts in fresh fruits and green vegetables, to a less extent in root vegetables and tubers. It is present in small amount in fresh meat and milk, and has not been detected in yeast, fats, cereals, pulses. The antiscurvy food factor is sensitive to high temperatures and suffers destruction when the living tissues in connection with which it is produced are disorganised by drying and other methods of preservation.[4]

'A SUFFICIENT EXPLANATION OF THE ANOMALY'

The experimental inquiry was undertaken by Hariette Chick, Margaret Hume and Ruth Skelton, with a vital historical inquiry by Alice Henderson Smith. They wrote:

> . . . the literature upon this subject appearing in the 18th and early 19th century is full of the praises of 'lime juice' and there appears to be every reason for believing that the use of so-called lime juice was responsible for the disappearance of scurvy from the British Navy in the first decade of the 19th century.[5]

However, they recognised there had been a change in attitude to lime juice in recent years, both in the Navy and in polar expeditions. The records of two polar voyages provided startling evidence for the lack of success of lime juice.

In January 1850 HMS *Investigator*, commanded by Captain Robert McClure, had left England and entered the ice the following summer. The Irish-born McClure was one of the great Arctic explorers; he later received an award from Parliament, and was promoted to admiral and knighted, for discovering the North-West Passage. This was yet another expedition in search of Franklin. *Investigator* had returned from Arctic waters the previous year after a search led by Sir James Clark Ross. Scurvy had been a serious problem, and the quality of the lemon juice had been suspect. For McClure, steps were taken to ensure improved quality of the fresh fruit, and to amend the methods of production of the juice, which it was decreed should in future be undertaken by the Navy at Deptford Dockyard.[6] Alexander Armstrong was the surgeon on board ship, and although he recognised that scurvy was by then unusual in the Navy, he was aware that polar expeditions appeared to be susceptible. He was a strong believer in the use of lemon juice:

> Lemon juice is in my opinion the sovereign remedy in the treatment of this disease, where fresh fruits and vegetables are not available. I have never seen it fail in any form of the disease, when I could command an unlimited supply of it.[7]

He ensured that the expedition was well supplied with lemon juice squeezed and prepared under rigorous new supervision at Deptford:

> The lemon juice with which we were supplied was of the most excellent quality, and consisted of two kinds, one of which was prepared by adding a tenth part of brandy, and the other was the acid simply boiled, and containing no spirit. The juice was kept in bottles, each containing 64 fl. ozs., with a stratum of olive oil, about half an inch in thickness, on its surface, and the bottles were carefully corked and sealed.
>
> Previous to my departure, I received instructions from the then Director-General of the navy to adopt whatever means might seem to me most judicious, whereby I might be able to report on the relative merits of the two kinds of acids, and their efficacy as antiscorbutic agents.[8]

The second version should have been less effective, due to vitamin C destruction by heat, but Armstrong did not distinguish one as being therapeutically preferable to the other. Since the boiled version deposited a cloudy sediment he chose the fortified one. He did not note the fact that the fortified version froze at a lower temperature. His intention was that one ounce of the juice be issued daily to each man individually, to be drunk in view of an officer. He had some of the juice tested after the expedition, and was emphatic in his belief of its efficacy:

> The lemon juice on board the *Investigator* was subject to every possible vicissitude of temperature from the highest degree of Equatorial heat, to the lowest of Polar cold, being under the influence of the latter for upwards of three years; and when I examined it at the end of this period, I found it as good and pure as on the day we left England, and its power of neutralising alkalis was not in the slightest degree impaired.[9]

'A SUFFICIENT EXPLANATION OF THE ANOMALY'

Armstrong was diligent in his intentions and forthright in ensuring that they were adhered to in practice. However, given the history, and the comparison with a later expedition of 1875, and the analysis of both voyages that would be undertaken in 1918, it is interesting and frustrating to witness Armstrong's confusion or disregard. In both his own written accounts and in his evidence to the later official enquiry, he constantly falls into the habit of using the terms 'lemon juice' and 'lime juice' indiscriminately, as if they were identical. Indeed, in the space of two sentences in his 1858 book, he uses both terms:

> I have already alluded to the mode in which lemon-juice should be given, and I have mentioned the good results which attended the mode adopted in the *Investigator*. I would again strongly urge that the same practice should be strictly carried out on board all ships, whenever the exhibition of lime-juice becomes necessary during a voyage.[10]

In his official log of the 1850 expedition, Armstrong gives medical and surgical details on individuals, and extensive general medical reports; there are also detailed meteorological reports and descriptions of the physical landscape and natural history.[11] Although from his personal account it appears uncertain whether he means lemon or lime juice, victualling records suggest that the McClure expedition was supplied with lemon juice.

Investigator sailed round Cape Horn, to Honolulu, up the American coastline and along the north coast of Alaska until, in October, she became ice-bound in Prince of Wales Strait, having failed in the secondary objective of finding a North-West Passage. Hunting parties shot considerable quantities of game, and scurvy grass was gathered, activities that were to make invaluable additions to the otherwise well-provisioned expedition. Throughout the winter and spring of 1851, when sledging parties were active, there was not a single case of scurvy. In the autumn, food rations were reduced by one third as it became clear that they would remain ice-bound for another winter. Only in the summer of 1852 did a case of scurvy occur, after being away from home for twenty-seven months and on reduced rations for seven months. Soon after, however, the ration of lemon juice had to be reduced, and by the end of the third winter it was issued only to those most at risk. In May 1853, Armstrong informed McClure that the health of the crew:

> . . . is such as renders them utterly unfit to undergo the rigours of another winter. There exists in all of them at present well-marked evidence of scurvy and debility in various stages of development.[12]

It was not until August 1853 that the crew was rescued by a party from HMS *Resolute*, which was searching for evidence of Franklin further east. In one sense, by making the trek across the ice to reach *Resolute* and *Intrepid*, McClure's party completed a North-West Passage, although the sea route did not become a reality until 1906, when it was discovered by Amundsen. (Ironically, this centuries-old holy grail of sailors and explorers may become a political and commercial confrontation zone in the next ten years as new sea routes emerge due to global warming.) McClure's expedition spent four winters and five summers on the ice, and during that period of the most severe conditions and deprivation there were only three deaths from scurvy, which all occurred at the end of their ordeal and just before rescue arrived. The determination to make the best possible use of lemon juice was regarded as the main reason for that successful outcome. The experiences on board the *Investigator* were found on later inquiry to be matched by those of other expeditions of the period that had been supplied with lemon juice from Deptford.

Little more than twenty years later, in May 1875, HMS *Alert* and HMS *Discovery* sailed with 122 men under the command of Sir George Nares, intending to reach the North Pole via Smith Sound. There was no expectation that scurvy would be a problem. The 1850 McClure expedition had been well-provisioned, and if anything Nares' ships were even better supplied in terms of diet. Alexander Armstrong was now Sir Alexander, and Medical Director-General of the Navy. In written instructions of 30 April 1875 he insisted that lemon juice be issued to *Alert* and *Discovery* in exactly the manner that had been used for *Investigator* twenty-five years earlier; in addition, he instructed that lemon juice be sent with the sledging parties. Three paragraphs from his official instructions are significant:

> I attach the greatest possible importance to the daily administration of lemon juice, to commence on the day after the fresh vegetables cease on leaving England, but this must be carried out on the most rigid principles, on which it was, without one day's interruption carried out on board the *Investigator*, on my representation, of its absolute necessity, *viz.*, by having the aggregate allowance of acid, one ounce per man, with a proportionate quantity of sugar and water, mixed in a tub and drank on deck in the presence of the officer of the watch.
>
> I cannot overrate the importance I attach to the importance of a similar course in the present expedition, and would urge its being carried out in the strictest manner. By doing so there will be positive evidence that every man in the ship is fortified with an antiscorbutic agent of undoubted efficacy; whereas in the course usually adopted of sending the lemon juice to the several messes for consumption, there is no evidence whatever of any man taking it, and so valuable an agent should not be left to the whim or caprice of individuals, but rigidly enforced as an element of their safety.
>
> The use of lemon juice when travelling should be enforced in the same manner as already recommended for the men on board the ship.[13]

Armstrong may have been thwarted or deceived, or he may himself have been heedless, because what was issued as lemon juice was actually West Indian lime juice, supplied by Evans of

Liverpool, bottled with the addition of 10 per cent rum. Although Armstrong specified lemon juice, at no point did he specifically reject lime juice. The easy and incompetent conflation of the two fruits was still not recognised as a disastrous problem. *Alert* was issued with 4,240 lbs and returned 1,012 lbs, and *Discovery* had 3,960 lbs and returned 1,290 lbs to stores.[14]

It was intended that the two ships should make winter in Northern Greenland not more than 200 miles apart. Stores were to be laid during the north-bound voyage, with a view to providing a possible line of retreat in emergency. Lengthy sledging expeditions were to penetrate further northwards from the ships' winter bases in the spring. The official records of provisions, special clothing, medicines and drugs supplied to the expedition (and later returned to stores as surplus) which were printed in the report of the government inquiry show that both ships were extremely well supplied. In addition, live sheep were carried for slaughter, and hunting parties provided puffin, guillemot, arctic hare, eider duck, geese and musk oxen. The winter station of *Alert* was a much worse one from which to hunt than that of *Discovery*, and the former was consequently less well supplied with fresh meat. To all intents and purposes, both the 1850 and 1875 expeditions were provisioned to similar standards. However, when Sir Alexander Armstrong was questioned about this in the 1877 enquiry, he was adamant that the 1850 expedition was better victualled in every respect. Of the 1875 Nares expedition he said:

> The quantity of meat was three-quarters of a pound; the vegetables, which were only of two kinds, potatoes and carrots, were also less, and the diet in all other respects regarding the issue of antiscorbutic articles of food was very much inferior.[15]

There were modest sledging expeditions carried out before the winter of 1875, and these trips resulted in considerable frostbite, leading to several amputations. In all affected cases, healing was

'A SUFFICIENT EXPLANATION OF THE ANOMALY'

extremely slow. The following April, long sledge journeys were undertaken in three different directions. These were arduous, heavily laden treks which lasted from two to three months, and placed the men under great stress and physical exertion. Sledging rations were entirely lacking in any vitamin C content, and lime juice was carried in small quantities solely for placing in depots rather than for consumption. Almost immediately, several men had to be returned to ship with early signs of scurvy, and soon there were fourteen men on board ship with the disease.

Nares countermanded Armstrong's instructions for the supply of lime juice to the sledging parties. The reasons for that decision were that the weight of the juice would be prohibitive; it would freeze; and the weight of the fuel required to melt the juice and the accompanying water for its consumption would further add to the weight problem. Every item carried on a sledge had to earn its place, but Nares' decision was to prove fatal. Fleet Surgeon Thomas Colan recorded in his journal his own worries, based on experience, that items such as lime juice, pickles, preserved fruits, vinegar and beer would freeze if they were landed for the use of sledge parties, or for emergency stores. He concluded of lime juice, 'It would not be for want of greater ease in issuing this acid, that any evil would result.'[16] On 16 October 1875, a reduced scale of victualling was introduced, although the level of lime juice and sugar aboard ship was maintained at one ounce per man per day. Surgeon Colan gave an account of the victualling from then onwards in his journal:

> Under this scale preserved meat was issued every second day at the rate of 1lb per man per diem, and soft bread was given three days out of four, instead of two days as formerly. On the 26th October 1875 half a gill of spirit was issued in the evening throughout the winter except on beer days. On the 7th October 1875 the rations of rhubarb and gooseberries were increased from two to six ounces. From the 4th March until the 3rd April 1876 an extra allowance of lime juice was issued to those who wished to have it; forty men and thirteen officers

took advantage of this offer. Fruit was issued daily after clearing the ice on the 8th September until arrival in England. On the return of sledge parties to the ship, in general each man received an extra ration of beer, lime-juice, coffee and preserved meats for from two to five days.[17]

Three sledge parties set out in early April. The Eastern Sledge Party under Lieutenant Beaumont comprised two crews of eight men with two five-man sledges in support; it averaged six miles per day in terrible conditions under which there was a severe breakdown in health as scurvy took a hold. Two months later the position was desperate, with men prostrate on the sledge and others able only to crawl for twenty yards at a time before lying down. The main party met up with support sledges at Polaris Bay, where two men died, two others were desperately ill and all others were affected by scurvy. Luckily, there were at that depot two 32-gallon casks of lime juice that had been left by a US expedition three years earlier; an experienced local Inuit hunter also kept the men well supplied with fresh meat.[18] Sledging was abandoned, and after a slow partial recovery, the survivors made an arduous trek across moving sea ice back to the *Discovery*.

A Northern Party under Commander Albert Markham of the *Alert* fared even worse. One man died of scurvy, five more were incapacitated on the sledge and the party was only saved because Lieutenant Parr trekked thirty-five miles alone to the *Alert* to raise the alarm and bring out a rescue party with emergency lime juice. Markham has been criticised for obsessively continuing as ordered, to get further north than anyone ever before, rather than turning back to safety.[19] The Western Party of Lieutenant Aldrich suffered severe scurvy but lost no men. By the time the sledging parties were safe on board ship forty out of sixty-two from *Alert* and twenty out of sixty from *Discovery* had severe scurvy. In June, Captain Nares had only nine men in good health, and the inevitable decision was made that the entire expedition would have to be abandoned a year early.

Although the public was encouraged to regard the expedition

as having been a great national event, and the Admiralty sent a letter of warm congratulations to Nares, Parliament set up an official Committee of Enquiry into the debacle in January 1877. The chairman of what became known as the British Scurvy Commission was Admiral Sir James Hope; he sat with Admiral Sir Richard Collinson, Vice-Admiral Edward Inglefield, Dr James Donnett the Inspector-General of RN Hospitals and Fleets and Dr Thomas Fraser. After what must have been a prodigious effort, involving the analysis of extensive written and oral evidence, including over 10,000 direct questions and answers, the committee produced a detailed 400-page report after only two months. Some of the issues dealt with in great depth were the provision of food (especially the quantity and quality of meat and vegetables); the supply of lime juice; ventilation and heating aboard ship; the effects of the lack of daylight; work rates for sledge parties, and exercise on board the two ships. There was constant comparison with the 1850 McClure expedition.

The two medical men on the committee submitted a 25-page paper on scurvy in which they speculated, somewhat hesitantly, on the cause of scurvy:

> The evidence is all but unanimous that the want of fresh vegetable food, or of some of the constituents that compose fresh vegetable, and probably also fresh animal food is the cause of scurvy.[20]

They noted the fact that since lemon juice was introduced in 1795, scurvy, which had been the scourge of the Navy, had become virtually extinct. They confirmed that the most valuable agents in the prevention and treatment of scurvy were fruits such as the orange, lemon and lime, and that was clearly still the official view:

> ... lemon or lime juice is generally used in Merchant Ships and in the Navy during Polar Service in a ration of one ounce daily, and it is found effectual in this quantity, even during the

existence of many conditions favourable to the development of the disease.[21]

Despite this strong continuing commitment to the value of lime juice, there was a willingness to admit that no-one knew quite what conferred the efficacy:

> Although there is no difference of opinion as to lime juice being the best of all known antiscorbutics, when vegetable food is absent or deficient in quantity, it has not yet been decided upon which of its constituents this valuable property depends.[22]

The constituents identified were citric acid, malic acid, tartaric acid, sugar, vegetable albumen, mucus, mineral substances and 80–90 per cent water. The predominating citric acid was thought likely to be the valuable ingredient, but, 'this supposition has not yet been satisfactorily proved'.

Experiments into the best form of concentrated lime juice were conducted for the Committee by John Bell and Company of Oxford Street, London. The crucial point was to find out which form would withstand freezing, and it was found that a version to which glycerine had been added was the most encouraging. The production of solid lozenges and impregnated biscuits was also investigated. Joseph Cooper of London had patented a method of producing lozenges, and had prepared lime in that form for Dr John MacDonald, the Deputy Inspector-General of Hospitals and Fleets. Four such tablets were the equivalent of the daily ration of juice, and their advantage was their small bulk, portability and freedom from spoiling.[23] Alexander Armstrong was in favour of such lozenges, but would accept no alternative to lime juice until their efficacy had been proven. On the same basis, he was also in favour of the impregnation of pemmican with lime juice. The question of the propensity of lime juice to freeze was settled with discussion of the fact that the two 32-gallon casks discovered at Polaris Bay by the Eastern

Sledging Party had been buried in snow and ice for five years, 'and was found at the end of that time to possess most marked antiscorbutic properties.' Armstrong regarded this incident as a significant vindication of his strong views in favour of lime juice.

Witnesses were questioned on what the essential antiscorbutic factor in lime juice might be. Most opinion was that it was citric acid, and it was stated that in some cases a separated form of citric acid had been used instead of the juice. However, it had generally been found to be less efficacious than natural, or concentrated lime juice, which was still the prime choice. Armstrong had written after the 1850 expedition:

> I have treated and cured the disease with the pure citric acid, exhibiting it in the same manner as the lemon juice, and in proportionate quantity (estimated from the relative power of the two in neutralising alkalis), but in no instance was the remedial power of the acid equal to that of the lemon juice. But as a preventative or curative agent in this disease, I know none so well adapted to occupy a second place as citric acid.[24]

Only one witness, Dr Coppinger of the *Discovery*, offered any argument against the efficacy of lime juice. While he regarded it generally as an excellent prophylactic, he gave several instances in which he had used it liberally to treat scorbutic men to no good effect. There was no discussion of the fact that lime juice had been used instead of lemon juice, or of what possible difference that might have made. The Committee declared that:

> The fully established value of lime-juice and the conveniences attending its use render it greatly superior to all other suggested antiscorbutic remedies.[25]

There was some argument about whether Armstrong's recommendations on lime juice, which had been requested by the Admiralty, constituted an official order. However, it was accepted that they were referred to in the official Sailing Orders signed by the Admiralty Secretary, and therefore carried mandatory status. Armstrong, furious that his orders had been ignored on Nares' expedition, had written to the committee in November 1876 saying:

> I considered this departure from instructions so grave and unaccountable that I called on the Senior Medical Officers of the *Alert* and *Discovery* respectively for an explanation of the omission of this most valuable antiscorbutic agent from the daily diet of the sledge parties.[26]

The same month, Sir George Nares wrote to the committee from Winchester,

> Doctor Colan was always very particular in representing the advantages of a continuous supply of lime juice. I alone am responsible for the sledge crews not being supplied with it.[27]

The main conclusion of the Committee of Enquiry was that the cause of the scurvy was attributed to the fact that the sledging parties had not been supplied with lime juice. They blamed Nares for issuing improper provisioning orders; in particular he was culpable of ignoring the orders on lime juice given to him by the Admiralty from Armstrong. There were other deficiencies identified relating to the lack of fresh meat and the deployment of depots, but it was clear that they saw the principal cause of the disaster as the lack of antiscorbutics, although there was the usual uncertainty about what the 'antiscorbutic factor' might be.

There was an outcry of objection from certain quarters. *The Times* supported the Committee of Enquiry's findings, and accused Nares of 'a lamentable failure of judgement'. However, it printed letters from Dr Black of Bart's Hospital, and two Arctic-experienced admirals, suggesting the true cause of scurvy was the lack of adequate fresh meat and vegetables. Black was a proponent of the idea, which was gaining some ground among polar experts, that the Inuit diet, which was rich in blubber and reindeer meat, was the best remedy for scurvy.[28] Rear-Admiral Richards, who had given evidence to the committee, rapidly produced a pamphlet on the matter in which he condemned the outcome and quoted several cases, anecdotes and unattributed opinion as to the uselessness of lime juice. He also claimed that lime juice had not been given by McClure to sledging parties on the 1850 expedition since McClure had regarded it highly and would not spare it from the ship.[29]

The man who led the Northern Sledging Party, Commander Markham, had a cousin who was Secretary of the Royal Geographical Society. Sir Clements Markham published a bitter pamphlet in 1877 refuting the views of the Enquiry and claiming that lime juice was useless against scurvy. On the first page, he described the 400-page report, with its analyses and verbatim evidence from all the witnesses, as 'meagre in the extreme'. He complained that there were not enough 'Old Arctic Officers' examined as witnesses, and condemned the fact that there were too many 'Medical Men who have not seen Arctic service'. He stated again and again that no other expedition had ever used lime juice for sledging parties, and detailed his view of how the committee had misunderstood the outbreaks of scurvy:

> ... the Autumn sledge parties took no lime juice and had no sign of scurvy; most of the officers, during the spring travelling, had no scurvy, although they never touched lime juice; while the men who were attacked in the spring were the same men who were exempt in the autumn. This is a proof that the outbreak was not caused by the absence of lime juice. Further, there were nine cases of men being attacked on board while taking lime juice regularly, and two cases during the sledge travelling with lime juice rations.[30]

Markham went on to say that 'it must not be supposed that the medical profession is agreed either upon the cause or cure of scurvy.' He noted a list of eminent medical men who had views on what some of these 'other causes' of scurvy, such as mineral deficiency, cold, fatigue, etc., might be. He complained that none of these men had been called to give evidence, and noted for good measure that, 'In the United States the use of lime juice as an antiscorbutic is utterly scorned, and it is not used in the American mercantile marine.[31]

In his book written in 1858, Armstrong had been scathing about some of the alternative theories:

> With regard to the opinions that have been advanced by some writers, that scurvy is caused by a deficiency of one or more of the mineral constituents of the blood, such as sulphur, phosphorus, lime, etc, it is unnecessary here to notice such a theory, further than to state that it is entirely unsupported by any trustworthy evidence to warrant such a conclusion. No refutation of this opinion is necessary, except in stating that by supplying those substances (phosphorus or sulphur) in proportions corresponding to the deficiency existing in the blood, we shall utterly fail in curing the disease.[32]

Markham's final assault on the committee's report took the form of a bitter personal attack on Sir Alexander Armstrong in which Markham essentially blamed him for the scurvy fiasco. He claimed that Armstrong's recommendations for the use of lemon juice did not constitute official orders, and that his reference to the enforcement of lemon juice on sledging parties was 'a mere slipshod hint'. Markham made much of this, and claimed with irrational hypercriticality that men on the sledge parties could not possibly have taken the lime juice 'in the same manner as the men on board ship' since the men on board ship were instructed to drink it 'on deck in the presence of the officer of the watch'. Markham insisted that Armstrong

> . . . knew, or ought to have known, that frozen lime juice in bottles could not be used. He confesses that it could not have been eaten in a frozen state. He has since suggested that it

might have been mixed with pemmican. But it is too late to make suggestions now. He ought to have explained the means of meeting all these difficulties before the expedition sailed, if he attached so much importance to it. In not doing so he is answerable for the consequences.[33]

Three years later Commander Markham (described elsewhere as being a moody, irritable and defensive character) published his own account of these events, in which he rather desperately blustered his way to a justification of events by recalling the Admiralty's letter of congratulations to Nares:

> ... the Lords of the Admiralty were pleased to express their satisfaction at the manner in which the expedition had been conducted by our leader.[34]

This extraordinary end to the 1875 expedition was to prove a remarkable catalyst. It was quickly observed by the researchers at the Lister Institute in 1918 that the inquiry had failed to recognise that the 1850 expedition had been supplied with Mediterranean lemon juice, and the Nares expedition with West Indian lime juice. This strong clue was followed up with diligence when the Lister team began work on antiscorbutics.

The laboratory work started after a range of samples of crude and preserved juices from fruit grown in various parts of the world had been prepared by L. Rose & Company, who also kept the laboratory regularly supplied with fresh fruit. The researchers recorded that, 'without this assistance the research would have been impossible.' After evaluating the various fresh, crude and preserved juices, experiments began with guinea pigs, which were fed a range of diets including one or other of four principal preserved lime juices. There were two purified juices of West Indian limes preserved with 14 per cent rum, one with no preservative, and a fourth preserved with salicylic acid and alcohol. Similar experiments were carried out on preparations of lemon juice, and the results analysed. The next stage involved the designing of a similar series of experiments, this time using monkeys:

> ... with young, growing monkeys, of 2,000–3,500 grammes weight, daily rations varying from 2.5 ccs–10 ccs of lemon juice never failed to prevent scurvy over periods of time as long as 4 to 7 months. The animals were in excellent health and spirits, and grew in a normal manner.[35]

However, using a range of lime juice preparations both the final analysis and the general state of health of the animals were distinctly inferior. Daily rations of 5 ccs resulted, in every case, in scurvy of a serious degree. In one case where the ration was 10 ccs, the animal died of the disease. The monkey results confirmed those using guinea pigs; the value of fresh lemon juice was four times that of fresh lime juice.

In parallel with the clinical experiments, the available Admiralty and other records were examined, from the earliest times until the McClure and Nares expeditions in particular:

> ... by comparing the experience of the ships provided with the pure lemon juice in 1850 with that of the first Arctic expedition that took out West Indian lime-juice we get a very satisfactory human experiment, demonstrating the relative value of the two fruits. The setting of the comparison is made more precise than is generally to be looked for in historical evidence.
>
> The two expeditions were so near to one another in time that the general conditions of diet etc, were very similar; but the later one did enjoy certain improvements of diet suggested by accumulated experience, including double vegetable and fruit rations, additional meat, sugar, etc., and a reduction in the amount of alcohol allowed.[36]

The researchers considered that the details of the two expeditions could hardly have been better arranged for the purposes of comparison. It was felt that what differences there were should have favoured the Nares expedition. Yet the historical comparisons, when analysed along with the clinical experimental work, were not only clear but emphatic. Fresh lime juice possessed about a quarter of the potency available in the same volume of fresh lemon juice. Preserved lime juice as a preventative of scurvy was proved to be useless. The confusion that began at the beginning of the nineteenth century and produced the eventual suspicion of the efficacy of lime juice was at last rationalised:

> A sufficient explanation of the anomaly will be found to lie in the fact that at this early date the term 'lime-juice' included the juice of lemons from the Mediterranean, whereas for the last 50 or 60 years it has been applied to the preserved juice of the West Indian lime.[37]

It seems incredible that it took almost a century for anyone to realise that two different fruits were involved in the confusion. However, the final step in the long trek to the end of the scurvy story was about to be taken. The identification of the 'vitamine', the mysterious *je ne sais quoi* of Lieutenant Saumarez during Anson's circumnavigation was at last in sight.

Other chemists were still trying to develop a method of providing 'an efficient, portable, and palatable antiscorbutic'. Surgeon-Admiral Bassett-Smith was working at the Royal Naval College in Greenwich using guinea pigs, and paying close attention to developments at the Lister Institute. Others had been attempting to produce a viable dried orange juice made in the same manner as dried milk by mixing the juice with corn syrup and injecting the mixture as a fine spray into a heated chamber. However, this method appeared to suffer as a result of using heat during the process.[38] Bassett-Smith himself had tried evaporation, de-acidification, impregnation on filter paper and rapid drying. He finally decided on a solid lozenge made with lemon juice. These lozenges were produced by evaporation of the juice in a vacuum with sulphuric acid, and the resulting syrup converted to a stiff paste with various gums. The process, which Bassett-Smith described as being 'similar to that used for the preparation of Nestlé's condensed sweetened milk' took five days, and each lozenge contained the equivalent of 24ccs of lemon juice.[39] He stated that the tablets kept well for over twelve months, and continued to be effective when used on experimental guinea pigs. He also claimed that separate experiments with tinned tomatoes, both as a cure and a preventative of scurvy, had been successfully carried out on the animals.[40]

By 1920, the laboratory work which would identify the mysterious factor that conveyed antiscorbutic protection was almost complete. In the early 1900s Axel Holst, professor of hygiene at Oslo's University of Christiania in Norway, had worked on the deficiency disease beriberi. In collaboration with a paediatrician, Dr Theodor Frölich, who had an interest in infantile scurvy, he discovered an anomaly in the reactions of guinea pigs to the course of dietary experiments. To their surprise, the animals appeared to show the effects of scurvy. There were three prevailing theories then underlying ideas of the disease; infection, toxification and faulty diet. They proposed that only the latter condition could apply, and devised an extended series of dietary experiments.[41] They discovered that some foods could prevent scurvy, while at the same time losing their efficacy when heated. This was nothing new, except that they were discovering and testing the extended theories by experiment, precisely as Lind had done in a more elementary way 160 years earlier.

In 1907, Holst and Frölich published results of further experiments which appeared to prove conclusively that scurvy was caused by diet and could be cured by diet. Their results in relation to scurvy were similar to what they had learned about beriberi. Both were now known with certainty to be dietary deficiency diseases which were caused by the lack of still unknown substances. Despite these significant steps forward, Holst and Frölich's work was ended in 1913 by lack of funding, and possibly by the hostility of Host's superiors, who adhered to the ideas of ptomaine poisoning.[42]

The previous year, Casimir Funk, a Polish chemist at the Lister Institute, devised the term 'vitamine' for the unknown substances. He identified four dietary deficiency diseases: scurvy, beriberi, pellagra and rickets, each of which he proposed was caused by a discrete factor in the diet, a 'vital amine' or compound of nitrogen. By the end of the First World War this entire area of research was extremely complex and active, with groups seeking the answer in London and Cambridge, Vienna, and in the USA at Yale, Chicago and in Wisconsin.

Two researchers at the Lister Institute, Arthur Harden and Sylvester Zilva, next began to separate citric acid from other acids in lemon juice. They found in 1918 that citric acid was useless as an antiscorbutic, but that one of the unknown residues was highly effective.[43] Further experiments were conducted with animals on the separated residues, which were referred to as the A, B and C factors. It was the last that proved to be the one with a high antiscorbutic effect. This was named in 1919 by J.C. Drummond as 'Water Soluble C'.[44]

The race was now on to synthesise the new 'vitamin C' on demand. A Hungarian-born American biochemist named Albert Szent-Györgyi, working on another matter in Cambridge, decided to isolate the compound from animal tissues. In 1928 he announced his discovery of what he called hexuronic acid. Although this was similar to what had been identified as vitamin C, he did not claim it as such. There was some controversy over this, and Zilva in London (who had spent many years seeking the compound) declared that it was not the vitamin. Szent-Györgyi produced more of the compound, this time using Hungarian paprika (the red pepper which is a potent source of vitamin C). He isolated a considerable amount of the compound, and submitted it for testing at a number of other laboratories.[45] Zilva again said in 1932 that, although there was an effect similar to that shown by his own preparation of vitamin C, the two were not identical.[46] However, Waugh and King, two

American researchers working at the University of Pittsburg, announced that they had isolated the compound from lemon juice and that it was identical in all respects to hexuronic acid. During 1932 it became widely accepted that vitamin C and hexuronic acid were one and the same; the following year the compound was renamed ascorbic acid.

In the 1930s, the new field of organic chemistry developed with startling rapidity. It was accompanied by a new characteristic of intuitive 'queue-jumping', logic that was different from the traditional dogged experiment and analysis of the laboratory. The change that had taken place since James Lind's ground-breaking clinical trial of 1747 could hardly have been greater. Sylvester Zilva was beaten to the finishing line by someone new in the field. Axel Holst, who had set the vitamin race running, died two years before the finish without any credit; and Szent-Györgyi won a Nobel Prize in 1937 for his continuing work on vitamin C and its role in cell respiration. With a sharp eye on the future, the chemical company Hoffman-La Roche acquired the patents for the commercial production of vitamin C. The world had suddenly moved on.

* * *

At long last, the identity of what Anson's Lieutenant Saumarez had called in 1740 the mysterious *je ne sais quoi* had been proved. A century later, Gilbert Blane had been 'at a loss to determine' how the superior efficacy of citrus juice worked. The work at the Lister Institute was the culmination of forty years of research on scurvy that finally vindicated the methods and conclusions of James Lind.

Working by candlelight at sea, Lind had provided the later magicians with the basis of their success. Without the benefit of financial support, he had battled against confused history, ignorance and bureaucratic prejudice to clarify the practical means of bringing to an end one of the most destructive of diseases. With the help of his later disciples Blane and Trotter,

'A SUFFICIENT EXPLANATION OF THE ANOMALY'

he achieved intellectual and practical success, yet this modest man recognised that his work did not constitute a conclusion:

> . . . though a few partial facts and observations may, for a little, flatter with hopes of greater success, yet more enlarged experience must ever evince the fallacy of all positive assertions in the healing art.[47]

James Lind was one of those giants on whose shoulders the midwives of organic chemistry stood. Their enlarged experience and imaginative strides certainly took Lind's work further forward and improved the 'healing art'. That progress notwithstanding, scientific enquiry is probably still awaiting further conclusions.

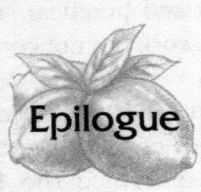

Epilogue

FOR the past 250 years, the search for a cure for scurvy has offered a confusing puzzle. Humans cannot produce vitamin C, and must acquire it in the diet, or by supplement. Conventional wisdom has it that the 'balanced diet' is the ideal, but when differing ethnic groups are considered, that rule seems to change. The Inuit consumed almost exclusively meat and fish, some of it raw, with very little incidence of scurvy. Some other communities, such as nomadic Arabs of North Africa, may be able to acquire or conserve ascorbic acid in unusual ways. Other puzzles have arisen in more developed communities. In the 1960s, scurvy became a significant problem in the infant population of countries such as the USA, Canada and Australia. Evidence even suggested that relatively wealthy, educated communities were worst affected.

Just as William Stark conducted experiments on himself in the mid-eighteenth century, similar practical investigations have been done on scurvy well into the twentieth century. In 1939, the Harvard surgeon John Crandon conducted experiments over a seven-month period. His severely deteriorated condition was reversed by injections of ascorbic acid. Lengthy and complex dietary experiments were conducted on volunteer conscientious objectors in Sheffield during the Second World War, and twenty years later on civil prisoners in Iowa City, USA. Both series of experiments verified the course of the disease in relation to specific dietary manipulation and also the certain efficacy of ascorbic acid in rapidly restoring health.

Scurvy today is generally confined to the very young and the very old, although it remains a major problem in refugee communities across the world. The World Health Organisation states that outbreaks of scurvy have increased in frequency during the last decade.[1] There have been numerous instances – in particular in Somalia in the 1980s and 1990s – when the problem became disastrous. Administrators were then accused of failing to consult nutritionists adequately in the planning of appropriate food supplies and supplements.

The incidence of scurvy in most developed countries is very low indeed. However, cultural changes can easily produce what appear to be anomalies to the normal situation. One such example is that in children the vitamin C intake now seems to be coming from processed fruit drinks rather from fresh fruit and vegetables. Another abnormality is that individuals who smoke appear to require almost twice the normal daily intake of vitamin C in order to maintain optimum levels.

The popularity of the use of vitamins as dietary supplements has become highly controversial. One report that appeared in the year 2000 from the fringes of medicine in the United States, where overexcitement about vitamin C is rife, claimed that scientists working on the human genome project maintained that they had identified a 'scurvy gene'. Suggestions were made that at-risk individuals should be regularly screened. The same source reported a five-day seminar to discuss 'The War on Scurvy', at which it was somewhat surprisingly claimed that the cure was 'just around the corner'.[2] The director of the National Scurvy Institute denied that there was any link between vitamin C and scurvy, and claimed that the vitamin was on their list of 'unproven remedies'. In the past thirty years, the report claimed, $30 billion have been spent on scurvy research; and eighty new drugs are in development to combat the disease. The extraordinary declaration was made that half a million Americans die from scurvy every year. These assertions appear to manifest a contemporary rendering of the eighteenth-century 'anti-fruiters'.

Nearly 200 years after Lind began the search that would lead to the isolation of vitamin C, Linus Pauling began research into its beneficial effects on heart disease and cancer. One of America's towering twentieth-century scientific geniuses, he was involved as a young man in the race to discover the structure of DNA that was eventually won by Crick and Watson in England. He went on to study and experiment in quantum mechanics as applied to molecular structures and proteins, and took a special interest in sickle-cell anaemia. He was renowned for his ability to make use of intuitive guesswork, which he called the stochastic method, from the Greek 'apt to divine the truth by conjecture'.

The deeply humanitarian Pauling won the Nobel Prize for Chemistry in 1954 for his work on proteins, and in 1962 he was awarded the Nobel Prize for Peace for his work towards a nuclear test ban treaty. He became interested in the possibilities of using large doses of vitamin C after reading accounts of the power of vitamins in combating scurvy, beriberi, pellagra, and other deficiency diseases. Pauling himself took 300 times the recommended dietary allowance of vitamin C for several years as part of his ongoing studies. He collaborated with Ewan Cameron, a Scottish surgeon who joined him in California in 1971. Together they developed their theories on the efficacy of vitamin C, much against the initial hostility and ridicule of the medical establishment, some of whom now felt able to attack Pauling politically. This time not only the disaffected Right was against him, as he began to lose support in more mainstream medicine, where he was accused of a fanaticism that his peers found intolerable.

Gradually however, opinion shifted somewhat towards Pauling's theories, and today there is more of an acceptance of the potential of vitamin C in complex treatments. Research is being conducted into the value of anti-viral activity in vitamin C, and work is also being taken up again into the so-called 'vitamin P' (so-called for the protected permeability of capillaries). This was a plant phenolic, never properly a vitamin and now known as a bioflavonoid, which was discovered by Dr Albert Szent-Györgyi. These compounds exist in many plants and fruits, and the proposition was that they could protect and enhance the absorption of vitamin C in the human body. They may also have antibacterial and antiviral benefits.

EPILOGUE

Linus Pauling died in California at the age of ninety-four in August 1994, almost 200 years to the day from the death of James Lind, who had faithfully picked up the gauntlet thrown down by Sir Richard Hawkins in the late sixteenth century, to become the 'learned man [who] would write of it'. He could have little realised the length of time that would pass before his proof of the efficacy against scurvy of 'sower Oranges and Lemmons' was accepted and brought into universal use. However, he had the ability to understand that the evidence of later experience was a cardinal feature of scientific endeavour. The protracted and disputed period during which the mystery of the 'unknown factor' perplexed and frustrated medicine was probably as inevitable as the two centuries of confused history that preceded Lind's own prodigious efforts.

> Forth then issued Hiawatha,
> Wandered eastward, wandered westward,
> Teaching men the use of simples
> And the antidotes for poisons,
> And the cure of all diseases.
> Thus was first made known to mortals,
> All the mystery of Medamin,
> All the sacred art of healing.
>
> 'The Song of Hiawatha',
> Henry Wadsworth Longfellow, 1855

Notes and References

Files from the Public Record Office, London are prefixed PRO; those from the National Maritime Museum, Greenwich NMM; and from the National Archives of Scotland in Edinburgh, NAS. *Dictionary of National Biography* is abbreviated to *DNB*.

INTRODUCTION

1. J. Lind, Preface to *A Treatise of the Scurvy*, Edinburgh, 1753, p. v.
2. M. Lister, 'Sex Exercitationes Medicinales' (1694), quoted in 'Some Pre-Lind writers on Scurvy' by Anthony Lorenz in *Proceedings of the Nutrition Society*, May 1953, p. 308.
3. C. Lloyd and J.L.S. Coulter, *Medicine and the Navy, 1200–1900*, 1958, vol. 3, p. 302; and C.C. Lloyd, 'The Conquest of Scurvy' in *British Journal of the History of Science*, 1963, p. 360.
4. Sir G. Blane, *A Brief Statement of the progressive improvement of the health of the Royal Navy at the end of the eighteenth century and the beginning of the nineteenth century*, London, 1830, pp. 12–13.

ONE: 'DEATH'S DIRE REVENGE'

1. *Oxford English Dictionary*, quoting from R. Hakluyt, 'Divers voyages . . .', London, 1582.
2. Sir W. Scott, *Peveril of the Peak*, 1st pub. 1823; quoted in *Oxford English Dictionary*, 2nd edn, 1989.
3. Boyne incident quoted in J. Lind, *A Treatise of the Scurvy*, Edinburgh, 1753, p. 435.
4. *Ibid.*, p. 341.
5. A.J. Lorenz, 'Some Pre-Lind writers on Scurvy', *Proceedings of the Nutrition Society*, May 1953, pp. 306–24.
6. J. Lind, *A Treatise of the Scurvy*, Edinburgh, 1753, p. 55
7. *Ibid.*, p. 131.

NOTES AND REFERENCES

8. Ibid., pp. 341–2.
9. Ibid., p. viii.
10. A.S. Hess, *Scurvy Past and Present*, J.B. Lippincott, Philadelphia, 1920, p. 7.
11. Luis de Camoëns, *The Lusiad, or the Discovery of India*, an epic poem translated from the original Portuguese of Luis de Camoëns by William Julius Mickle, Oxford, 1776, book V, p. 224.
12. R. Hakluyt, *Principal Navigations*, London, 1598–1600, vol. 3, ch. 13, pp. 225–6.
13. Ibid., p. 227.
14. Ibid., p. 227.
15. J. Lind, *A Treatise of the Scurvy*, Edinburgh, 1753, p. 222.
16. Account published by L'Escabot in 1604; quoted in J. Lind, *A Treatise of the Scurvy*, pp. 351–2.
17. J. Woodall, *The Surgeon's Mate*, 1639, p. 163.
18. J. Coltbatch, 'A Collection of Tracts, Surgical and Medical', 1699, quoted in *Editorial Review*; 'The Role of Diet in the cause, prevention and cure of dental diseases' in *The Journal of Nutrition*, January 1931, p. 442.
19. Incidence of land scurvy in A.S. Hess, *Scurvy Past and Present*, J.B. Lippincott, Philadelphia, 1920, p. 4.
20. J.J. Keevil, *Medicine and the Navy*, 1958, vol. 2, p. 209.

Two: 'Soe Many of the Best Chirurgeons'

1. T. Smollett, *Roderick Random*, 1748, Penguin Classics, 1995, p. 34. (A 'clyster' is an enema.)
2. See H.G. Graham, *The Social Life of Scotland in the Eighteenth Century*, 1st pub. 1899; 5th edn, 1969, p. 474.
3. Smollett served most of his short naval career in the 80-gun HMS *Chichester*, sailing with the fleet to Port Royal, Jamaica. He was involved in the disastrous attack on Cartagena in 1741, and later wrote an account of the affair which sent him to prison for a time in 1760. He left the Navy about 1743, and set up practice as a physician in Downing Street, until the success of *Roderick Random* enabled him to give up medicine.
4. T. Smollett, *Roderick Random*, p. 82. (A 'third rate' ship had nothing to do with quality in any sense; it referred to the number of guns, in this case between seventy and eighty-four. Bribery of officials was

obviously common; a 'three pound twelve piece' was probably a Portuguese gold coin.)
5. *Ibid.*, pp. 91–2.
6. Regulations quoted in C. Lloyd and J. Coulter, *Medicine and the Navy*, vol. 3, E. & S. Livingstone, Edinburgh, 1958, p. 22.
7. T. Smollett, *Roderick Random*, p. 154.
8. See W. Laird Clowes, *The Royal Navy: A History from the earliest times to the present*, vol. 4.
9. *Medicine and the Navy*, vol. 3, p. 33.
10. See N.A.M. Rodger, 'Stragglers and Deserters from the Royal Navy During the Seven Years' War', in *Bulletin of the Institute of Historical Research*, vol. 57, 1984.
11. See D. Baugh, 'The eighteenth-century navy as a national institution 1690–1815', ch. 5 in *The Oxford Illustrated History of the Royal Navy*, ed. J.R. Hill, Oxford University Press, 1995, p. 137.
12. N.A.M. Rodger, *The Wooden World: An Anatomy of the Georgian Navy*, 1988, p. 257.
13. Privy Council order to Barber-Surgeons' Company, quoted in *Medicine and the Navy*, vol. 2, p. 82.
14. Samuel Pepys, better known as the diarist, was, thanks to patronage, appointed to several Admiralty posts before becoming Secretary to the Admiralty in 1672. He was sacked and imprisoned in 1679 after allegedly being involved in what was known as 'The Popish Plot'; he was later reinstated, but again sacked.
15. Letter to Samuel Pepys, quoted in *Medicine and the Navy*, vol. 2, p. 84.
16. *Medicine and the Navy*, vol. 3, pp. 20–1, 113.
17. Letter from John Cockburne to Clerk of Penicuik, 2 June 1726, NAS, Clerk of Penicuik Papers: GD18/4153.
18. Letter from John Drummond to Clerk of Penicuik, 11 March 1729, NAS, Clerk of Penicuik Papers: GD18/5368.
19. *Medicine and the Navy*, vol. 3, p. 38.
20. Dr Samuel Johnson (March 1759), in Boswell's *Life of Johnson*, March 1759, Clarendon Press, 1934, vol. 1, p. 348.
21. Letter of Sir Walter Raleigh to Sir John Gilbert, 31 March 1592, in *The Letters of Sir Walter Raleigh*, 1999, p. 303.
22. J. Nicol, *The Life and Adventures of John Nicol*, 1822, pp. 162–3.
23. NAS: Melville Castle Papers: GD51/16/107.
24. *The Life and Adventures of John Nicol*, pp. 172–3.

NOTES AND REFERENCES

25. Vernon's letter to George II, quoted in G. Treasure, *Who's Who in Early Hanoverian Britain*, 1992, p. 58.
26. *The Oxford Illustrated History of the Royal Navy*, 1995, p. 146.
27. DNB/*The Oxford Illustrated History of the Royal Navy* 1995, p. 144.
28. *The Life and Adventures of John Nicol*, pp. 35–6.
29. J. Lind, preface to *An Essay on the most effectual Means of preserving the Health of Seamen in the Royal Navy*, London, 1757, pp. x–xi.
30. Anonymous pamphleteer quoted in C. Gill, *The Naval Mutinies of 1797*, 1913, p. 292.
31. Captain Martin quoted in *Medicine and the Navy*, vol. 2, p. 213.
32. Victualling Board quoted in G. Williams, *The Prize of all the Oceans*, HarperCollins, 2000, p. 22.
33. Basic ship's weekly provisions, *Medicine and the Navy*, vol. 3, p. 81.
34. Figures modified from those in S. Gradish, *The Manning of the British Navy during the Seven Years' War*, Royal Historical Society, London, 1980, p. 144.
35. C.C. Lloyd, 'The Conquest of Scurvy', in *British Journal of the History of Science*, 1963, p. 359.
36. *The Journals of Captain Cook* (Monday, 7 December 1778), Penguin Classics, 1999, p. 595.
37. W. Thompson, 'Appeal to the Public . . . to prevent the Navy being supplied with pernicious provisions', 1761, quoted in *Medicine and the Navy*, vol. 3, p. 84.
38. Surgeon Leonard Gillespie's Journal, PRO, ADM/101/102/4.
39. *Medicine and the Navy*, vol. 3, p. 98.
40. Figures from *The Oxford Illustrated History of the Royal Navy*, 1995, p. 140.

THREE: 'THE VAIN AND CHIMERICAL BELIEF'

1. J. Lind, *An Essay on the most Effectual means of Preserving the Health of Seamen in the Royal Navy*, London, 1757, edited in *The Health of Seamen – Selections from the works of Dr James Lind, Sir Gilbert Blane and Dr Thomas Trotter*, Navy Records Society, 1965, p. 80
2. J. Lind, summary from the 3rd edn of *A Treatise of the Scurvy*, 1772, in bicentenary edn, 1953, p. 368.
3. See *Medicine and the Navy*, vol. 1, p. 18.
4. H.G. Graham, *The Social Life of Scotland in the Eighteenth Century*; A. & C. Black, London, 1969 edn, p. 49.

LIMEYS

5. R. Crosfield, *Remarks on the Scurvy etc.*, 1797.
6. J. Lind, *A Treatise of the Scurvy*, Edinburgh, 1772, p. 367.
7. *The Skilful Physician* first published by Theo. Maxey, London, 1656; 1997 edn, Harwood Academic Publishers, Amsterdam, p. 58.
8. Bachstrom quoted in J. Lind, *A Treatise of the Scurvy*, Edinburgh, 1753, p. 411.
9. A. Moellenbrok, *Cochlearia Curiosa*, 1676, pp. 112–13; quoted in A.J. Lorenz, 'Some Pre-Lind writers on Scurvy' in *Proceedings of The Nutrition Society*, vol. XII, 1953, p. 323.
10. From J.J. Bechorus, *Parnassus Medicinus Illustratus*, p. 324, quoted by Moellenbrok (1676) and A.J. Lorenz, in *Proceedings of The Nutrition Society*, vol. XII, 1953, p. 322.
11. Figures given in *Mauve*, by Simon Garfield, Faber & Faber, London 2000, p. 32.
12. Sir R. Hawkins, *The Observations of Sir Richard Hawkins*, 1622, 1933 edition, Argonaut Press, p. 40.
13. *Ibid.*, p. 41.
14. *A Worthy Treatise of the Eyes* by J. Guillemeau, 1588, quoted in *Medicine and the Navy*, vol. 1, p. 102.
15. Sir R. Hawkins, *The Observations of Sir Richard Hawkins*, p. 56.
16. *Ibid.*, p. 42.
17. Sir J. Lancaster quoted in K.J. Carpenter, *A History of Scurvy and Vitamin C*, Cambridge University Press, 1986, p. 17.
18. *Ibid.*
19. See G. Milton, *Nathaniel's Nutmeg*, Sceptre, 1999, p. 79.
20. *Medicine and the Navy*, J.J. Keevil, vol. 1, pp. 108, 112; and K.J. Carpenter, *A History of Scurvy and Vitamin C*, pp. 18, 27–8.
21. Sir H. Platt, 'Certaine Philosophical Preparations of Foode and Beurage for Sea-men, in their Long Voyages', 1607, quoted in *Medicine and the Navy*, vol. 1, p. 108.
22. *Ibid.*
23. Platt quoted in K.J. Carpenter, *A History of Scurvy and Vitamin C*, p. 18.
24. J. Woodall, *The Surgeon's Mate*, 1639 edition, p. 175.
25. *Ibid.*, p. 161.
26. *Ibid.*, p. 160.
27. *Ibid.*, p. 161.
28. *Ibid.*, p. 165.
29. *Ibid.*

NOTES AND REFERENCES

30. *Ibid.*
31. R. Stockman MD, 'James Lind and Scurvy', *Edinburgh Medical Journal*, June 1926, pp. 329–50.
32. J. Woodall, *The Surgeon's Mate*, 1639 edition, p. 170.
33. *Ibid.*, p. 160.
34. *A Counterblast to Tobacco, to which is added a learned discourse written by Dr Everard Maynwaringe, proving that tobacco is a procuring cause of the scurvy . . .* by King James VI of Scotland, London, 1672.
35. *Ibid.*
36. J. Lind, *A Treatise of the Scurvy*, p. 390.
37. J. Fryer, 1672, quoted in *Medicine and the Navy*, vol. 2, pp. 164–5.
38. J. Moyle, *Chirurgus Maritus*, 1693, p. 23, quoted in *Medicine and the Navy*, vol. 2, p. 164.
39. *Medicine and the Navy*, J.J. Keevil, vol. 1, p. 110
40. General Robert Venables, quoted in *Medicine and the Navy*, vol. 2, p. 60.
41. T. Dover, *The Ancient Physician's Legacy to his Country*, 1773, quoted in *Medicine and the Navy*, vol. 2, p. 228.
42. Goldsmith story, see *DNB* and G. Treasure, *Who's Who in Early Hanoverian Britain*, 1992, p. 192
43. Dr James quoted in *Medicine and the Navy*, vol. 3, p. 333.
44. *Chemist and Druggist*, 25 June 1927.

FOUR: 'A LEARNED MAN'

1. *Medicine and the Navy*, vol. 3, p. 109.
2. See *Medicine and the Navy*, vol. 3, p. 110
3. J. Lind, *An Essay on the most effectual means of preserving the health of Seamen in the Royal Navy*, London, 1762, pp. 122–3.
4. *Medicine and the Navy*, vol. 3, p. 40
5. PRO: ADM/106/2178, Navy Board to Admiralty, 13 June 1740.
6. G. Williams, *The Prize of All the Oceans*, 1999, p. 43.
7. 'A Discourse on The Scurvy' by Richard Mead, p. 444; printed in S. Sutton, *An Historical account of a new method for extracting the foul air out of ships*, London, 1749.
8. L. Dulieu, 'Pierre Chirac et les maladies des équipages des vaisseaux', 1984, quoted in K.J. Carpenter *A History of Scurvy and Vitamin C*, Cambridge University Press, 1986, p. 46.
9. PRO: ADM/106/916, Letter from Anson to Admiralty, 6 July 1740.

10. PRO: ADM/106/916, Letter from Anson to Admiralty, 15 July 1740.
11. PRO: ADM/106/916, Letter from Anson to Admiralty, 22 July 1740.
12. *A voyage round the World in the years 1740–4*. Compiled from papers and other materials of the Rt Hon. George, Lord Anson, and published under his direction, by Richard Walter MA. London, 1748, introduction, p. 6.
13. *Ibid.*, p. 100.
14. P. Thomas, *A True and Impartial Journal*, 1745, pp. 21–2.
15. Saumarez, quoted in Sir J. Watt, 'The Medical bequest of disaster at sea: Commodore Anson's circumnavigation 1740–44', *Journal of the Royal College of Physicians*, vol. 32, no. 6, November/December 1998, p. 574.
16. Surgeon Ettrick, quoted in G. Williams, *The Prize of All the Oceans*, p. 44.
17. *A voyage round the World in the years 1740–44*, p. 101.
18. *Ibid.*, p. 102.
19. P. Thomas, *A True and Impartial Journal*, 1745, pp. 142–3.
20. *A voyage round the World in the years 1740–44*, p. 102.
21. Sir J. Watt, 'The Medical bequest of disaster at sea: Commodore Anson's circumnavigation 1740–44', *Journal of the Royal College of Physicians*, vol. 32, no. 6, November/December 1998, p. 575.
22. *A voyage round the World in the years 1740–44*, p. 113.
23. J. Lind, *A Treatise of the Scurvy*, p. 102.
24. P. Thomas, *A True and Impartial Journal*, 1745, pp. 143–4.
25. *Ibid.*, p. 144.
26. Abstract of a Journal by Philip Saumarez (Macao, December 1742) quoted in 'Documents relating to Anson's Voyage round the World, 1740–44', ed. G. Williams; *Navy Records Society*,. vol. 109, 1967, p. 168.
27. P. Thomas, *A True and Impartial Journal*, 1745, p. 148.
28. R. Mead, *The Medical Works of Richard Mead MD*, London, 1762, pp. 443–4.
29. *Ibid.*, p. 444.
30. Account of Huxham's proposals in *Medicine and the Navy*, vol. 3, p. 297.
31. J. Lind, *A Treatise of the Scurvy*, p. 104.

NOTES AND REFERENCES

FIVE: 'I SHALL CONFIRM ALL BY EXPERIENCE AND FACTS'

1. *A voyage round the World in the years 1740–44*, p. 102.
2. J. Wesley, *Primitive Physic*; 13th edn, 1768.
3. J. Lind, *A Treatise of the Scurvy*, 1753, p. 202.
4. Surgeon Hammond, letter to Admiral Steuart in *Naval Administration, 1715–50*, ed. D. Baugh, Navy Records Society, 1977, pp. 149–51.
5. J. Lind, *A Treatise of the Scurvy*, p. 103.
6. *Ibid.*, p. 107.
7. *Ibid.*, pp. 107–8.
8. *Ibid.*, pp. 89–90.
9. *Ibid.*, pp. 203–4.
10. *Ibid.*, pp. 204–5.
11. *Ibid.*, pp. 199–200, Surgeon Murray's letter.
12. *Ibid.*, p. 109.
13. *Ibid.*, p. 190.
14. National Bioethics Advisory Commission in *Ethical Considerations in the Design and Conduct of International Clinical Trials*, www.bioethics.gov/clinical/
15. Years later, in investigating fevers in the West Indies, Lind conducted another series of experiments which unwittingly came close to defining the basis of immunology. (Sir Sheldon Dudley, 1953.)
16. D.P. Thomas MD, D.Phil. 'Experiment versus Authority', *The New England Journal of Medicine*, vol. 281, no. 17, 23 October 1969, pp. 932–3.
17. J. Lind, *A Treatise of the Scurvy*, p. 190.
18. J. Lind, *A Treatise of the Scurvy*, p. 170. (Strontianite, the mineral which led to the use of the radioisotope Strontium-90, was discovered here in 1764 by Sir Humphrey Davy.)
19. J. Lind, *A Treatise of the Scurvy*, pp. 191–3.
20. *Ibid.*, p. 196.
21. *Ibid.*, p. 187.
22. H.D. Rolleston, 'James Lind, Pioneer of Naval Hygiene', *Journal of the Royal Naval Medical Service*, 1915, vol. 1, p. 181.

SIX: 'THE PROVINCE HAS BEEN MINE'

1. J. Lind, *A Treatise of the Scurvy*, p. 76.
2. R. Boyle, 'Medicinal Experiments; or a Collection of Choice and Safe Remedies, etc.' (1696), quoted in *Some Pre-Lind writers on Scurvy* by A. Lorenz, in *Proceedings of The Nutrition Society*, May 1953, p. 310.
3. J. Colbatch, 'Collection of Tracts, Chirurgical and Medical', 1700, quoted in *Some Pre-Lind writers on Scurvy* by A. Lorenz, in *Proceedings of The Nutrition Society*, May 1953, p. 316.
4. *Ibid.*
5. *Ibid.*
6. Kramer, quoted in J. Lind, *A Treatise of the Scurvy*, pp. 205–6.
7. *The Practitioner*, vol. 56, 1896, p. 622.
8. J. Lind, *A Treatise of the Scurvy*, preface, p. xi.
9. K.J. Carpenter, *A History of Scurvy and Vitamin C*, 1986, p. 54.
10. J. Lind, *A Treatise of the Scurvy*, p. 273.
11. *Chambers Biographical Dictionary*.
12. Allan and Schofield, *Stephen Hales, Scientist and Philanthropist*, Scolar Press, London, 1980. p. 91.
13. J. Lind, *A Treatise of the Scurvy*, p. 229.
14. *Ibid.*, pp. 232–3. (A loggerhead was an iron instrument with a long handle and a ball or bulb at the end, used for melting pitch or heating liquids in a fire.)
15. *Ibid.*, p. 90.
16. *Ibid.*, pp. 207–8.
17. *Ibid.*, pp. 211–12. (Arrack was a fermented drink made from dates: it later referred to any fermented drink.)
18. *Ibid.*, p. 267.
19. *Ibid.*, p. 210.
20. Table based on those in K.J. Carpenter, *A History of Scurvy and Vitamin C*, p. 227, *British Journal of The History of Science*, 1963, pp. 357–63, *The Conquest of Scurvy*, C.C. Lloyd, and *Medicine and the Navy*, vol. 3, C. Lloyd and J.L.S. Coulter, p. 302.
21. J. Lind, *The Scots Magazine*, vol. xvii, May 1754, pp. 227–9.
22. *Ibid.* (Quotation from anonymous correspondent.)
23. J. Lind, quoted in C. Lloyd and J.L.S. Coulter, *Medicine and the Navy*, vol. 3, p. 333.
24. Letter from Sick and Hurt Board to Admiralty, 6 March 1754, NMM: ADM/F/11.

NOTES AND REFERENCES

25. *Ibid.*
26. *Ibid.*
27. See C.E. Jones, 'Tobias Smollett, the Doctor as Man of Letters', *Journal of the History of Medicine and Allied Sciences*, July 1957, vol. 12, pp. 337–48.
28. French surgeon H. Rey, *Étude analytique et critique sur le traité du scorbut de Lind*, 1867, quoted in K.J. Carpenter, *A History of Scurvy and Vitamin C*, p. 57.
29. See 'James Lind and the cure of scurvy, an experimental approach', by R.E. Hughes in *Medical History*, vol. 19, 1975, pp. 342–51.
30. J. Lind, *Essay on the most effectual means of preserving the Health of Seamen in the Royal Navy*, 1757, p. 123.

SEVEN: 'BUT THE POWER IS IN OTHERS'

1. Admiralty Secretary's Register of Commissioned and Warrant Ranks, 1742–58, quoted in Surgeon Lieutenant-Commander J. Glass, 'James Lind MD, 18th Century Medical Hygienist', *Journal of the Royal Naval Medical Service*, vol. 35, January and April 1949.
2. *Ibid.*.
3. Remarks by Surgeon William Barton, quoted in L.H. Roddis, *James Lind, Founder of Nautical Medicine*, Heineman Medical Books, London, 1950, p. 131.
4. Letter of James Lind, dated 3 September 1758, published in L.H. Roddis, *James Lind*, 1950, p. 127.
5. Surgeon Ives, *Voyage from England to India*, 1773, quoted in *Medicine and the Navy*, vol. 3, p. 113.
6. Sir G. Blane, *A Brief Statement of the progressive improvement of the health of the Royal Navy at the end of the eighteenth century and the beginning of the nineteenth century*, London, 1830, p. 13.
7. J. Lind in C. Lloyd (ed), *The Health of Seamen*, Navy Records Society, vol. CVII, 1965, p. 121.
8. Commodore Byron in John Hawkesworth, *An Account of the Voyages undertaken. . . . For making discoveries in the Southern Hemisphere, etc, etc'*, London, 1773, vol. 1, p. 93.
9. *Ibid.*, p. 114.
10. *Ibid.*, p. 116.
11. Lady Anson quoted in N.A.M. Rodger, *The Wooden World: An Anatomy of the Georgian Navy*, Fontana, 1988, p. 102.

12. R. Mead, 'A Discourse on the Scurvy' in S. Sutton, *An Historical Account of a new method for extracting the foul air out of ships*, London, 1749, p. 443.
13. K.J. Carpenter, *A History of Scurvy and Vitamin C*, p. 63; and Charles Bissett, *Medical Essays and Observations*, 1766.
14. J. Leake, *A Dissertation on the properties and efficacy of the Lisbon Diet-Drink in the cure of venereal disease and scurvy, etc, etc*, London, 1762.
15. J. Profily MD, *An Easy and Exact Method of curing The Venereal Disease in all its different Appearances; with an Account of its Nature, Causes and Symptoms . . . and likewise a Method of curing The Scurvy, Gleets, Whites, Etc, Illustrated with Curious Copper-Plates*, London, 1748.
16. Experiment described in *Medical History*, vol. 20, 1976, pp. 80–1, 'Copper Boilers and the occurrence of Scurvy: An Experimental Approach' by E. Jones and E. Hughes.
17. K.J. Carpenter, *A History of Scurvy and Vitamin C*, pp. 64, 240.
18. Research on copper at Southampton University, reported in Glasgow *Herald*, August 2001.
19. N. Hulme, *A Safe and Easy Remedy, etc*, 1778. (Joseph Priestley was a theologian and experimental chemist of great significance. He discovered oxygen, sulphur dioxide and half a dozen other gases, and studied the fermentation processes in brewing vats and devised an industrial method of dissolving this 'fixed air' or carbon dioxide.)
20. D. MacBride, *Experimental Essays* 'No. 4 – On the Scurvy', London, 1764.
21. *Ibid.*
22. A. Lorenz in 'Some Pre-Lind writers on Scurvy', *Proceedings of The Nutrition Society*, May 1953, p. 312.
23. Sir J. Watt, 'Medical aspects and consequences of Cook's voyages' in R. Fisher and H. Johnston (eds), *Captain James Cook and his Times*, University of Vancouver Press, 1979, p. 144.
24. *Ibid.*
25. D. MacBride, *Experimental Essays*, 'No. 4 – On the Scurvy', London, 1764.
26. *Ibid.*
27. K.J. Carpenter, *A History of Scurvy and Vitamin C*, p. 65.
28. Admiralty Board Minutes, 1 July 1762, PRO: ADM 3/70.
29. *Medicine and the Navy*, vol. 3, p. 308.

NOTES AND REFERENCES

30. J. Lind, *Treatise*, 3rd edn, 1772, quoted in K.J. Carpenter, *A History of Scurvy and Vitamin C*, p. 69
31. J. Lind, *Treatise*, 3rd edn, 1772, quoted in bicentenary edition, 1953, p. 368.
32. *Ibid*.
33. Letter, Sick and Hurt Board to Admiralty, 1 July 1767, NMM: ADM/FP/10.
34. See *Medical History*, vol. 19, 1975, R.E. Hughes, 'James Lind and the Cure of Scurvy: An Experimental Approach'.
35. J. Lind, *Treatise*, 3rd edn, 1772, quoted in bicentenary edition, 1953, p. 366.
36. From 'Introduction of Soyabean to North America by Samuel Bowen in 1765' by T. Hymowitz and J.R. Harlan, *Economic Botany* 39(4), 1983, New York, pp. 371–9.
37. *Ibid*.
38. H.W. Wiltshire, 'Germinated Beans in the Treatment of Scurvy', *The Lancet*, 14 December 1918, pp. 811–13.
39. Admiralty Orders to Commanders, 10 June 1768, PRO: ADM/2/94.
40. Admiralty Orders to Commanders, 30 July 1768, PRO: ADM/2/94.
41. Surgeon Clerk, *Observations on the Diseases of Hot Climates*, 1773, quoted in *Medicine and the Navy*, vol. 3, p. 309.
42. K.J. Carpenter, *A History of Scurvy and Vitamin C*, p. 77.
43. Surgeon F. Thomson, *An Essay on the Scurvy*, 1790, pp. 91–2.
44. Surgeon Clerk, *Observations on the Diseases of Hot Climates*, 1773, in *Medicine and the Navy*, vol. 3, p. 309.
45. Captains' letters to Admiralty, 12 July 1771 (James Cook enclosing letter from Surgeon Perry), PRO: ADM/1/1609, pt 1.
46. *Ibid*.
47. *Ibid*.
48. *Ibid*.
49. J. Banks, *Journal*, 1896 edn, p. 71.
50. *Ibid*., pp. 71–2.
51. *Ibid*., Letter of 1 August 1768 from Hulme to Banks.
52. *Ibid*.
53. W. Stark quoted in 'An Eighteenth Century Experiment in Nutrition' by J.C. Drummond and A. Wilbraham, © *The Lancet*, 24 August 1935, pp. 459–62.
54. J.C. Drummond and A. Wilbraham, 'An Eighteenth Century Experiment in Nutrition', © *The Lancet*, 24 August 1935,

pp. 459–62. (See also Commentary by Guthrie and Meiklejohn (p. 398) in 1953 bicentenary edn of *A Treatise of the Scurvy*, J. Lind.)
55. Cook's Journal, 25 December 1771, *The Journals of Captain Cook*, selected and edited by P. Edwards, Penguin Classics, p. 224.
56. *Ibid.*, p. 227.
57. Cook, quoted in 'Beer and Scurvy' by A. Henderson Smith, © *The Lancet*, 14 December 1918, p. 813.
58. Sir J. Watt, 'Medical aspects and consequences of Cook's voyages' in *Captain James Cook and his Times*, 1979, p. 135.
59. Cook's report to the Royal Society quoted in K.J. Carpenter, *A History of Scurvy and Vitamin C*, p. 82.
60. Cook, quoted in *Medicine and the Navy*, vol. 3, p. 315.
61. Cook's report to the Royal Society quoted in K.J. Carpenter, *A History of Scurvy and Vitamin C*, p. 82.
62. Pringle in *Medicine and the Navy*, vol. 3, p. 315.
63. Cook in *Medicine and the Navy*, vol. 3, p. 316.
64. J. Lind, *Treatise*, 3rd edn, 1772; quoted in bicentenary edn, 1953, p. 368.

EIGHT: 'MY ATTENDANCE WAS NEVER AGAIN ASKED'

1. N.A.M. Rodger, *The Wooden World*, 1988, p. 276.
2. W. Laird Clowes, *History of the Royal Navy from the Earliest Times to 1900*, vol. 3, p. 19.
3. See N.A.M. Rodger, *The Admiralty*, Lavenham, 1979, p. 72.
4. Anonymous letter, 25 November 1794, NMM: ADM/F/25.
5. Letter from George Clode, 10 December 1794, NMM: ADM/F/25.
6. *Surgeon Gillespie's Journal*, PRO: ADM/101/102/4.
7. *Medicine and the Navy*, vol. 4, p. 105.
8. Letter by Edward Thompson from HMS *Stirling Castle* at Antigua, in 1756; quoted in W. Laird Clowes, *History of the Royal Navy from the Earliest Times to 1900*, vol. 3, p. 23.
9. Sir R. Hawkins, *The Observations of Sir Richard Hawkins* (1622), Argonaut, 1933 edn, p. 56.
10. J. Lind, appendix from *An Essay on Diseases incidental to Europeans in Hot Climates*, London, 1768.
11. *Ibid.*
12. Royal Society Journal Book, May 1762, p. 384. (The address to the

NOTES AND REFERENCES

Royal Society appears in Lind's *Essay on the most effectual means of preserving the Health of Seamen in the Royal Navy*, 1757, pp. 85–7.)

13. J. Lind quoted in H.D. Rolleston, 'James Lind, Pioneer of Naval Hygiene' in *Journal of the Royal Naval Medical Service*, vol. 1, 1915, pp. 181–90.
14. J. Lind, Appendix from *An Essay on Diseases incidental to Europeans in Hot Climates*.
15. 'James Lind MD, Eighteenth-Century Medical Hygienist', by Surgeon Lieutenant-Commander J. Glass in *Journal of the Royal Naval Medical Service*, vol. 35, no. 1, January 1949, pp. 1–20, and no. 2, April 1949, pp. 68–86.
16. Poissonnière, 'Maladies des Gens de Mer', 1767, quoted in *Medicine and the Navy*, vol. 3, p. 303.
17. Surgeon Frederick Thomson, *An Essay on The Scurvy*, 1790, p. 88.
18. J. Hawksworth, *An account of the Voyages undertaken ... for making discoveries in the Southern Hemisphere ... by Commodore Byron, Captain Wallis, Captain Carteret and Captain Cook, drawn from the Journals which were kept by the several commanders, and from the papers of Joseph Banks Esq.*, London, 1773, pp. 515–16.
19. C. Irving, in *A Voyage towards the North Pole* by Constantine John Phipps RN, London, 1774, appendix, p. 207.
20. Surgeon Vice-Admiral Sir Sheldon Dudley, 'The Lind Tradition in the Royal Naval Medical Service' in Lind's *Treatise of Scurvy*, bicentenary edn, 1953, 1953 edn., p. 371.
21. J. Lind, in *Medicine and the Navy*, vol. 3, p. 91.
22. W. Laird Clowes, *The Royal Navy – a History from the earliest times to the present*, London, 1898, vol. 3, p. 337.
23. C.J. Phipps RN, *A Voyage towards the North Pole*, London, 1774.
24. Cook in *Medicine and the Navy*, vol. 3, p. 313.
25. Cook's report to the Royal Society quoted in K.J. Carpenter, *A History of Scurvy and Vitamin C*, p. 82.
26. Sir J. Watt, 'Medical aspects and consequences of Cook's voyages' in R. Fisher and H. Johnston (eds), *Captain James Cook and his Times*, University of Vancouver Press, 1979, pp. 129–58.
27. Surgeon Davis quoted in L.H. Roddis, *James Lind, Founder of Nautical Medicine*, Heinemann Medical Books, London, 1951, p. 102.
28. C. Fletcher, 'Health for Seamen', 1786, quoted in *James Lind, Founder of Nautical Medicine*, p. 103.

29. Letter from Joseph Black NAS: Melville Castle Papers: GD51/2/73/1/1.
30. Notes by Joseph Black NAS: Melville Castle Papers: GD51/2/73/2/1.
31. Letter of 4 August 1804 from Richard Younger NAS: Melville Castle Papers: GD51/2/193.
32. Quote from 'Health Report 1837' in *Medicine and the Navy*, vol. 4, p. 105.
33. Assistant Surgeon Cree, 1840, in *The Cree Journals*, M. Levien (ed.), Webb & Bower, Exeter, 1981, p. 66.
34. *Medicine and the Navy*, vol. 4, p. 105.
35. Sir J. Watt, 'Medical aspects and consequences of Cook's voyages', in *Captain James Cook and his Times*, 1979, p. 144.
36. Surgeon Vice Admiral Dudley in his laudatory address at the James Lind Bicentenary Symposium, Edinburgh, May 1953, *Proceedings of The Nutrition Society*, May 1953, p. 203.
37. W. Laird Clowes, *History of the Royal Navy from the Earliest Times to 1900*, vol. 3, p. 337.
38. K.J. Carpenter, *A History of Scurvy and Vitamin C*, p. 84.
39. *Ibid.*, p. 91.
40. Letter from the Sick and Hurt Board to Admiralty, 6 June 1783, PRO: ADM/98/14.

NINE: 'POLICY AS WELL AS HUMANITY CONCUR'

1. C. Lloyd (ed.), introduction to *The Health of Seamen – Selections from the works of Dr James Lind, Sir Gilbert Blane and Dr Thomas Trotter*, Navy Records Society, vol. CVII, 1965, p. 132.
2. Surgeon Robertson in C. Lloyd and J.L.S. Coulter, *Medicine and the Navy*, vol. 3, p. 130.
3. Sir G. Blane, preface to *Observations on the Diseases of Seamen*, in C. Lloyd (ed.), *The Health of Seamen – Selections from the works of Dr James Lind, Sir Gilbert Blane and Dr Thomas Trotter*, Navy Records Society, vol. CVII, 1965, p. 136.
4. *Ibid.*, p. 138.
5. Sir G. Blane, *A Short Account of the Most Effectual Means of Preserving the Health of Seamen*, August 1780.
6. *Medicine and the Navy*, vol. 3, p. 131.
7. April 1782, between Guadeloupe and Dominica, from W. Laird Clowes, *The Royal Navy, a History*, 1898, vol. 3, p. 533.

NOTES AND REFERENCES

8. Letter from Kempenfelt to Middleton, *Barham Papers*, Navy Records Society, vol. 1, p. 327.
9. *Ibid.*, p. 329.
10. Admiral Hawke, quoted in *Medicine and the Navy*, vol. 3, p. 126.
11. *Barham Papers*, Navy Records Society, vol. 1 p. 329.
12. *Ibid.*, p. 331.
13. *Ibid.*, p. 75.
14. *Ibid.*
15. Surgeon Bedford, in *Medicine and the Navy*, vol. 3, p. 134.
16. 23 April 1781, letter from Sir Samuel Hood, G. Barnes and J. Owen (eds), *The Private Papers of John, Earl of Sandwich*, vol. 4, Navy Records Society, 1988, pp. 45–7.
17. *Ibid.*, 20 June 1781, letter from Admiral Darby.
18. *Ibid.*, 14 July 1781, letter from Admiral Darby.
19. *Ibid.*, 19 August 1781, letter from Surgeon Northcote, pp. 178–9.
20. Sir G. Blane, preface to *Observations on the Diseases of Seamen*, Navy Records Society, vol. CVII, p. 171.
21. *Ibid.*, pp. 168–9.
22. Letter from Sick and Hurt to Admiralty, 18 December 1781, PRO: ADM/98/14.
23. *Ibid.*
24. Letter from Surgeon Patten, from Sick and Hurt to Admiralty, 18 December 1781, PRO: ADM/98/14.
25. Letter from Sick and Hurt to Admiralty, 18 December 1781, PRO: ADM/98/14.
26. Letter from Sick and Hurt to Admiralty, 18 December 1781, PRO: ADM/98/14.
27. Sir G. Blane, preface to *Observations on the Diseases of Seamen*, Navy Records Society, vol. CVII, p. 148.
28. Rodney, quoted in *DNB*.
29. Sir G. Blane, *A Brief Statement of the progressive improvement of the health of the Royal Navy at the end of the eighteenth century and the beginning of the nineteenth century*, London, 1830, pp. 24–5.
30. *Ibid.*
31. Sir G. Blane, 12 April 1782, quoted by Surgeon Vice-Admiral Sir Sheldon Dudley in 'The Lind Tradition in the Royal Naval Medical Service' in Lind's *Treatise of Scurvy*, bicentenary edn, 1953, p. 379.
32. Guthrie and Meiklejohn (eds), Lind's *Treatise of Scurvy*, 1953, p. 400.
33. Sir G. Blane, *Observations on the Diseases of Seamen*, p. 161.

34. 'Salep', another version of 'saloop', was powdered orchid root, used as a thickener in making broth.
35. Sir G. Blane, *Observations on the Diseases of Seamen*, pp. 159–60.
36. Letter from Sick and Hurt to Admiralty, 28 March 1786, PRO: ADM/98/15.
37. Captain W. Bligh, in O. Rutter, *Turbulent Journey*, 1936, p. 94.
38. F. Thomson, preface to *An Essay on The Scurvy*, 1790, p. xv.
39. Sir G. Blane, *Diseases of Seamen*, in A. Henderson Smith, 'Beer and Scurvy', © *The Lancet*, 14 December 1918, pp. 813–15.
40. Letter from Sick and Hurt to Admiralty, 13 December 1793, PRO: ADM/98/16.
41. *Ibid.*
42. Sir G. Blane, *Observations on the Diseases of Seamen*, p. 178.
43. Surgeon Leonard Gillespie, quoted in *Medicine and the Navy*, vol. 3, p. 322.
44. T. Trotter, *Observations on Scurvy*, p. 223, quoted in *Medicine and the Navy*, vol. 3, p. 323.
45. *Medicine and the Navy*, vol. 3, p. 322.
46. *Ibid.*, T. Trotter, p. 324.
47. *Ibid.*
48. Letter from Collingwood to Admiralty, 15 June 1795, NMM: ADM/F/26.
49. Letter from Sick and Hurt to Admiralty, 19 June 1795, NMM: ADM/F/26.
50. Letter from Sick and Hurt to Admiralty, 31 August 1795, NMM: ADM/F/26.
51. Memorandum by Lord Spencer, 25 August 1795, *Barham Papers*, vol. 3, p. 2.
52. *Ibid.*, p. 4. (Cornwallis was blockading Brest, and Warren was at Quiberon, near the islands of Hédic and Houat in the Bay of Biscay, off the French coast near St Nazaire).
53. Sir G. Blane, *A Brief Statement of the progressive improvement of the health of the Royal Navy at the end of the eighteenth century and the beginning of the nineteenth century*, London, 1830, pp. 12–13.
54. D. Paterson, *A Treatise on the Scurvy*, 1795.
55. D. McBride, *An Account of the Most Important Discovery . . . made for the restoration and preservation of Health, in all complaints of the Stomach and Bowels, Fevers, Fluxes, Scurvy, Dropsy, Debility, Etc.*, London, 1798, pp. 62–4.

NOTES AND REFERENCES

56. *Ibid.*
57. Letter from Jervis to Spencer, March 1796, *Spencer Papers*, vol. 2, Navy Records Society, p. 19.
58. Letter from Sick and Hurt to Admiralty, 25 May 1796, NMM: ADM/F/27.
59. T. Trotter, *Medicina Nautica*, vol. 1, 1791–1803, p. 423, in *Medicine and the Navy*, vol. 3, p. 325.
60. Letter from Sick and Hurt to Admiralty, 5 September 1796, NMM: ADM/F/27.
61. Sir G. Blane, *A Brief Statement of the progressive improvement of the health of the Royal Navy at the end of the eighteenth century and the beginning of the nineteenth century*, London, 1830, pp. 23–4.
62. Letter from G. Blane to Admiralty, 19 October 1796, NMM: ADM/F/27.
63. Letter from Sir R. Bickerton to Sick and Hurt Board, 15 September 1796, NMM: ADM/F/27.
64. Letter from Hyde Parker to Spencer, December 1796, *Spencer Papers*, vol. 3, p. 242.
65. *Ibid.*, pp. 257–8.
66. R. Crosfield MD, *Remarks on the Scurvy as it appeared among the French prisoners in France, in the year 1795; with an account of the effects of opium in that disease, and of the methods proper to render its use more extensive and easy (written during his confinement in the Tower)*, London, 1797.
67. *Ibid.*
68. *Medicine and the Navy*, vol. 3, p. 325.
69. Letter from Sick and Hurt to Admiralty, 19 July 1799, NMM: ADM/F/30.
70. Sir G. Blane, *A Brief Statement of the progressive improvement of the health of the Royal Navy at the end of the eighteenth century and the beginning of the nineteenth century*, p. 16.
71. *Ibid.*, p. 18.
72. Sir G. Blane, *Observations*, in *Medicine and the Navy*, vol. 3, p. 320.
73. H. Spencer, *Study of Sociology*, London, 1876, p. 163.

TEN: 'EVERY SHIP SHALL HAVE ON BOARD A SUFFICIENT QUANTITY'

1. Sir G. Blane, *Observations on the Diseases incident to Seamen*, 1789, pp. 502–16, quoted in *Medicine and the Navy*, vol. 3, p. 319.

2. K.J. Carpenter, *A History of Scurvy and Vitamin C*, p. 233.
3. A.F. Hess, *Scurvy Past and Present*, p. 9.
4. *Medicine and the Navy*, vol. 3, p. 321.
5. T. Trotter, *Medicina Nautica*, vol. 3, p. 387, in R. Stockman, 'James Lind and Scurvy', *Edinburgh Medical Journal*, June 1926.
6. Table based on figures given by Lind and Blane in *Medicine and the Navy*, vol. 3, p. 371.
7. Sir G. Blane, *A Brief Statement of the progressive improvement of the health of the Royal Navy at the end of the eighteenth century and the beginning of the nineteenth century*, pp. 12–13.
8. Dr Beatty, in Alfred Jay Bollet, *Plagues and Poxes: The Rise and Fall of Epidemic Disease*, New York, 1987, pp. 1–8.
9. Nelson; figures and quote in *Medicine and the Navy*, vol. 3, p. 150. (See Wellcome Historical Medical Library for Nelson MSS.)
10. Surgeon Leonard Gillespie, letter of January 1805 in *Medical Magazine*, 1895, p. 10, in *Medicine and the Navy*, vol. 3, p. 152.
11. T. Trotter, *Medicina Nautica* 2nd edn, 1804, quoted in K.J. Carpenter, *A History of Scurvy and Vitamin C*, p. 234.
12. Letter from Sick and Hurt to Admiralty, 14 July 1800, NMM: ADM/F/31.
13. T. Trotter, *Medicina Nautica*, 1803, in *Medicine and the Navy*, vol. 3, p. 326.
14. *Ibid.*, p. 327.
15. Letter, 2 August 1800, from Surgeon Baird enclosed with Sick and Hurt to Admiralty, 7 August 1800, NMM: ADM/F/31.
16. Letter from Trotter to Melville, 4 June, 1804, NAS: Melville Castle Papers: GD51/2/1091 (bundle no. 9, letter no. 48).
17. J.S. Taylor, *U.S. Naval Medical Bulletin*, 14, 1920, p. 563.
18. Surgeon Peter Henry, in B. Lavery (ed.), *Shipboard Life and Organisation, 1731–1815*, Navy Records Society, 1998, p. 528.
19. Letter from Sick and Hurt to Admiralty, 16 May 1803, NMM: ADM/F/34.
20. Letter from Harness to Middleton, *Barham Papers*, Navy Records Society, 1910, vol. 3, pp. 131–6.
21. *Medicine and the Navy*, vol. 3, p. 5.
22. Dr J. Weir to Lord Melville, January 1822, NAS: Melville Castle Papers: GD51/2/640/1–2.
23. Letter from Sick and Hurt to Admiralty, 4 February 1807, PRO: ADM/98/24.

NOTES AND REFERENCES

24. Letter from Sick and Hurt to Admiralty, 6 July 1807, PRO: ADM/98/24.
25. Letter from Sick and Hurt to Admiralty, 10 May 1808, PRO: ADM/98/24.
26. Dr R. Brooke, June 1808, PRO: T1/1061/165–167.
27. A.G. Course, *The Merchant Navy, A Social History*, Frederick Muller Ltd., London, 1963, p. 107.
28. Quotation from Surgeon Bowler's Journal in *Medicine and the Navy*, vol. 4, pp. 138–9.
29. Quotation from Mercantile Marine Act 1851, in *Medicine and the Navy*, vol. 4, p. 115.
30. Dr Barnes, quoted in *Medicine and the Navy*, vol. 4, p. 114.
31. Board of Trade Notice, September 1865, PRO: M187/1866.
32. PRO: MT9/25.
33. PRO: MT9/57.
34. Board of Trade statement in *Pall Mall Gazette*, 26 January 1871, PRO: MT9/57.
35. Letter from Sick and Hurt to Admiralty, 30 December 1812, PRO: ADM/98/27.
36. Letter from Admiralty to Sick and Hurt, 12 March 1816, PRO: ADM/97/1.
37. Sick and Hurt Board quoted by Alice Henderson Smith in © *The Lancet*, 14 December 1918, pp. 813–15.
38. K.J. Carpenter, *A History of Scurvy and Vitamin C*, p. 237.
39. *Medicine and the Navy*, vol. 3, p. 301.
40. Account given by naval surgeon W.E. Home in *The Lancet*, 'Etiology of Scurvy', 4 August 1900, p. 322.
41. Dr W. Budd, article on scurvy in *Tweedie's System of Practical Medicine*, 1840, quoted in *Medicine and the Navy*, vol. 4, p. 114.
42. Dr Busk, evidence to Committee of Enquiry, 1877, p. vi.
43. K.J. Carpenter, *A History of Scurvy and Vitamin C*, p. 237.

ELEVEN: 'LIME JUICE AND WINE MERCHANTS'

1. Edinburgh and Leith Post Office Directories.
2. Collins *Biographical Dictionary of Scientists*, HarperCollins, 1994.
3. P. Durand, British Patent No. 3,372 of 25 August 1810, 'Preserving animal and vegetable food and other articles from decay.'
4. Lauchlan Rose, British Patent No. 3,499 of 9 December 1867.

5. PRO: BT31/1456/4365.
6. *Royal Album of Arts and Industries of Great Britain*, London, 1898, pp. 198–203.
7. *Ibid.*
8. PRO: BT31/4003/25469.
9. D. Simmons, *Schweppes – the first 200 Years*, pp. 98–100.
10. *Ibid.*, p. 101.
11. L. Rose & Company, from *Green Gold*, 1959.
12. J. Ayto, *Twentieth Century Words*, OUP, 1999, p. 91. (© by permission of Oxford University Press).
13. H. Rawson, *A Dictionary of Invective*, Hale, 1991, pp. 238–9.
14. *Ibid.*

TWELVE: 'THE BRITISH ARMY WERE ALLOWED TO ROT OF SCURVY'

1. A. Lorenz, 'Scurvy in the Gold Rush', in *Journal of the History of Medicine and Allied Sciences*, vol. 12, 1957, p. 475.
2. K.J. Carpenter, *A History of Scurvy and Vitamin C*, pp. 109–12.
3. F. Galton, *The Art of Travel, or shifts and contrivances available in wild countries*, John Murray, London, 1867, quoted in A. Lorenz, 'Scurvy in the Gold Rush', p. 477.
4. W.S. Greever, *Bonanza West: The Story of the Western Mining Rushes 1848–1900*, p. 57.
5. K.J. Carpenter, *A History of Scurvy and Vitamin C*, p. 111.
6. A. Lorenz, 'Scurvy in the Gold Rush', in *Journal of the History of Medicine and Allied Sciences*, vol. 12, 1957, p. 488.
7. K.J. Carpenter, *A History of Scurvy and Vitamin C*, p. 112.
8. A. Lorenz, 'Scurvy in the Gold Rush', in *Journal of the History of Medicine and Allied Sciences*, vol. 12, 1957, p. 506.
9. P. Guedalla, *The Two Marshalls*, 1943, quoted in *The Dictionary of War Quotations*, Justin Wintle (ed.), Hodder & Stoughton, 1989, p. 274.
10. K.J. Carpenter, *A History of Scurvy and Vitamin C*, p. 113.
11. Report of official inquiry, *The Times*, 3 February 1857, p. 6.
12. Florence Nightingale was so incensed by this situation that she published her own account of the consequences of such administrative ineptitude after the war: 'Notes on matters affecting the Health, Efficiency and Hospital Administration of the British Army'.
13. *Medicine and the Navy*, vol. 4, pp. 145–6

14. Report of official inquiry, *The Times*, 6 February 1857, p. 10.
15. *Ibid.*
16. K.J. Carpenter, *A History of Scurvy and Vitamin C*, p. 118.
17. *Ibid.*, p. 116.
18. *Ibid.*, p. 123.
19. Stephen B. Oates, *A Woman of Valour: Clara Barton and The Civil War*, p. 328
20. See website, www.spartacus.schoolnet.co.uk/USACandersonville.htm
21. D. Hamilton, *The Healers: a History of Medicine in Scotland*, pp. 191–2.
22. K.J. Carpenter, *A History of Scurvy and Vitamin C*, p. 103.
23. *Ibid.*, pp. 105–9.
24. *The Lancet*, 5 March 1904, p. 657; and 18 June 1904, pp. 1714–17.
25. A.S. Hess, *Scurvy Past and Present*, 1920, p. 6.
26. K.J. Carpenter, *A History of Scurvy and Vitamin C*, p. 186.
27. A.S. Hess, *Scurvy Past and Present*, 1920, p. 6

THIRTEEN: 'THE TRUE ANTISCORBUTIC IS PURITY OF FOOD'

1. A. Henderson Smith, 'Beer and Scurvy', *The Lancet*, 14 December 1918, p. 813.
2. P.C. Newman, *Company of Adventurers*, Penguin, pp. 49–50.
3. K.J. Carpenter, *A History of Scurvy and Vitamin C*, p. 137.
4. P.C. Newman, *Company of Adventurers*, Penguin, pp. 206–15.
5. *Narrative of the Sufferings of the Crew of the Dee*, 1887, in *The Ice-bound Whalers*, ed. James A. Troup, Orkney Press, 1987, pp. 60–1.
6. Anonymous surgeon, *Dundee, Perth and Cupar Advertiser*, 28 December 1836, quoted in *The Ice-bound Whalers*, James A. Troup (ed.), Orkney Press, 1987, pp. 35–6.
7. 'Outbreak of Scurvy in the South African Native Labour Corps', *The Lancet*, 19 October 1918, pp. 513–15.
8. A. Henderson Smith, 'Beer and Scurvy', *The Lancet*, 14 December 1918, p. 814.
9. Alexander Armstrong, *Observations on Naval Hygiene and Scurvy*, 1858, pp. 106–7.
10. *Medicine and the Navy*, vol. 4, p. 110.
11. A. Henderson Smith, 'Beer and Scurvy', *The Lancet*, 14 December 1918, p. 814.
12. McClintock, *Voyage of the Fox*, 1908, p. 6, quoted in *Medicine and the Navy*, vol. 4, p. 110.

13. Peter C. Newman, *Company of Adventurers*, Penguin, p. 421.
14. Forensic details from Prof. J. Lenihan, *The Crumbs of Creation*, Adam Hilger, 1988, pp. 99–100.
15. A. Armstrong, *Observations on Naval Hygiene and Scurvy*, 1858, p. 80.
16. *The Geographical Journal*, London, vol. 1, 1893, p. 367.
17. Jackson and Harley, 'An Experimental Inquiry into Scurvy', *The Lancet*, 28 April 1900, p. 1184.
18. 'Scurvy in the Arctic Regions', in *The Practitioner*, 1896, quoted in © *The Lancet* 28 April 1900, p. 1184.
19. Almroth Wright in 'On the pathology and therapeutics of Scurvy', 25 August 1900, © *The Lancet*, pp. 565–7.
20. Account of blood testing in A. Cherry-Garrard, *The Worst Journey in the World*, Chatto & Windus, 1965.
21. *Medicine and the Navy*, vol. 4, p. 120.
22. Ibid., p. 120
23. Jackson and Harley, 'An Experimental Inquiry into Scurvy', 28 April 1900, © *The Lancet*, pp. 1184–8.
24. 25 August 1900, editorial, © *The Lancet*, p. 589.
25. 28 April 1900, © *The Lancet*, pp. 1184–8. (This is the full text of Jackson and Harley's paper to the Royal Society.)
26. Surgeon Home, 4 August 1900, © *The Lancet*, p. 321–2.
27. Ibid.
28. A. Armstrong, *Observations on Naval Hygiene and Scurvy*, 1858, p. 111.
29. A. Turnbull, 'Discussion on the Prevention of Scurvy', *British Medical Journal*, 1902, ii, p. 1023.
30. Ibid.
31. Ibid.
32. Ibid.

FOURTEEN: 'A SUFFICIENT EXPLANATION OF THE ANOMALY'

1. M. Coplans, 'On the Etiology of Scurvy', 18 June 1904, © *The Lancet*, pp. 1714–17.
2. Report in *Journal of the Royal Navy Medical Service*, 1919, p. 319, quoted in *Medicine and the Navy*, vol. 4, p. 121.
3. R. Alexander, *The Cruise of the Raider Wolf*, 1939, p. 250, *Medicine and the Navy*, vol. 4, p. 122.
4. Chick, Skelton and Smith, 'The Antiscorbutic principle in limes and lemons', 30 November 1918, © *The Lancet*, pp. 735–8.

NOTES AND REFERENCES

5. *Ibid.*
6. *Medicine and the Navy*, vol. 4, p. 112.
7. A. Armstrong, *Observations on Naval Hygiene and Scurvy*, Churchill, London, 1858, p. 98.
8. *Ibid.*, pp. 17–18.
9. *Ibid.*, p. 93.
10. *Ibid.*, pp. 91–2.
11. Armstrong's Journal of the 1850–3 expedition, PRO: ADM/101/250.
12. A. Armstrong, *Observations on Naval Hygiene and Scurvy* quoted in *Medicine and the Navy*, vol. 4, p. 113.
13. Armstrong's instructions on lemon juice, paragraphs 3, 4 and 11, quoted in Rear-Admiral Richards, *The Arctic expedition of 1875–76: a reply to its critics*, Stanford, London, 1877, pp. 29–30.
14. Useful sources for the Nares expedition include Dr E. Kendall, 'Scurvy during some British Polar Expedition, 1875–1917', in *The Polar Record*, Scott Polar Research Institute, Cambridge, vol. 7, September 1955, pp. 467–85; and A. Henderson Smith in *The Lancet*, 30 November 1918, pp. 737–8; and 'Report of the Committee appointed by the Lords Commissioners of the Admiralty to enquire into the causes of the outbreak of scurvy in the recent Arctic expedition', *Parliamentary Papers* (1877) LVI.
15. Sir A. Armstrong, Evidence to Scurvy Committee: report p. 292.
16. Fleet Surgeon Colan's Journal, PRO: ADM/101/270.
17. *Ibid.*
18. Dr E. Kendall, 'Scurvy during some British Polar Expedition, 1875–1917', *The Polar Record*, vol. 7, September 1955, p. 473.
19. Years later, as Rear-Admiral, Albert Markham again rigidly obeyed orders, with catastrophic results. Aboard HMS *Camperdown* in the Mediterranean on 22 June 1893, he obeyed an insane order from Vice-Admiral Sir George Tryon which led to *Camperdown* colliding with HMS *Victoria*, Tryon's flagship. *Victoria* sank with the loss of Tryon and 358 men.
20. Report to the Scurvy Committee by Drs Donnet and Fraser, 1877, p. vi.
21. *Ibid.*, p. xxiii.
22. *Ibid.*, p. xxvii.
23. Dr J. MacDonald, Evidence to Scurvy Committee, report p. 161.

24. A. Armstrong, *Observations on Naval Hygiene and Scurvy*, Churchill, London, 1858, p. 100.
25. Report to the Scurvy Committee, p. xxviii.
26. Letter from Armstrong to Committee of Enquiry, 13 November 1876, report appendix no. 32, 1877.
27. Letter from Captain Nares to Committee of Enquiry, 10 November 1876, report appendix no. 32, 1877.
28. *The Times*, 19 May 1877.
29. Rear-Admiral Richards, *The Arctic expedition of 1875–76: a reply to its critics*, Stanford, London, 1877.
30. C.R. Markham, *A Refutation of the Report of the Scurvy Committee*, Griffin & Co., Portsmouth, 1877, pp. 10–11.
31. *Ibid.*, p. 13.
32. A. Armstrong, *Observations on Naval Hygiene and Scurvy*, Churchill, London, 1858, pp. 77–8.
33. C.R. Markham, *A Refutation of the Report of the Scurvy Committee*, Griffin & Co., Portsmouth, 1877, p. 21.
34. Commander Markham, quoted in *A History of Scurvy and Vitamin C*, p. 143.
35. Chick, Skelton and Smith, 'The Antiscorbutic principle in limes and lemons', 30 November 1918, © *The Lancet*, pp. 735–8.
36. *Ibid.*
37. *Ibid.*
38. Harden and Robison, 'The antiscorbutic properties of concentrated fruit juices', *Biochemical Journal*, April 1920.
39. Bassett-Smith, 'Scurvy, with special reference to prophylaxis in the Royal Navy', *The Lancet*, 22 May 1920, pp. 1102–5.
40. Bassett-Smith, 'Further experiments on the preservation of lemon juice and the prevention of scurvy', *The Lancet*, 13 August 1921, pp. 321–2.
41. L.G. Wilson, 'The Clinical Definition of Scurvy and the Discovery of Vitamin C', *Journal of Medicine and Allied Sciences*, vol. 30, 1975, pp. 40–60.
42. K.J. Carpenter, *A History of Scurvy and Vitamin C*, p. 178.
43. Harden and Zilva, 'The antiscorbutic factor in lemon juice', *Biochemical Journal*, vol. 12, 1918, pp. 259–69.
44. J.C. Drummond, 'Note on the role of the antiscorbutic factor in nutrition', *Biochemical Journal*, vol. 13, 1919, pp. 77–80.
45. K.J. Carpenter, *A History of Scurvy and Vitamin C*, p. 191.

46. Harris and Mills, 'The chemical identification of Vitamin C', *The Lancet*, 30 July 1932, pp. 235–7.
47. J. Lind, *Treatise*, 1772 edn, p. vi.

EPILOGUE

1. 'Scurvy and its prevention and control in major emergencies', WHO/NHD/99.11.
2. Reuters report from Washington DC, USA, on the National Scurvy Institute: www.internetwks.com/pauling/haha.html

Bibliography

BOOKS

Allan, D., and Schofield, R., *Stephen Hales, Scientist and Philanthropist*, Scolar Press, London, 1980.

Anson, G., *A Voyage Round the World in the Years 1740–4*, compiled from papers and other materials of the Rt Hon. George, Lord Anson, and published under his direction, by Richard Walter, London, 1748.

——, *A Voyage Round the World in the Years 1740–4*, ed. Glyndwr Williams, Oxford University Press, 1974.

Armstrong, A., *Observations on Naval Hygiene and Scurvy*, Churchill, London, 1858.

Balaban, C., Erlen, J., and Siderits, R. (eds), *The Skilful Physician*, Harwood Academic Publishers, Amsterdam, 1997. (1st pub. Theo. Maxey, London, 1656.)

Banks, Sir J., *Journal . . . During Captain Cook's first voyage in HMS Endeavour*, Sir J. Hooker (ed.), MacMillan, London, 1896.

Barnes, G., and Owen, J. (eds), *The Private Papers of John, Earl of Sandwich*, vol. 4, Navy Records Society, 1988.

Baugh, D., (ed), *Naval Administration 1715–1750*, Navy Records Society, 1977.

Baynham, H., *Before the Mast: Naval Ratings of the Nineteenth Century*, Hutchinson, 1971.

Beattie, O., *Frozen in Time – The Fate of the Franklin Expedition*, Bloomsbury, London, 1993.

Bissett, C., *Medical Essays and Observations*, Newcastle upon Tyne, 1766.

Blane, Sir G., *A Brief Statement of the progressive improvement of the health of the Royal Navy at the end of the eighteenth century and the beginning of the nineteenth century*, London, 1830.

Bollet, A.J., *Plagues and Poxes: The Rise and Fall of Epidemic Disease*, Demos Medical Publishing, New York, 1987.

Boswell, J., *Boswell's Life of Johnson*, Clarendon Press, Oxford, 6 vols, 1934.

BIBLIOGRAPHY

Carpenter, K.J., *A History of Scurvy and Vitamin C*, Cambridge University Press, 1986.

Cartwright, F.F., and Biddiss, M.D., *Disease and History*, Hart-Davis, London, 1972.

Cherry-Garrard, A., *The Worst Journey in the World*, Chatto & Windus, London, 1965.

Clowes, W.L., *The Royal Navy – A History From the Earliest Times to the Present*, 5 vols, Sampson Low, Marston & Co., London, 1898.

Colledge, J.J., *Ships of the Royal Navy*, 2 vols, David & Charles, 1969.

Committee on Scurvy; *Report to the Committee appointed by the Lords Commissioners of the Admiralty, to enquire into the causes of the outbreak of scurvy in the recent Arctic expedition*, HMSO, 1877.

Cook, J., *The Journals of Captain Cook*, Philip Edwards (ed.), Penguin Classics, 1999. (1st pub. in 4 vols by the Hakluyt Society, 1955–67.)

Course, Captain A.G., *The Merchant Navy, a Social History*, Frederick Muller, London, 1963.

Crosfield, R.T., *Remarks on the Scurvy*, London, 1797.

de Camoëns, L., *The Lusiad, or the Discovery of India, an Epic Poem translated from the original Portuguese of Luis de Camoëns by William Julius Mickle*, Oxford, 1776.

Defoe, D., *A Journal of the Plague Year*, Anthony Burgess and Christopher Bristow (eds), Penguin, 1986. (1st pub. 1722.)

Dictionary of National Biography, Oxford University Press, 1975.

Fisher, R. and Johnston, H. (eds), *Captain James Cook and his Times*, University of Vancouver Press/Croom Helme, London, 1979.

Ford, D., *Admiral Vernon and the Navy*, London, 1907.

Garfield, S., *Mauve*, Faber & Faber, London, 2000.

Gill, C., *The Naval Mutinies of 1797*, Manchester University Press, 1913.

Graham, H.G., *The Social Life of Scotland in the Eighteenth Century*, 1st pub. 1899; reprinted with introduction by Eric Linklater, A. & C. Black, London, 1969.

Greever, W.S., *Bonanza West – the Story of the Western Mining Rushes, 1848–1900*, University of Idaho Press, Moscow, Idaho, 1993.

Hakluyt, R., *Principal Navigations, voiyages, traffiques and discoveries of the English nation, made by sea or overland, to the remote quarters of the earth, at any time within the compasse of these 1500 yeeres*, London, 1598.

Hamilton, D., *The Healers – A History of Medicine in Scotland*, Canongate, Edinburgh, 1981.

Harding, R., *The Evolution of the Sailing Navy, 1509–1815*, St Martin's Press, New York, 1995.

Hawkesworth, J., *An Account of the Voyages undertaken . . . for making discoveries in the Southern Hemisphere . . . by Commodore Byron, Captain Wallis, Captain Carteret and Captain Cook, drawn from the Journals which were kept by the several commanders, and from the papers of Joseph Banks, Esq.*, 3 vols, London, 1773.

Hawkins, Sir R., *The Observations of Sir Richard Hawkins, Knight, in his Voyage into the South Sea, 1593*. Edition of 1622, James A. Williamson (ed.), Argonaut Press, London, 1933.

Hess, A.S., *Scurvy Past and Present*, J.B. Lippincott, Philadelphia, 1920.

Hill, J.R. (ed.), *Oxford Illustrated History of the Royal Navy*, Oxford University Press, 1995.

Hough, R., *Captain James Cook*, Coronet Books, Hodder & Stoughton, London, 1995.

Hulme, N., *A safe and easy Remedy proposed for the relief of the stone and gravel, the scurvy, gout etc.*, London, 1778.

Huntford, R., *The Last Place on Earth – Scott and Amundsen's Race for the South Pole*, Abacus, 2000.

James VI of Scotland, *A Counterblast to Tobacco, to which is added a learned discourse written by Dr Everard Maynwaringe, proving that tobacco is a procuring cause of the scurvy . . .*, London, 1672.

Johnston, R., *The Arctic Expedition of 1875–76; compiled from official sources*, Frederick Warne, London, 1877.

Keay, J., *The Honourable Company: A History of the English East India Company*, HarperCollins, London, 1993.

Keevil, J.J., *Medicine and the Navy, 1200–1900*, vols 1–2, vols 3–4 by Lloyd, C., and Coulter, J.L.S., E. & S. Livingstone Ltd, Edinburgh, 1958.

Kennedy, P., *The Rise and Fall of British Naval Mastery*, Penguin Press, 1976, Penguin Classic, 2001.

Kennedy, W.J.D., *On the Plains with Custer and Hancock – the Journal of Isaac Coates, Army Surgeon*, Johnson Books, Boulder, Colorado, 1997.

Landes, D.S., *Revolution in Time*, Belknap Press, Harvard University, 1983.

Latham, A., and Youings, J. (eds), *The Letters of Sir Walter Raleigh*, University of Exeter Press, 1999.

Laughton, Sir J. (ed.), *Letters and Papers of Charles, Lord Barham, 1758–1813*, Navy Records Society, 3 vols, 1906–10.

BIBLIOGRAPHY

Lavery, B. (ed.), *Shipboard Life and Organisation, 1731–1815*, Navy Records Society, 1998.

Leake, J., *A Dissertation on the properties and efficacy of the Lisbon Diet-Drink in the cure of venereal disease and scurvy, etc, etc*, London, 1762.

Lenihan, Professor J., *The Crumbs of Creation*, Adam Hilger, Bristol, 1988.

Levien, M. (ed), *The Cree Journals; the voyages of Edward Cree, Surgeon RN, as related in his private journals, 1837–1856*, Webb & Bower, Exeter, 1981.

Lewis, M., *England's Sea-Officers, The Story of the Naval Profession*, Allen & Unwin, London, 1939.

Lind, J., *An Essay on Diseases incidental to Europeans in Hot Climates*, London, 1768.

——, *An Essay on the most effectual means of preserving the health of Seamen in the Royal Navy*, London, 1762.

——, *A Treatise of the Scurvy*, Kincaid and Donaldson, Edinburgh, 1753.

——, *Lind's Treatise of Scurvy*. A reprinted edn of Lind's *Treatise* of 1753, with notes; C.P. Stewart and D. Guthrie (eds), Edinburgh University Press, 1953.

Lloyd, C.C. (ed.), *The Health of Seamen – Selections from the works of Dr James Lind, Sir Gilbert Blane and Dr Thomas Trotter*, Navy Records Society, vol. CVII, 1965.

Lyon, D., *The Sailing Navy List: All the ships of the Royal Navy, built, purchased and captured, 1688–1860*, Conway Maritime Press, London, 1993.

MacBride, D., *Experimental Essays*, London, 1764.

Magnusson, M. (ed.), *Chambers Biographical Dictionary*, W. & R. Chambers, Edinburgh, 1990.

McBride, D., *An Account of the Most Important Discovery . . . made for the Restoration and Preservation of Health, in all Complaints of the Stomach and Bowels, Fevers, Fluxes, Scurvy, Dropsy, Debility, Etc.*, London, 1798.

Manning, Captain T.D., and Walker, Captain C.F., *British Warship Names*, Putnam, London, 1959.

Markham, C.R., *A Refutation of the Report of the Scurvy Committee*, Griffin & Co., Portsmouth, 1877.

Milton, G., *Nathaniel's Nutmeg*, Sceptre, Hodder & Stoughton, London, 1999.

Morse, H.B., *The Chronicles of the East India Company Trading with China, 1635–1834*, 5 vols, Oxford, 1926.

Newman, P.C., *Company of Adventurers*, Penguin, 1987.

Nicol, J., *The Life and Adventures of John Nicol, Mariner*, Edinburgh, 1822.
Nikiforuk, A., *The Fourth Horseman – a short history of epidemics, plagues and other scourges*, Phoenix (Orion Books), London, 1993.
Oates, S.B., *A Woman of Valour: Clara Barton and The Civil War*, Free Press, New York, 1994.
Oxford Dictionary of Quotations, Oxford University Press, 1981.
Pack, Captain J., *Nelson's Blood; The Story of Naval Rum*, Royal Naval Museum, Sutton, 1982.
Pakenham, T., *The Boer War*, Abacus, 1992, 1st pub. 1979.
Paterson, D., *A Treatise on the Scurvy*, 1795.
Phipps, Captain C.J., *A Voyage Towards the North Pole*, London, 1774.
Picard, L., *Dr Johnson's London*, Phoenix Press, London, 2001.
Porter, R., *The Greatest Benefit to Mankind: A Medical History of Humanity from Antiquity to the Present*, Fontana Press, London, 1999.
Profily, J., *An Easy and Exact Method of curing The Venereal Disease in all its different Appearances; with an Account of its Nature, Causes and Symptoms . . . and likewise a Method of curing The Scurvy, Gleets, Whites, Etc, Illustrated with Curious Copper-Plates*, London, 1748.
Richards, Rear-Admiral Sir F., *The Arctic Expedition of 1875–76; a Reply to its Critics*, Stanford, London, 1877.
Richmond, Admiral H.W. (ed.), *The Private Papers of George, 2nd Earl Spencer*, vols 2–3, Navy Records Society, 1914–23.
Roddis, L.H., *James Lind, Founder of Nautical Medicine*, Heinemann Medical Books Ltd, London, 1951.
Rodger, N.A.M., *The Admiralty*, Lavenham, 1979.
———, *The Wooden World: An Anatomy of the Georgian Navy*, Fontana, London, 1988.
Royal Album of Arts and Industries of Great Britain, London, 1887.
Rutter, O., *Turbulent Journey, a life of William Bligh, Vice-Admiral of the Blue*, Ivor Nicholson and Watson, 1936.
Sainty, J.C., *Admiralty Officials 1660–1870*, Athlone Press, London, 1975.
Serafini, A., and Asimov, I., *Linus Pauling – A Man and his Science*, i-Universe.Com Inc., 2000.
Simmons, D., *Schweppes, The First 200 Years*, Springwood Books, 1983.
Sherrow, V., *Linus Pauling – Investigating the Magic Within*, Raintree Steck-Vaughan, 1994.
Smollett, T., *Roderick Random*, Penguin, 1995, 1st pub. 1748.
Sobel, D., *Longitude*, Fourth Estate, London, 1998.
Spencer, H., *A Study of Sociology*, Henry S. King & Co., 1874.

BIBLIOGRAPHY

Sutton, S., *An Historical Account of a new method for extracting the foul air out of ships*, London, 1749. (Containing 'A Discourse on the Scurvy' by Richard Mead.)

Thomas, P., *True and Impartial Journal*, London, 1745.

Thomson, F., *An Essay on the Scurvy*, London, 1790.

Treasure, G. (ed.), *Who's Who in Early Hanoverian Britain*, Shepheard-Walwyn, 1992.

——, *Who's Who in Late Hanoverian Britain*, Shepheard-Walwyn, London, 1997.

Troup, J.A. (ed.), *The Ice-Bound Whalers*, The Orkney Press & Stromness Museum, 1987.

Wesley, J., *Primitive Physic, or an easy and natural method of curing most diseases*, 13th edn, Bristol, 1768.

Williams, G. (ed.), *Documents relating to Anson's Voyage round the World, 1740–1744*, Navy Records Society, vol. 109, 1967.

——, *The Prize of All the Oceans*, HarperCollins, London, 1999.

Williams, T. (ed.), *Collins Biographical Dictionary of Scientists*, HarperCollins, 1994.

Periodicals and Other Documents

British Medical Journal (various issues).

Dunn, P.M., 'James Lind (1716–94) of Edinburgh and the treatment of Scurvy', *Archives of Diseases in Childhood*, 1997, 76, pp. 64–5.

Economic Botany, New York, 39(4), 1983.

Geographical Journal, London, vol. 1, 1893, p. 367.

Glass, Surgeon Lieutenant-Commander J., 'James Lind MD, Eighteenth-Century Medical Hygienist', *Journal of the Royal Naval Medical Service*, vol. 35, no. 1, January 1949 (pp. 1–20) and no. 2, April 1949 (pp. 68–86).

Hughes, R.E., 'James Lind and the Cure of Scurvy: An Experimental Approach', *Medical History*, vol. 19, 1975, (Wellcome Institute).

Jones, E., and Hughes, E, vol. 20, 1976, 'Copper Boilers and the occurrence of Scurvy: An Experimental Approach', *Medical History*.

Journal of the History of Medicine and Allied Sciences (various issues).

Kendall, Dr E.J.C., *Scurvy during some British Polar expeditions, 1875–1917* in *The Polar Record*, Scott Polar Research Institute, Cambridge, September 1955, pp. 467–85.

Lancet, The (various issues).

Lloyd, C.C., 'The Conquest of Scurvy', *British Journal of The History of Science*, 1963.

McBride, W., '"Normal" Medical Science and British Treatment of the Sea Scurvy, 1753–75', *British Journal of the History of Medicine and Allied Sciences*, 1991.

'Proceedings of The Nutrition Society', Lind Bicentenary Symposium, Edinburgh, May 1953.

'Proprietaries of Other Days', in *Chemist and Druggist*, 25 June 1927.

Risse, G.B., 'Britannia Rules the Seas: The Health of Seamen, Edinburgh, 1791–1800', *British Journal of the History of Medicine and Allied Sciences*, 1988, pp. 426–46.

Rodger, N.A.M., 'Stragglers and Deserters from the Royal Navy During the Seven years War', *Bulletin of the Institute of Historical Research*, vol. 57, 1984, pp. 56–79.

Rolleston, H.D., 'James Lind, Pioneer of Naval Hygiene', *Journal of the Royal Naval Medical Service*, vol. 1, 1915, pp. 181–90.

'Scurvy, and its prevention and control in major emergencies', *World Health Organisation*, WHO/NHD/99.11.

Stockman, R., 'James Lind and Scurvy', *Edinburgh Medical Journal*, June 1926, pp. 329–50.

'Studies on the destruction of Vitamin C in the boiling of milk', *Journal of Nutrition*, vol. II, March 1930, p. 325.

'The role of diet in the cause, prevention and cure of dental diseases', *Journal of Nutrition*, vol. III, January 1931, p. 433.

Thomas, D.P., 'Experiment versus Authority', *New England Journal of Medicine*, vol. 281, no. 17, 23 October 1969, pp. 932–3.

Watt, Sir J., 'The Medical bequest of disaster at sea: Commodore Anson's circumnavigation 1740–44', *Journal of the Royal College of Physicians*, vol. 32, no. 6, November/December 1998.

Wyatt, H.V., 'James Lind and the Prevention of Scurvy', *Medical History*, vol. 20, 1976, (Wellcome Institute).

Index

American Civil War; scurvy
    during, 233–4
Appert, Nicholas; preservation
    of foodstuff, 220
Appleby, Joshua: 151
Anson, Commodore George;
    19
  prepares for 4-year voyage,
    61–8
  the circumnavigation, 68–79
  captures Spanish treasure
    galleon, 78–9
  Lind dedicates *Treatise* to, 100
  probable sponsor of Lind,
    115–116
Antarctic exploration,
    1901–1917; incidence of
    scurvy, 250–2
'Anti-fruitism', 65, 245
Arctic expedition of 1875;
    258–62
Armstrong, (Sir) Alexander;
  on the use of beer, 241
  promotes ships' bands, 243–4
  on the potato, 248–9
  on use of lemon juice in 1850
    expedition, 255–8
  medical orders for 1875
    expedition, 259–61
  fury at violation of his
    instructions, 266
  condemns alternative scurvy
    theories, 268
Ascorbic acid
  Tables of content in food
    items, 107–8
  Vitamin-C defined as, 274
Atkinson, Dr. Edward; uses
    blood litmus tests for
    scurvy, 245–6

Bachstrom, J.F; 45–6
Baird, Surgeon Andrew; on
    success of citrus remedy,
    202–3
Banks, (Sir) Joseph; 20,
  on lemon juice, 137–8
  on scientific aspects of Cook's
    voyages, 140
Barnes, Dr; accuses ship-owners,
    209–10
Bassett-Smith, Surgeon-Admiral;
    experiments on solid
    tablets, 271–2
Bates, Dr. John; at
    Andersonville, Georgia,
    234
Beatty, Dr. (Sir) William, 200

Beer and alcohol against scurvy,
        181–2
    As substitute for lemon juice,
        212
    As antiscorbutic, 240–1
Bedford, Surgeon Nathaniel; use
        of lime-juice gargle,
        169–170
Bembridge, Isle of Wight; 148
Berkeley, Rear-Admiral George;
        complains of lack of
        lemons, 194
Bickerton, Sir Richard; 192
Bioflavonoids; 278
Bissett, Dr. Charles; treatise on
        scurvy, 122
Black, Joseph; on water
        purification, 158
Blane, (Sir) Gilbert, 6–7
    education and entry to Royal
        Navy, 163–6
    memorandum to Admiralty
        Board, 172–3
    campaigns for citrus remedy,
        176
    leaves Navy for private
        practice, 177
    follows Lind's conclusions,
        178–9
    appointed to Sick & Hurt
        Board, 184
    national prosperity results
        from citrus remedy, 188
    relationships with colleagues,
        191–2
    on success of citrus remedy,
        200
    his death, 215–16
Bligh, Captain William; views on
        scurvy, 180
Blood-letting; 11, 43, 63
Blood poisoning; 244–5
Boer War; scurvy during, 233,
        253
Boerhaave, Hermann; 22
Bowen, Samuel; and soya beans,
        132
Boyle, Robert; 97
British Scurvy Commission;
        examines 1875 Arctic
        expedition, 263–6
    aftermath and outcry,
        266–269
Brooke, Dr. Richard; his quack
        scurvy cure, 207–8
Budd, Dr. William; on the
        'mystery factor', 216
Burial; as a remedy for scurvy,
        44, 230
Byron, Commodore John; 120–1

Cactus juice; mixed with whisky,
        229
de Camöens, Luis; 14
Carrot marmalade; use on
        Cook's 2nd voyage,
        141
Carteret, Lt. Philip; 129
Cartier, Jacques; the best early
        description of scurvy at
        sea, 14–16
Cider; 86, 93, 172
Citric acid; 225, 265
Citrus juice; botanical

INDEX

misunderstanding, 212–13
limes preferred to lemons for commercial reasons, 213–14, 216–17
confusion in supply for Arctic, 259–60
Citrus remedy; first recommendation by Sick & Hurt Board, 182–3
successful use on voyage to India, 183
demands from home fleets, 192–3
general orders throughout Navy, 194–7
reasons for success unknown, 198
logistics of supply, 206–7
and Merchant Navy, 205–8
and lemon-lime confusion, 212–14, 216–17
incompetent supply ravaged British Army in Crimea, 231–2
Clerk, Surgeon John; 134, 136
Clinical trials; 89–90
Clowes, William; 49
Clutton, Joseph; 57
Cocoa-nuts; use against scurvy, 120–1
Cockburn, Dr. William; recommends vinegar, 63–4 66, 76, 79, 87, 103
Cockburne, John; 29
Cocoa-nut milk; successful use of as antiscorbutic, 120–1
Colan, Surgeon Thomas; on diet during 1875 Arctic Expedition, 261–2
Collingwood, Commodore Cuthbert; 33
demands lemon juice, 185
Coltbatch, Dr. John; 17, 97–8
'conditioned deficiencies'; modern understanding relates early theories to action of vitamin C, 101
Cook, Captain James; 5, 38–9, 126–7
treatment of scurvy on his South Sea voyages, 133–44
his remarks on malt wort, 137
rates sauerkraut and portable soup, 142
his 'holistic' view of health at sea, 143
on water provision, 157
Copper poisoning; 54, 123–4, 214
Crimean War; scurvy during, 230–3
Crandon, John; scurvy self-experimentation, 276
Cree, Assistant Surgeon Edward; on putrid water, 159–60
Crosfield, Surgeon Robert; 44
Suggests use of opium, 193–4

Darby, Admiral George; warns of effects of scurvy, 170

Davis, Surgeon; on distilled water, 157
Diet; human anomalies and experiments, 276
Dover, Dr. Thomas; 56
Drummond, J.C.; names 'water soluble C', 273
Dudley, Vice-Admiral Sir Sheldon; on Lind's conquering of scurvy & typhus, 160–1
Dundas, Henry (Viscount Melville); 158–9
Durand, Peter; food canning, 220

East India Company; 18, 21, 25, 27, 27, 31, 47, 49, 51, 54–5, 65, 179
Edinburgh; in the early 18th century, 21–3
Edinburgh Medical School; 22
Eugalenus; on scurvy, 96
Evans & Sons; lime-juice suppliers, 222, 259

First World War; scurvy during, 237, 250
'Fixed Air' theory; 124–8
Fletcher, Charles; 157–158
Franklin, Benjamin; 139
Franklin, Lady Jane; mounts Arctic expedition, 242–3
Franklin, Sir John; fatal arctic expedition, 241–3
Frölich, Dr. Theodor; proves dietary link to scurvy, 272
Fryer, Surgeon John; 54–5
Funk, Casimir; uses term 'vitamine', 273

Galton, Francis; on scurvy among travellers, 229
Garth, Sir Samuel; 58
Gilbertus de Aquila; 43
Gillespie, Surgeon Leonard; on water supplies, 39, 148
on use of citrus remedy, 183
on improving health at sea, 201
Gold Rush; scurvy during, 228–30
Grainger, Surgeon James; 91
Guedalla, Philip; 230

Haddock, Admiral Sir Nicholas; 60
Hales, Dr. Stephen; on ventilation, 102
on water purification, 151
Hall, Dr. John; first suggestion of specific antiscorbutic, 53–4
Hammond, Surgeon John; 85–6
Harden, Arthur; separates the 'C' factor, 273
Harley, Prof. Vaughan; experiments with monkeys, 246–7
Harness, Dr. John; claims credit for use of lemon juice, 205–6

INDEX

enquires into fraud in lemon juice supply, 207
Harrison, John; 72, 140
Haslar Hospital; Lind appointed, 115–18
Hawke, Admiral Edward; 167–8
Hawkins, Sir Richard; wishes for 'a learned man' on scurvy, 47–9
uses early water distillation system, 149
Henna; use against scurvy, 244
Henry, Surgeon Peter; on success of citrus remedy, 204
Hess, Alfred; 237
Hill, Surgeon; responds to Lind's *Treatise*, 110–12
Hippocrates; recognised scurvy, 13
Hogarth, William; 57
Holmes, Oliver Wendell; 133
Holst, Prof. Axel; proves dietary link to scurvy, 272
Home, Surgeon William; 248
Hood, Sir Samuel; 170
Hudson's Bay Company; 25, 239
Hulme, Surgeon Nathaniel; ideas on scurvy, and 'fixed air', 124–5
on 'rob' of lemons, and beer, 138
his 'fizzy drink', 174
Huxham, Dr. John; 81

Investigator, HMS; the 1850 Arctic expedition, 255–8
Irving, Surgeon Charles; plagiarises Lind's water process, 154–7
Ives, Surgeon Edward; 91, 119

Jackson, Frederick; believed only in purity of food, 246
James, Dr. Robert; his infamous Powders, 57
responds to Lind's *Treatise*, 110–11
his Powders demanded by Cook's surgeon, 141
Powders preferred to citrus by Sick & Hurt Board, 174
Jervis, Admiral Sir John (Earl St. Vincent); protests about incidence of scurvy, 190
Johnson, Dr. Samuel; 30

King James VI; 54
Kempenfelt, Rear-Admiral Richard; 167–8
Koettlitz, Dr. Reginald; 246, 250
Kramer, Dr; 98–9

Lancaster, Sir James; understands preventative use of citrus juice, 49–50
Langlands, George; 23–24
Lead poisoning; Lind on, 109–10
as cause of Franklin disaster, 243
Leake, Dr. John; his quack remedy, 122–3

Leith; Edinburgh's sea port, 218–19
Lemon juice (see also 'rob' of lemons); naval suppliers, 205
   specified for 1850 Arctic expedition, 255–8
   produced in lozenge form, 271–272
Lime juice; produced in capsule form, 251
   produced in lozenge form, 271–2
'Limeys'; origins of the expression, 226–7
Lind, James; the origins of scurvy, 13–14
   family, education and training, 20, 22–5
   on Cartier, 16
   his motivation, 19
   at sea, 59–61, 74, 83–5
   learns of Anson's medical disaster, 81–2
   on the health of seamen, 34–5, 42–4
   on typhus, 60–1
   on scurvy, 87–91
   his experiment at sea, 92–4
   leaves the Royal Navy, 95
   on the early writers on scurvy, 96–9
   his character, 99
   publishes his *Treatise*, 99–107
   on ventilation as cause of scurvy, 102
   on salt as cause of scurvy, 103
   on the efficacy of vegetables, 104
   on the 'rob' of lemons, 105–6
   on dangerous 'medicines', 106–7
   on use of limes, 107
   on sauerkraut, 107
   on lead poisoning, 109–10
   his later writing, 110
   Admiralty reactions to his *Treatise*, 110–112
   his *Treatise* criticised, 113–14
   describes Haslar Hospital, 117–19
   his 'store-ship-proposals adopted, 119–20
   revises his *Treatise*, 129–32
   additional recommendations on scurvy, 131–2
   loses patronage with death of Anson, 144
   water distillation, 150–60
   Admiralty orders publication of his distillation process, 152
   and Irving's water process, 155
   later contributions to naval medicine, 160–2
   retires from Royal Navy, 162
   dies at Gosport, 187
Lind, James (cousin); 20–1, 140
Lind, Dr. John (son); appointed at Haslar. 162
Lister Institute; experiments on antiscorbutic food

INDEX

properties, 254–5, 269–71
compares citrus provision in two polar expeditions, 270–1
explains the lemon-lime anomaly, 271
Lister, Martin; 3
Lorenz, Anthony; 126, 230

MacBride, Dr. David; his malt wort theory, 125–9
MacBride, Captain John; 129
McClintock, (Sir) Francis Leopold; commands Lady Franklin's expedition, 242
McClure, Captain Robert; commands 1850 Arctic expedition, 255–8
Magellan, Ferdinand; 44
Malt Wort, 127–9
trials on Cook's voyages, 133
report by Cook, 142–3
recommended by Sick & Hurt Board, 175
condemned by Trotter, 184
use discontinued, 191
Markham, Sir Clements; condemns British Scurvy Commission, 267–9
blames Armstrong for 1875 disaster, 268–9
Maynwaringe, Dr. Everard; 54

Mead, Dr. Richard; 64, 79–81, 87, 102, 122

Moellenbrok, Dr. Andreas; 46
Molasses; use against scurvy, 11, 138, 178, 242
Montagu, John (4th Earl of Sandwich); 126–7
Moyle, Surgeon John; 55
Murray, Surgeon; 88–9

Nansen, Fridtjof; on 'ptomaine poisoning', 244
Nares, Sir George; commands 1875 Arctic expedition, 258
ignores Armstrong's medical orders, 261
absolves expedition surgeon, 266
Naval Surgeons; 4, 26–30
Nelson, Admiral Horatio; on waste of life due to disease, 201
Nicol, John; 32–33
Nightingale, Florence; condemns incompetence, 231
Northbrooke, John; 12
Northcote, Surgeon William; letter to First Lord about scurvy, 171–2

Oglethorpe, Sir Theophilus; 151

Paris; 1870 scurvy outbreak, 236
Parker, Sir Hyde; seeks holistic approach, 192–3
Paterson, Surgeon David; his

treatise causes mischief, 188
Patronage; 126–7, 145–7, 161–2
Patten, Surgeon; condemns 'rob' of lemons, 175
Pauling, Dr Linus; 277–9
Perry, Asst. Surgeon William; on Cook's use of antiscorbutics, 136–7
Peruvian Bark ('Jesuits' Bark'); 47, 211–12
Phipps, Constantine John (Lord Mulgrave); 156
Platt, Sir Hugh; his 'secret' method of producing citrus juice, 50–1
Pliny; on scurvy, 96
Poissonnière, Dr; 152–3
Polar expeditions; 240–262
Portable Soup; 35, 129, 175
Potato; as antiscorbutic, 234–6, 248–9
Priestley, Joseph; 126, 140
Pringle, Sir John; 126, 139–40
Profily, Dr. John; 123
'Ptomaine Poisoning' theory; 244–248, 273

Quack medicines; 56–8, 63, 106–7

Raleigh, Sir Walter; 30–1
Richards, Rear-Admiral Sir Frederick; condemns lime juice, 267
'Rob' of lemons;
Lind's method, 105–6
Admiralty investigates, 130–1
Cook ordered to make trials, 133
Cook gets meagre supply, 141
condemned by Cook, 143
cost of production, 175
logistics of supply, 190
Blane suspects heat causes impairment, 198
Robertson, Surgeon Robert; 165, 211
Rodney, Admiral George; 164–5
demands antiscorbutics, 173
praises Blane's achievements, 175–6
Ronsseus of Gonda; 16
Rose & Company; lime-juice producers, 218–26
lime growing estates, 223
assist Lister Institute, 269
Rose, Lauchlan; devises preservation method, 219–21
Royal Navy; recruiting, 28–9
conditions, 30–3
disease, 40–1
'Hosier's Ghost', 40
organisation, 145–7
Royal Society of London; Lind's water process, 151
Rush, Benjamin; 90–1

'*Salisbury*' HMS; 83, 119
Salop (also 'saloop' and 'salep'); 129, 178
Salt and scurvy; 34–5, 103, 122
Sauerkraut; 11, 84, 175, 184

INDEX

Saumarez, Lt. Philip; 70, 77
Scott, Robert Falcon; 250
Scott, Sir Walter; 12
SCURVY;
  Admiralty attitudes, 18–19, 85, 128–9, 194–5, 196–7
  Avoidance of during naval actions, 199–201
  'anti-fruitism', 55–6
  early use of citrus remedy, 16–17, 47–53, 55, 80–1, 84–5, 88–9, 97–8
  Cook's 'blunderbuss' approach, 142
  descriptions, 12–18
  diet, proof of as cause, 272
  OUTBREAKS;
    during Vasco da Gama's voyage, 14
    during Jacques Cartier's voyage, 14–16
    land epidemics, 17–18
    during Anson's circumnavigation, 69–78
    in the Mediterranean, 119–20
    in the Magellan Straits, 120–1
    in the English Channel, at New York and in the West Indies, 166–73
    at Haslar Hospital 1758–1809, 199
    increasing despite use of lime juice, 215
    during the Californian Gold Rush, Crimean War, American Civil War Boer War and First World War, 228–37, 253
    in the whaling industry, 239–40
  'ptomaine poisoning' theory, 230, 244–8, 273
  remedies attempted, 11, 17–18, 42–58, 85, 193, 229–30, 233, 239, 244
  quack remedies, 122–3, 189, 207–8
  role of salt, 34–5, 103, 122
  variant spellings, 11–12
Scurvy-grass; 45–7, 49, 85, 97
Selkirk, Alexander ('Robinson Crusoe'); 56, 72
Shackleton, Ernest; 250–1
Shovell, Admiral Sir Clowdisley; 36, 63
Sick & Hurt Board;
  advises refusal of scurvy treatment, 173–4
  condemns use of citrus fruit, 179
  agrees use of citrus fruit, 182
  limits use of citrus fruit, 185–6
  reorganisation, 206
Smellie, Dr. William; 112, 125
Smith, Alice Henderson; on the lime-lemon anomaly, 255
Smollett, Tobias; 23–7, 59–60, 112–13
Soya beans; used against scurvy, 132

Spencer, George, 2nd Earl;
  issues Admiralty order on lemon juice, 186
  fails to see scurvy case at Haslar, 194
Spencer, Herbert; on Admiralty perversity, 196–7
Spruce beer; 11, 44–5, 238–9
Stark, William; fatal scurvy experiment, 139–40
Stockman, Prof. Ralph; 53
Strontian, Argyllshire; 92
Sturge & Company; 214, 221–3
Sulphuric acid; used against scurvy, 11, 48, 64, 71, 85, 92–3, 141, 174, 184
Sydenham, Dr. Thomas; 97
Szent-Györgyi, Albert; work to isolate vitamin C, 273–4

Tamarinds, 65
Thomas, Pascoe; describes scurvy during Anson's voyage, 70–2
  condemns Cockburn's ideas on indolence, 75–7
Thomson, Surgeon Frederick; conditions on Cook's voyages, 135
  on water distillation, 153
  his Treatise on scurvy, 180–1
Thompson, William; 39
Trotter, Surgeon Thomas; support for Lind's proposals, 183–7
  on use of lemon crystals, 201–2

resigns from Navy, 203–4
Travis, Dr. John; 123–124
Tulloch, Col. Alexander; on Crimea disaster, 231–2
Turnbull, Surgeon Alexander; condemns citrus juice, 249–50

Vasco da Gama; the first description of scurvy at sea, 14
Venables, General Robert; 55–6
Vernon, Admiral Edward; 33, 40
Victualling; 35–9
Vinegar; used against scurvy, 11, 63–4, 229
vitamin C: 12, 50, 101, 107–8, 124, 131, 213–14, 246, 251, 273–4, 276–9
'vitamin P'; 278

Wager, Admiral Sir Charles; 62, 80
Walter, Rev. Richard; 67, 69, 71, 83–4
Ward, Dr. Joshua; 55–6
  his 'Pill and Drop', 57–8, 65, 75
Water; 39–40, 159–60
  distillation and purification, 148–60
Watt, Sir James; 126, 157
Weir, Dr; 211–12
Wesley, John; 85
Whalers; 239–240
White, Surgeon James; 56
Willis, Prof. Thomas; 96

INDEX

Woodall, Surgeon John; 17–18, 51–3, 222, 253
World Health Organisation; 276–7
Wright, Sir Almroth; 245

Young, (Admiral Sir) George; 168–9
Younger, Richard; 159

Zilva, Sylvester; 273–4